Perinatal Palliative Care

Erin M. Denney-Koelsch
Denise Côté-Arsenault
Editors

Perinatal Palliative Care

A Clinical Guide

Springer

Editors
Erin M. Denney-Koelsch, MD, FAAHPM
Strong Memorial Hospital
University of Rochester
Rochester, NY
USA

Denise Côté-Arsenault, PhD, RN, CPCL, FNAP, FAAN
School of Nursing
Saint Louis University
Saint Louis, MO
USA

ISBN 978-3-030-34750-5 ISBN 978-3-030-34751-2 (eBook)
https://doi.org/10.1007/978-3-030-34751-2

This Springer imprint is published by the registered company Springer Nature Switzerland AG
The registered company address is: Gewerbestrasse 11, 6330 Cham, Switzerland

Foreword

When I first heard Drs. Denney-Koelsch and Côté-Arsenault in 2015 present data from interviewing parents who had experienced carrying a fetus with a lethal diagnosis, I knew the field of perinatal palliative care was entering a new phase. For the prior two decades, a variety of practitioners had been quietly supporting families who learned their fetus had a life-limiting condition. Hospice nurses, obstetricians, neonatologists, palliative care doctors, social workers, and others were all working at a grassroots level trying to do better for these grieving families. Sometimes, they worked in teams, but often, they practiced alone. All were operating from first principles – bring compassion and the ideals of palliative care into the perinatal space. No one knew for sure if their approach would ease the grief families were experiencing, but it was clear there was a need to do better.

Erin Denney-Koelsch and Denise Côté-Arsenault had captured something fundamental. A major driver of decision-making was a desire to avoid regret. For me, it was a "eureka moment." Families were in fact struggling with the challenges we thought they were. It was validating to hear that families wanted what we were providing – a safe space to explore what it meant to be a parent under the hardest circumstances and a compassionate ear to help them think through how best to care for their baby. Since hearing that talk, qualitative research and published experience have grown tremendously. Perinatal palliative care has become a field in its own right with an early evidence base. Formal teams have been created, best practices are being shared, and families are becoming more aware that help is available.

The very existence of this book is affirmation for those of us who have engaged in this work. It is filled with crystal clear summaries of evidence-based practice, as well as practical advice for addressing everything from psychosocial needs to pain management and from spiritual care to care coordination. By its very nature, perinatal palliative care deals with the rare, so having a source to turn to that covers such a wide range of special circumstances will be invaluable. This book's publication is an opportunity for all of us to improve our care. Have we engaged everyone who should be a part of our teams? Do we have all of the components in place that create a high-quality experience for our families? Are we still making it up as we go along, or is there something we should learn from other's experience and published research?

I am confident that the leaves of my copy of this book will become well-worn in short order, and I will be sharing several chapters with the neonatology fellows in our training program at the Children's Hospital of Philadelphia. For those who wish to enter the field by joining a perinatal palliative care team or who are considering starting a program from scratch in a hospital without one, a road map has now been provided.

All of you who meet these expectant mothers, their partners, and their families already know there is something profoundly satisfying in this work. These families embody courage, compassion, and beauty while wrestling with the most difficult existential challenges. Just as these families often feel alone, so, too, have the providers often felt alone. The power of this book is in the concrete demonstration of collective knowledge. Together, we will learn how to do this right.

Philadelphia, PA, USA David Munson, MD

Preface

Our work together, as research colleagues, began when we were both at the University of Rochester: Erin Denney-Koelsch as a Medicine-Pediatrics-Trained Palliative Care Fellow and Denise Côté-Arsenault a Maternal-Child Nurse Academic with research focused on parent experiences of perinatal loss and subsequent pregnancies. The field of perinatal palliative care (PPC) had not yet emerged in central New York, but the need for such care was becoming evident with parents choosing to continue their pregnancy after learning of their baby's life-limiting fetal condition (LLFC). The literature on PPC was thin, and research on the topic was scarce. From our shared interest sprang a pilot study – can we work together? Will parents talk to us?

Clearly, the answer to both questions was a resounding yes! And thus began our collaboration: nurse researcher and palliative care physician. Our research and the work of many others have expanded our understanding of what couples go through and what their needs are during their very challenging pregnancies. However, we have still found that there was a lack of adequate resources to guide the large number of people who care for these families. It is out of this inadequacy and the growing expertise that now exists in PPC that this book was formed.

We have put together a book that seeks to address the current evidence, expert opinions, and recommendations for the comprehensive care of families dealing with one of the worst moments of their lives. We turned to our esteemed colleagues from across the country to share their tremendous knowledge and wisdom so that care for families faced with LLFC is of the highest level and the field of PPC develops strong standards of care of the highest quality.

The organization of this book allows for reading the chapters in the order they are presented, while at the same time, each chapter stands on its own and will be a useful reference on the stated topic. The topical areas range from the theoretical to the clinical and practical levels. Chapters include tables and figures designed for easy reference. PPC is unique in that there are two patients: the mother and the fetus or baby. Because of this maternal-fetal dyad, there are multiple specialities and disciplines involved in their care. We have aimed to speak to all care team members caring for families with imperiled pregnancies, from obstetrics and maternal-fetal medicine, nursing, genetic counseling, neonatology, palliative care, social work, parent advocates, bereaved parents themselves, certified child life specialists, bereavement therapists, chaplains, legal experts, and ethicists. This book should be relevant to all who care for these families.

Part I provides the foundations upon which the entire field has grown. Chapter 1 is an overview of the field and what will be presented in the book. Chapter 2 presents several theories that are related to pregnancy, pregnancy with an LLFC, grief, loss, and trauma that provide strong and unique perspectives to enhance one's understanding of the issues facing families and care providers. Chapter 3 is an overview of ethical principles and their application to the perinatal period. Chapter 4 is from the parents' perspective on the experience of being diagnosed with an LLFC and how they make subsequent decisions, coping with the grief and loss, and work together as a couple.

Part II includes practical, clinical care across the multispecialty and interdisciplinary team. We will address prenatal care from both obstetrical (Chap. 5), genetics counseling (Chap. 6), and neonatology (Chap. 7) perspectives. We address obstetrical management including diagnostic testing, prenatal care, termination options, intrapartal care, fetal monitoring, and postpartum care (Chap. 5). We also address neonatal pain (Chap. 8) and symptom management (Chap. 9), including the challenges of differentiating pain and other forms of neonatal distress. These chapters provide practical clinical tips, doses, and indications for each medication. They guide the care of a neonate who is actively dying, either after withdrawal of life-sustaining treatment or when a family has chosen a comfort-oriented approach at the time of birth. The unique role of the palliative care specialist in counseling of families, birth planning, and expert symptom management is presented (Chap. 10). We address spiritual care in the perinatal period (Chap. 11) and perinatal bereavement care (Chap. 12).

Part III presents models of PPC. Chapters 13 and 14 discuss the evidence for different types of PPC program structures and processes (for hospital-based teams in Chap. 13 and for community-based teams in Chap. 14), the critical roles of the different members of the interdisciplinary team (IDT), and the importance of care coordinator. In both cases, the role of the IDT in coordinating care for the family and creating a unified birth plan that is consistent with their goals and values is discussed in Chap. 15.

Part IV focuses on some larger topics for the field. Chapter 16 discusses aspects of PPC from unique populations, such as racial, ethnic, and cultural implications for perinatal care, unique experiences of those who have struggled to conceive, LGBTQ families, and when the mother is the one who is seriously ill. Principles across the book apply to these populations, but this chapter elucidates some of the special care and considerations these populations deserve. Finally, the final chapters discuss how to build the field of PPC through education and training (Chap. 17) and the state of the field, current needs, and how to advance from the 30,000 foot view (Chap. 18). In the final chapter, the authors and other experts across the field (physicians, nurses, ethicists, and legal experts) weigh in on where we are, where we need to go, and how to get there.

We intend for this book to be highly useful for *anyone who works with families with LLFCs* – from palliative care specialists; obstetricians; midwifes; neonatologists; hospice providers; nurses in obstetrics, labor and delivery, NICU, and home care; doulas; social workers; chaplains; therapists; ethicists; child life specialists; and parent advocates. In short, we aim for this to be the guidebook for helping families in their journey through improving the care from every possible angle. Whether read cover to cover or in search of an answer to a specific question, we believe that this book will be useful, offering new insights for the reader. Tables and figures are intended to be quick references which are clinically relevant and easy to use and answer questions often asked by members of the IDT. Incorporated into each chapter are case studies that illustrate realistic scenarios that providers confront with application of principles or theories presented in that chapter. While we, as editors, sought to create a unified approach, philosophy, and "feel" of the book, any conflicting information or approaches are the purview of each author.

As editors, Dr. Denise Côté-Arsenault and Dr. Erin Denney-Koelsch are uniquely suited to edit this book. Dr. Denise Côté-Arsenault has a clinical background in childbearing family nursing having worked as a Staff Nurse in postpartum, newborn nursery, family-centered care, labor and delivery, and a center. She was a partner in a private nursing practice which provided childbirth education, bereavement counseling, and lactation consultation to numerous families. Perinatal loss education for nurses was their main focus working with healthcare professionals. From these clinical perspectives, combined with over 30 years as an academic in nursing, came 25 years of research which has focused on parent experiences of perinatal loss, subsequent pregnancy after loss, and most recently experiences of continuing pregnancy with life-limiting fetal diagnosis and perinatal palliative care program structure and processes. She brings nursing, research-based, and theoretical perspectives to this work.

Dr. Erin Denney-Koelsch is originally trained in Internal Medicine and Pediatrics. She is a Board-Certified Palliative Care Physician for all ages who has always been drawn to the magic of the mother-baby bond and has been practicing perinatal palliative care for 10 years. She developed and directs the Perinatal Supportive Care Program at the University of Rochester, which includes a prenatal consultation clinic for palliative care, neonatology, obstetrics, and social work to meet with families to develop a well-informed and values-aligned plan for birth and long-term follow-up through the neonatal period. She brings a physician's and practical patient care perspective to our research and scholarly work.

Drs. Côté-Arsenault and Denney-Koelsch have worked together for 10 years on a program of research to better understand the experiences and needs of families facing LLFCs, to understand the structure and process of PPC program across the country, and to help determine standards of care for PPC programs. We bring unique and complementary perspectives and life experiences to the designing and editing of this book, the first known clinical guide to perinatal palliative care. Through many hours on videoconference over these years, we have also developed a deep mutual respect, a highly productive working relationship, and a life-long friendship.

In the process of conceiving of, designing the content for, coaching the authors, and editing this book, we have learned on an even deeper level of the passion of the many amazing people working with families who are facing death of a baby. They describe their work as beauty amidst tragedy, meaning amidst loss, "sacred space," or even "the borders of heaven and earth." The work itself is hard, intense, exhausting, beautiful, meaningful, and, at times, transcendent. We all depend on each other for our unique expertise, advice, debriefing, and support. Like all good things in life, work like this takes a village. We are so grateful to the village that made this book possible. We sincerely hope the book is useful to you in your work of caring for families in need.

Rochester, NY, USA Erin M. Denney-Koelsch, MD, FAAHPM
St. Louis, MO, USA Denise Côté-Arsenault, PhD, RN, CPCL, FNAP, FAAN

Acknowledgments

We are deeply grateful to the many authors from across the country who have contributed their time, energy, expertise, and passion for care of parents and babies, as reflected in the chapters of this book. Their dedication to advancing the field of prenatal palliative care is evidenced by the excellent writing they have produced. We are keenly aware of the effort demanded, and we are grateful for their patience with the revision process.

We are also grateful to all the mothers and fathers who have shared their pregnancy and loss experiences with us and our research teams over the years. We want them to know that their willingness to participate in research has led to improved understanding of parent experiences and enhanced our ability to provide other families with the best possible care. Their stories are the reason this field exists.

We would also like to thank Stephanie Frost, our Developmental Editor, for being so approachable, responsive, and helpful and to Caitlin Prim for approaching us with the idea to write this book in the first place.

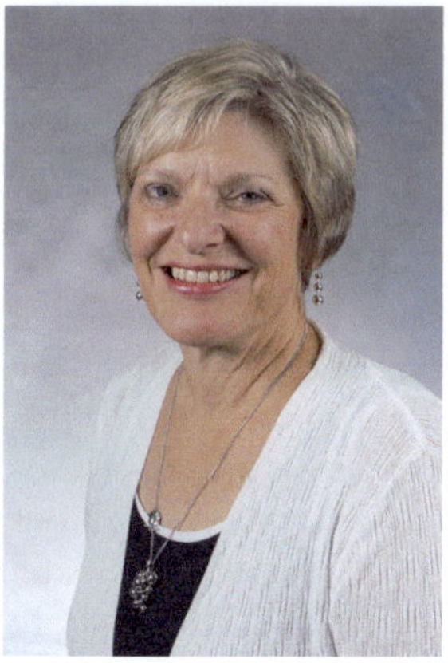

Denise Côté-Arsenault

First and foremost, I must thank Dr. Denise Côté-Arsenault who has been simultaneously coeditor, colleague, mentor, sister, mother, and friend. I could never have done it without you!!!

I also thank my career mentors and dear friends: Dr. Robert Horowitz, Palliative Care Division Chief, for being a steadfast supporter of my academic endeavors through allotment of time, encouragement to "go for it," and a welcome shoulder for emotional support; Dr. David Korones, my Pediatric Palliative Care Division Chief, for being my solid cheerleader and double chapter author; and Dr. Timothy Quill for being my forever mentor, palliative care pioneer, and humble leader.

Denise and I are both so grateful for the contributions of the brilliant scientific editor and conceptual genius (who is also my mother), Dr. Constance Baldwin, who transformed the rougher chapters with ease and took the good ones to a whole new level. Her babysitting expertise are also greatly appreciated! I'm forever grateful for the love, support, and pride of my father, Richard Denney, and stepmother, Karen Denney. I am almost frantically grateful that our healthy, creative, and fascinating children, Cora (9) and Evan (6), have never had to deal with any of what our patients and families have gone through. We try every day to teach them not to take their blessings for granted. And my greatest gratitude of all goes to my husband, Matthew Koelsch, my bedrock of support who tolerates the after-hours conference calls and editing deadlines with rarely a complaint, helps me to slow down, and keeps our homestead and family happy and thriving! I can do almost anything with you to come home to.

It's true that this work is a calling and that we work in sacred space. There could never be a more gratifying type of work than caring for those who need us the most. But I could never do it without all of you!

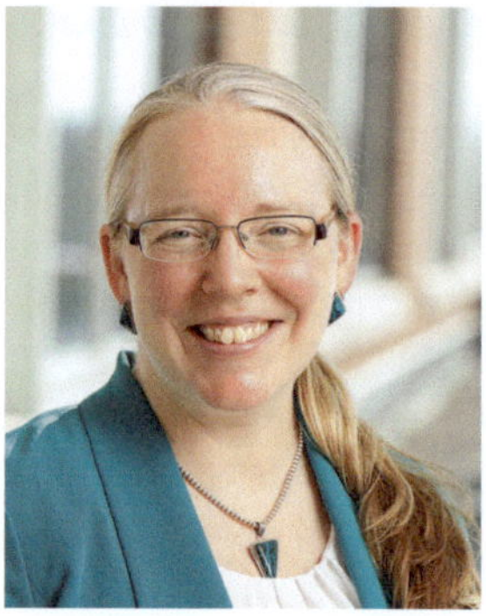

Erin Denney-Koelsch

I admit, I certainly was naïve about the time commitment this book project would require, but it has been so worthwhile. I have learned so much from each and every author, and I have no doubt that our readers will benefit from the treasures that this book holds.

When Erin Denney-Koelsch asked me whether we should consider undertaking this project, I did not hesitate because Erin and I work so well together. We have different skills and professional backgrounds, with a shared passion, commitment to excellence, and respect for each other: a winning combination. Thank you, Erin, for being my partner, colleague, and dear friend in this and all of our scholarly projects.

I would like to thank my father, Dr. Wilfred A. Côté, Jr., a world-renowned Wood Ultrastructure Scientist and Writer, who taught me the benefits of hard work and the importance of family and role modeled what excellence looks like. I miss you Dad.

Lastly, I want to acknowledge my family. I want to thank my husband, Peter J. Arsenault, Architect and Writer, who continues to encourage and support me and my dreams. His exquisite writing and editing skills have contributed to this book in untold ways. I am grateful that we journey side-by-side in our professional work as well as share the joy that our children and their spouses and our grandchildren bring us. I am so proud to all of them. And Marcel, our tiny baby boy whose life was hidden and brief, your life has empowered me and my work in ways beyond words.

Contents

Contributors

Rebecca Carter, MS, CGC McGovern Medical School at the University of Texas Health Science Center at Houston, Department of Obstetrics, Gynecology, and Reproductive Services, Houston, TX, USA

Marianne C. Chiafery, DNP, MS Clinical Ethics, PNP University of Rochester School of Nursing, Rochester, NY, USA

University of Rochester Strong Memorial Hospital and Golisano Children's Hospital, Department of Nursing and Bioethics/Humanities, Rochester, NY, USA

Melanie Chichester, BSN, RNC-OB, CPLC Christiana Care Health Services, Department of Labor & Delivery, Newark, DE, USA

Denise Côté-Arsenault, PhD, RN, CPCL, FNAP, FAAN St. Louis University, Trudy Busch Valentine School of Nursing, St. Louis, MO, USA

Carl T. D'Angio, MD Departments of Pediatrics and Medical Humanities & Bioethics, University of Rochester School of Medicine and Dentistry, Rochester, NY, USA

University of Rochester Medical Center, Department of Pediatrics, Rochester, NY, USA

Rita Dadiz, DO, FAAP Golisano Children's Hospital, University of Rochester Medical Center, Department of Pediatrics, Rochester, NY, USA

Barbara A. Dean, BSN Neonatal Intensive Care Unit (NICU), Christiana Care Health Services, Newark, DE, USA

Andrew S. Decker, PharmD Department of Pharmacy, University of Rochester Medical Center, Golisano Children's Hospital, Rochester, NY, USA

Erin M. Denney-Koelsch, MD, FAAHPM University of Rochester Medical Center/Strong Memorial Hospital, Department of Medicine, Division of Palliative Care, Rochester, NY, USA

Rachel E. Diamond, MD, MS University of Rochester Medical Center, Department of Pediatric Palliative Care, Rochester, NY, USA

Alyssa W. Gupton, LCSW, ACHP-SW Lifetime Care Home Health Care and Hospice, CompassionNet, Rochester, NY, USA

Natalia Henner, MD Divisions of Neonatology and Palliative Care, Ann and Robert H. Lurie Children's Hospital of Chicago, Northwestern University, Feinberg School of Medicine, Department of Pediatrics, Chicago, IL, USA

Laurie Hewlett-Miller, MSW, CSW Christiana Care Health Services, Department of Pediatrics, Newark, DE, USA

Stefanie J. Hollenbach, MD Department of Obstetrics and Gynecology, Division of Maternal-Fetal Medicine, University of Rochester Medical Center, Rochester, NY, USA

Maurice Hopkins, MDiv, BCC Golisano Children's Hospital at University of Rochester Medical Center/CompassionNet, Department of Pediatrics, Rochester, NY, USA

Patrick Hopkins, DNP, C-PNP, NNP-BC Golisano Children's Hospital, University of Rochester Medical Center, Department of Pediatrics, Rochester, NY, USA

Vanita D. Jain, MD High Risk Unit (PSCU) & Clinic, Division of Maternal Fetal Medicine, Christiana Care Health Services, Newark, DE, USA

Sidney Kimmel SOM, Thomas Jefferson University, Newark, DE, USA

Perinatal Special Care Unit, Clinic & Antenatal Step-Down, Christiana Care Health System, Department of Obstetrics & Gynecology, Division of Maternal Fetal Medicine, Newark, DE, USA

Karen Kavanaugh, PhD, RN, FAAN Children's Hospital of Wisconsin, Nursing Research, Milwaukee, WI, USA

Rebecca A. Kirch, JD National Patient Advocate Foundation, Policy Department, Washington, DC, USA

Kathie Kobler, PhD, APRN, PCNS-BC, CHPPN, FPCN, FAAN Advocate Children's Hospital, Center for Fetal Care, Park Ridge, IL, USA

David N. Korones, MD Lifetime Care Home Health Care and Hospice, CompassionNet, Rochester, NY, USA

Department of Pediatrics, University of Rochester Medical Center, Rochester, NY, USA

Amy Kuebelbeck, MA Editor, perinatalhospice.org, St. Paul, MN, USA

Stephanie K. Kukora, MD University of Michigan, Division of Neonatal-Perinatal Medicine, Department of Pediatrics, Ann Arbor, MI, USA

Center for Bioethics and Social Sciences in Medicine, University of Michigan, Ann Arbor, MI, USA

Emilie Lamberg Jones, BSW, RN, C-EFM, CPLC Children's Wisconsin, Fetal Concerns Center, Milwaukee, WI, USA

Steven R. Leuthner, MD, MA Medical College of Wisconsin, Department of Pediatrics and Bioethics, Wauwatosa, WI, USA

Children's Hospital of Wisconsin, Medical College of Wisconsin, Department of Pediatrics, Wauwatosa, WI, USA

Children's Wisconsin, Fetal Concerns Center, Milwaukee, WI, USA

Rana Limbo, PhD, RN, CPLC, FAAN Resolve Through Sharing®, Gundersen Medical Foundation, La Crosse, WI, USA

Jonna Marret, DO, FAAP Golisano Children's Hospital, University of Rochester Medical Center, Department of Pediatrics, Rochester, NY, USA

Baptist Healthcare Systems, Little Rock, AR, USA

Jeffrey M. Meyers, MD Department of Pediatrics, University of Rochester Medical Center, Rochester, NY, USA

Division of Neonatology, Golisano Children's Hospital, University of Rochester Medical Center, Department of Pediatrics, Rochester, NY, USA

David Munson, MD The Perelman School of Medicine at the University of Pennsylvania, Philadelphia, PA, USA

Harriet and Ronald Lassin Newborn/Infant Intensive Care Unit, The Children's Hospital of Philadelphia, Philadelphia, PA, USA

Barbra L. Murante, MS, RN Department of Pediatrics, University of Rochester Medical Center, Rochester, NY, USA

Ashley Pinkeney, LMFT, CT, MA Department of Pediatric Palliative Care, Golisano Children's Hospital, University of Rochester Medical Center, Rochester, NY, USA

Rhonda Rusinko, RN, BSN, CCRN Golisano Children's Hospital, University of Rochester Medical Center, Department of Pediatrics, Rochester, NY, USA

Michael L. Spear, MD, MSEdL St Christopher's Hospital for Children, Drexel University College of Medicine, Department of Pediatrics, Philadelphia, PA, USA

Pediatric Palliative Care, St Christopher's Hospital for Children, Philadelphia, PA, USA

Blair Stevens, MS, CGC McGovern Medical School at the University of Texas Health Sciences Center at Houston, Department of Obstetrics, Gynecology, and Reproductive Sciences, Houston, TX, USA

Loralei L. Thornburg, MD Department of Obstetrics and Gynecology, Division of Maternal-Fetal Medicine, University of Rochester Medical Center, Rochester, NY, USA

Chris Tryon, MS, CCLS Department of Child Life, Golisano Children's Hospital, University of Rochester Medical Center, Rochester, NY, USA

John W. Wax, MD Department of Family Medicine, Division of Palliative Medicine, Burlington, VT, USA

Elizabeth A. Westen, MD Department of Obstetrics and Gynecology, Division of Maternal-Fetal Medicine, University of Rochester Medical Center, Rochester, NY, USA

Danuta M. Wojnar, PhD, RN, MED, FAAN Seattle University, College of Nursing, Seattle, WA, USA

Lauren M. Zwetsch, BS, MS Lifetime Care Home Health Care and Hospice, CompassionNet, Rochester, NY, USA

Part I

Foundations of Perinatal Palliative Care

Introduction to Perinatal Palliative Care

1

Erin M. Denney-Koelsch and Denise Côté-Arsenault

Background

This book addresses one of the oldest of human experiences: the devastating loss of a baby. Despite the historical frequency of neonatal death, advances in medical care have made survival more common, and death is no longer an expectation in industrialized countries. As such, families are often unacquainted with anyone who has lost a baby and feel isolated and alone when they learn that their unborn baby is unlikely to survive [1]. However, it is still true today that the perinatal period has the highest rate of morbidity and mortality of pediatric patients, with an infant mortality rate of near 6 per 1000 infants [2]. Approximately 100,000 infants, or 2–3% of the near four million births a year in the USA, are born with a birth defect, with up to 1 in 5 of these not surviving infancy. For perspective, in 2018, in the USA, it is estimated that pediatric cancers accounted for approximately 15,590 newly diagnosed children annually from birth to 19 years of age and 1780 deaths from the disease, which is about 5–6 times fewer than from perinatal causes [3]. With the numbers of congenital anomalies, prematurity, and unpredictable perinatal events, perinatal clinicians are certain to encounter these cases, requiring at least a basic level of understanding of and competency and collaboration with palliative care.

The death of a baby disrupts the worldview of modern parents, their families, and health-care teams alike [4]. While parents' time together with their baby may be short, the loss is no less acute than the loss of any other loved one. With the loss of a baby comes the loss of the entire future the parents had envisioned with that wished-for

E. M. Denney-Koelsch (✉)
University of Rochester Medical Center/Strong Memorial Hospital, Department of Medicine, Division of Palliative Care, Rochester, NY, USA
e-mail: erin_denney@urmc.rochester.edu

D. Côté-Arsenault
St. Louis University, Trudy Busch Valentine School of Nursing, St. Louis, MO, USA
e-mail: denise.cotearsenault@slu.edu

E. M. Denney-Koelsch, D. Côté-Arsenault (eds.), *Perinatal Palliative Care*,
https://doi.org/10.1007/978-3-030-34751-2_1

child. Additionally, the number of mourners is likely quite small as newborns are not known within their family or community yet. It is a tragedy that is nearly unthinkable for those who have not experienced it or known someone who has. Parents faced with a life-limiting fetal condition (LLFC) in their baby are devastated, in shock, grieving, and overwhelmed with information and decisions to be made [4].

As the health-care system becomes more and more isolated in separate silos of highly specialized teams, each patient and family is foisted into the tangles of a complex system which often lacks the coordination and empathy that are essential to the family's well-being. Like all of palliative care, which seeks to lessen the burden of serious illness through expert symptom management and facilitation of improved care coordination and communication through an interdisciplinary model, perinatal palliative care (PPC) programs have risen organically across the country in many different sites to embrace the families who are suffering and need an extra layer of support [5]. However, there is significant variability in care models, lack of understanding among providers about the value of PPC involvement, and significant lag in available research to guide clinical practice and quality improvement [6, 7].

Caring for families who face a LLFC requires a comprehensive, interdisciplinary, multispecialty team of clinicians. The team must inform and guide them through complex medical information and options; understand the needs, goals, and values of the patient and family; and create a medically appropriate, value-aligned plan of care for birth and neonatal care [8]. They need care for mother, baby, and family beginning in the prenatal period and through the birth, neonatal period, and in some cases death of the baby and bereavement period.

With increasing ability to detect fetal anomalies early, PPC has arisen from the confluence of pediatric palliative care, perinatal hospice, and perinatal bereavement. Fetal surgery now allows some intervention for conditions that previously had no treatment options [9]. Pediatric palliative care clinicians saw a need to meet families earlier in their baby's disease course, even before birth, and began seeing prenatal consultations for families diagnosed with life-limiting fetal conditions (LLFCs). At the same time, perinatal bereavement specialists expanded their bereavement work from the unexpected miscarriage, stillbirth, or neonatal death to those families facing a prenatally diagnosed and therefore a long-anticipated loss [10]. While both are devastating, knowing of an LLFC for many weeks or months during pregnancy presents a fundamentally different experience than families who have a sudden event. With an LLFC, the long waiting period increases stress during pregnancy and anticipatory grief and also provides an opportunity for processing, understanding the diagnosis, spending time with baby, preparing for the birth and aftermath, and making decisions and memories throughout [4].

While PPC programs have been increasingly prevalent across the country (over 200 known as of 2019) [11], most programs arose through grassroot efforts by a few passionate people based on their own perception of an unmet need and what felt right to them. There has been little on which to guide program growth, no standard care models, no established structure or process of programs that is recommended, and no clear quality measures by which to measure outcomes [5]. This book aims to bring together what we know thus far and set a baseline for standards of care.

Terminology

A common misconception is the false equivalence of perinatal palliative care (PPC) with perinatal hospice. Hospice, by definition, is a philosophy of care provided through the Medicare insurance benefit (largely matched by most private insurances) that focuses on the comfort and quality of life of the patient who has chosen a purely comfort-oriented approach to care. While hospice can now be provided to children concurrently with life-prolonging care through the Concurrent Care Provision of the Affordable Care Act [12], it is still limited to those with a 6-month prognosis. The hospice model can be applied to the perinatal setting when the family has chosen a comfort-oriented approach for their baby.

However, palliative care is much broader and can be provided across the entire spectrum of care, from those choosing hospice and comfort care for their baby, those providing some life-prolonging treatment but also prioritizing quality of life (a middle-ground approach), or alongside intensive and life-prolonging therapies. Palliative care is a specialty that provides a second layer of support for families that focuses on the reduction of suffering, whether physical, psychological, spiritual, or existential [13]. Palliative care specialists are the experts in pain and symptom management, maximizing quality of life, improving communication between patients and their care team, and helping families to achieve value-aligned care. Due to the reality that the care of families with LLFCs involves both specialized obstetrical care for the mother and neonatology care for the baby, along with many other specialist's appointments, organizing and making arrangements may be very overwhelming for families. This book includes the current evidence-based state of the field of comprehensive care of families with LLFCs, not just *specialist* perinatal palliative care clinicians (those with specific palliative care training working on PPC teams), but *primary* perinatal palliative care clinicians (those who use basic palliative care skills in their own specialties) such as obstetricians, neonatologists, genetic counselors (GC), bedside nurses, social workers, and all the interdisciplinary team (IDT) members who care for these families. Care coordination from skilled communicators is ideal to ensure that all family needs are heard and addressed whenever possible.

Because PPC can be provided alongside life-sustaining and disease-directed treatments and can be provided by specialist PPC teams or as primary care, PPC is appropriate for a wide range of patients with a range of serious and life-limiting illnesses with prognostic or even diagnostic uncertainty. Because of prognostic uncertainty with many prenatally diagnosed conditions with some babies living much longer than expected, we have chosen to use the term "life-limiting fetal condition" (LLFC) throughout the book instead of "lethal fetal diagnosis."

Throughout the book, the terms "fetus" and "baby" are used in individual chapters when referring to the unborn child. After birth, "neonate," "baby," "infant," and "child" may be used. In all cases, respect for the baby as a unique and valued person is conveyed in language and meaning.

The Interdisciplinary Team

Because of the goal of reducing physical, psychosocial, and spiritual suffering, specialty PPC teams are by nature interdisciplinary. Specialty PPC interdisciplinary teams (IDT) often include the following team members [5]:

- Physician or nurse practitioner with palliative care training. This individual provides expert pain (see also Chap. 8) and symptom management (see also Chap. 9), can facilitate challenging goals of care conversations, and supports patients and families through their entire disease course. The role of the PPC specialist is discussed in Chap. 10, including how to run a family meeting and discuss difficult goals of care.
- Nurse or nurse practitioner, often as care coordinator. Nurses bring a holistic caring perspective to all patient care. The care coordinator acts as liaison to all the other team members, as a single point of contact for families, and supports families in their creation of a plan of care that honors their goals for themselves, their pregnancy, and the baby, often through a documented birth plan. The nurses' roles are discussed in Chaps. 13, 14, and 15.
- Social worker. The social worker may be a care coordinator or a facilitator of access to resources, such as insurance, housing, finances, and psychosocial support on all levels. The social worker role is discussed in Chaps. 13 and 14.
- Chaplain. The chaplain provides spiritual assessment and care. They may act as liaison to community spiritual and religious support people, facilitating rituals such as baptism, or just be a nonmedical, nonjudgmental ear for reflective listening. Spiritual Care in the Perinatal Period is discussed in Chap. 11.
- Certified child life specialist (CCLS). The CCLS primarily works with siblings or children in the affected family. They can provide developmentally appropriate ways to communicate, support, and facilitate conversations and emotional expression with the other children involved. The role of child life is discussed further in Chaps. 13 and 14.

Additional team members may also include the following:

- Obstetrician or maternal-fetal medicine (MFM) physician. The obstetrician or MFM provides all the direct maternity care: prenatal, labor and delivery, and postpartum care. They are often the team member who first learns of the abnormal finding and is the mother's first line of information. Their roles are discussed in Chap. 5.
- Genetic counselor (GC). The GC facilitates testing for any genetic or chromosomal etiologies for the abnormalities found. They use a nonjudgmental, nonguiding approach that allows families to learn information and make decisions on their own terms. The genetic counselor role is discussed in Chap. 6.
- Neonatologist. As the provider of the primary care for the baby, the neonatologist manages care whether a comfort-oriented approach or life-sustaining treatments the baby is receiving. They are the ones in the delivery room doing the initial neonatal assessment. Their role can be critical in prenatal counseling of what to

expect with the particular diagnosis and prognosis of the baby. The neonatologist's role in prenatal counseling is discussed in Chap. 7. Their roles in symptom management are discussed in Chaps. 8 and 9.
- Bereavement specialist. This could be a social worker with counseling background, a psychologist, or sometimes a bereaved parent with special training. The role of bereavement specialist is described in Chap. 12.
- Other specialists (cardiology, surgery, neurology, developmental specialist). Other specialists can be called in for consultation either prenatally or after birth, depending on the individual diagnosis.

More details on the team structure and function of individual team members are found in Chaps. 13 and 14.

The Care Coordinator

Because of the large number of team members and specialties involved in the care of a family dealing with a LLFC, it can be helpful to have a single point of family contact in the form of a care coordinator. This person (often a nurse or social worker) can develop a relationship with the family; come to know their pregnancy story, their needs, goals, and values; ensure the information they need and want to understand their baby's condition and treatment options; coordinate visits with other specialists as needed; and help them create and communicate a birth plan that honors their baby's life and wishes. The care coordinator role and processes will be discussed at length in Chap. 15.

Birth Planning

The process of planning for the birth often results in a written document outlining the families' preferences, goals, and wishes for the labor, delivery, and birth. The birth plan has a range of lengths, contents, and uses. In some cases, it is a medical plan of care; in other cases, it can be a worksheet for parents to review at home that allows them to think through their many decisions and then discuss with their providers. The process of birth planning is an important part of PPC and will be discussed extensively in Chap. 15. The process of making decisions for the pregnancy and their baby is a form of parenting, providing parents some control over a situation that often otherwise feels out of control [14].

Patient Population

To reach the greatest number of families who could benefit from the interdisciplinary palliative care approach, and the option of concurrent comfort-oriented and life-prolonging care, we propose the following populations as appropriate for PPC services:

1. Very likely lethal conditions (e.g., anencephaly, bilateral renal agenesis)
2. Probably lethal conditions with some hope of longer life (e.g., Trisomies 13 and 18)
3. Possibly lethal conditions with complex clinical course (e.g., hypoplastic left heart, congenital diaphragmatic hernia)
4. Any condition likely to have a complex and/or chronic course (e.g., multiple congenital anomalies, rare chromosomal conditions, brain anomalies, extreme prematurity, severe intrauterine growth restriction)

With those babies who survive past the neonatal period, their care can be seamlessly integrated into pediatric palliative care programs.

There are some populations of families who require special consideration. These include those traditionally underserved or with minority status; families with language or cultural differences; those who are lesbian, gay, bisexual, transgender, or queer (LGBTQ); or any who struggle to conceive for any reason who require a particularly sensitive patient- and family-centered approach. Additionally, the decision-making is even more challenging in the case of multiple gestation, especially in the event that one of the fetuses is affected with a LLFC and the other(s) are apparently healthy. In some cases, the mother's health may also be threatened, leaving challenging ethical decisions in balancing fetal and maternal best interests. These complexities are discussed in Chaps. 3 and 16.

The Option of Pregnancy Termination

There is some debate about the role of PPC in families who choose termination of pregnancy for fetal anomalies. Some families educate themselves about the fetal diagnosis, consider the condition that their baby will be born with, and feel that their baby will suffer in a way that they feel is not acceptable. Under these circumstances, these parents choose pregnancy termination or early induction with the sense that it is the best choice for them under terrible circumstances. They often feel tremendous grief over the loss of their normal pregnancy, a loved and desired baby, and their future with their child [15]. Some parents also desire to create memories and experience meaningful rituals including making memory boxes and photographs. The long-term effects of termination of pregnancy for lethal anomalies show that there can be grief, PTSD, and in some cases severe regret (2.7%), though the regret was found to be worse when there was poor support and less severe anomalies [16]. On the other hand, those who chose to continue their pregnancies also expressed a similar rate of regret, with 97% expressing no regrets about continuation of pregnancy [17].

There is no question that all families deserve expert, informed care and time to talk through their options, make the best values-aligned decision they can, and have expert bereavement care. There is clearly overlap in the needs of those who choose termination for LLFCs and those who choose to continue their pregnancy. In the ever-changing political landscape in which pregnancy termination availability and limitations vary widely by state, parents' options may or may not be limited. PPC will remain entwined with the abortion debate. Whether to call the care provided to families who terminate the pregnancy for LLFCs "perinatal palliative care" is debated by experts in the field.

In this book, we include some information about the process of termination in the obstetrical care and genetic counseling chapter so that all families can have their full spectrum of care options. Many families who decide to continue their pregnancies have been offered termination and choose to continue the pregnancy for a variety of reasons (religion beliefs, limitations on gestational age for which abortion is legal in their area, a sense of what is moral or right for them, etc.) [18]. Most patients who terminate never have the opportunity to meet with palliative care teams, so often this population never received specialist palliative care. Our philosophy on this issue aligns with palliative care principles in general: parents deserve to know their options and make the decision that is right for them. We want everyone to know that PPC is an option that many families have chosen, that it is a reasonable choice, that nearly no one who chooses it regrets that choice [17], and that many have gone on to experience a meaningful or even joyful birth [19].

Caring for the Caregivers

Because of the inherently emotional work of caring for grieving families, self-care and team care are essential aspects of a functional PPC team. Through mindful practice, debriefing opportunities, administrative supportive, and adequate time for training, self-reflection, and time away from work, the interdisciplinary team can thrive and continue to provide outstanding compassionate care to families in need. Care of the care team is discussed further in several chapters but most extensively in Chap. 15.

Growth of the Field of Perinatal Palliative Care

Education and training of both specialists and primary PPC providers are essential to meet the needs of patients and families facing LLFCs. Grounded in a relationship-based approach, existing experts in the field can increase the pool of trained professionals who can provide high-quality care to patients and their families through conferences, webinars, web modules, and literature (see also Chap. 17). Funding and training for research is also essential to increase the evidence base upon which the field aligns care with quality metrics. Advocacy at a local, state, and national level will also increase the public understanding of the need for care provision for this especially vulnerable population.

Conclusion

Perinatal palliative care is clearly a valuable option for parents who learn that their baby has a LLFC. While all parents have the right to make their own decision about their pregnancy, nonjudgmental presentation of options is critically important.

Once decision is made to continue pregnancy, then the interdisciplinary team and the expertise described in every chapter in this book become highly relevant. It is our goal to provide every reader a comprehensive description of all aspects of maternal, neonatal, and family perinatal palliative care within relationship-based, evidence-guided support. We see the ultimate goal for parents is to feel that they did everything possible for their baby, with no regrets about their parenting and choices. We want them to feel cared for and listened to. In addition, we hope that all members of the health-care team and community feel supported in their caregiving, from each other and their institutions, and practice mindful self-care to sustain this energy-laden yet incredibly meaningful work.

References

1. Côté-Arsenault D, Denney-Koelsch E. "My baby is a person:" parents experiences with life-threatening fetal diagnosis. J Palliat Med. 2011;14(12):1302–8. https://doi.org/10.1089/jpm.2011.0165.
2. Murphy SL, Xu J, Kochanek KD, Arias E. Mortality in the United States, 2017. U.S. Department of Health and Human Services, Centers for Disease Control and Prevention, National Center for Health Statistics. NCHS Data Brief No. 328, November 2018.
3. Siegel RL, Miller KD, Jemal A. Cancer statistics, 2015. CA Cancer J Clin. 2015;65(1):5–29. https://doi.org/10.3322/caac.21254.
4. Côté-Arsenault D, Denney-Koelsch E. "Have no regrets:" parents' experiences and developmental tasks in pregnancy with a lethal fetal diagnosis. Soc Sci Med. 2016;154:100–9. https://doi.org/10.1016/j.socscimed.2016.02.033.
5. Wool C, Côté-Arsenault D, Black B, Denney-Koelsch E, Kim S, Kavanaugh K. Provision of services in perinatal palliative care: a multicenter survey in the United States. J Palliat Med. 2016;19(3):279–85. https://doi.org/10.1089/jpm.2015.0266.
6. Denney-Koelsch E, Black B, Côté-Arsenault D, Wool C, Kim S, Kavanaugh K. A survey of perinatal palliative care programs in the US: structure, process, and outcomes. J Palliat Med. 2016;19(10):1080–6.
7. Wool C. State of the science on perinatal palliative care. J Obstet Gynecol Neonatal Nurs. 2013;42(3):372–82; quiz E54–5. https://doi.org/10.1111/1552-6909.12034.
8. Munson D, Leuthner SR. Palliative care for the family carrying a fetus with a life-limiting diagnosis. Pediatr Clin North Am. 2007;54(5):787–98, xii.
9. Matsui H, Gardiner H. Fetal intervention for cardiac disease: the cutting edge of perinatal care. Semin Fetal Neonatal Med. 2007;12(6):482–9.
10. Kobler K, Limbo R. Making a case: creating a perinatal palliative care service using a perinatal bereavement program model. J Perinat Neonatal Nurs. 2011;25(1):32–41; quiz 42–3. https://doi.org/10.1097/JPN.0b013e3181fb592e.
11. Perinatal Hospice and Palliative Care. List of programs. https://www.perinatalhospice.org/list-of-programs/. Accessed 8-9-19.
12. Your Child's Health Care and the Affordable Care Act (ACA): concurrent care for children. https://medicalhomeinfo.aap.org/tools-resources/Documents/ACA-ConcurrentCare%20FINAL.pdf/. Accessed 7/8/19.
13. WHO | WHO definition of palliative care. www.who.int/cancer/palliative/definition/en/.
14. Côté-Arsenault D, Krowchuk H, Hall WJ, Denney-Koelsch E. "We want what's best for our baby": prenatal parenting of babies with lethal conditions. J Prenat Perinat Psychol Health. 2015;29(3):157–76.
15. Sandelowski M, Barroso J. The travesty of choosing after positive prenatal diagnosis. J Obstet Gynecol Neonatal Nurs. 2005;34(3):307–18.

16. Korenromp MJ, Page-Christiaens GC, van den Bout J, Mulder EJ, Visser GH. Adjustment to termination of pregnancy for fetal anomaly: a longitudinal study in women at 4, 8, and 16 months. Am J Obstet Gynecol. 2009;201(2):160.e1–7. https://doi.org/10.1016/j.ajog.2009.04.007.
17. Wool C, Limbo R, Denney-Koelsch E. "I would do it all over again": cherishing time and the absence of regret in continuing a pregnancy after a life-limiting diagnosis. J Clin Ethics. 2018;29(3):227–36.
18. Wool C. Systematic review of the literature: parental outcomes after diagnosis of fetal anomaly. Adv Neonatal Care. 2011;11(3):182–92. https://doi.org/10.1097/ANC.0b013e31821bd92d.
19. Côté-Arsenault D, Denney-Koelsch E. "Love is a choice:" couple responses to continuing pregnancy with a lethal fetal diagnosis. Illn Crisis Loss. 2018;26(1):5–22.

Theoretical Perspectives to Guide the Practice of Perinatal Palliative Care

2

Denise Côté-Arsenault

Health-care practitioners from all disciplines use a variety of theories to guide their thinking while making assessments and decisions and considering interventions. However, some practitioners may not be aware that they are using theories, while others deliberately choose a theoretical framework to guide their work. The most commonly used scientific theories used in patient care come from the hard sciences or the social sciences. Utilization of theory elevates and improves the care that is provided, through adding systematic approaches to that care. In this chapter, several relevant and useful theories to perinatal palliative care (PPC) will be described as well as how they can be used to improve practice. A case study will be used to demonstrate how application of theory informs thinking and changes one's approach to improve PPC presented in table at end of chapter.

A theory has been defined as "a set of principles on which practice of an activity is based" (Google) and "a set of interpretative assumptions, principles, or propositions that help explain or guide action" [1, p. 11]. These definitions point to the inherent interconnection between theory and practice; they inform and feed each other (see Fig. 2.1). Physiologically based theories abound – germ theory and principles of infection, general adaptation theory (response to stress), and gate control theory of pain (non-painful input closes the nerve "gates" in the spinal cord to pain sensation) – just to name a few. Theories can be simple or complex, but because providing care for human beings is complicated, the most useful ones reflect complex, often abstract, concepts that are simplified to make them utilitarian. Theories aid our thinking about describing, explaining, or predicting phenomena or outcomes [2]. Theoretical thinking involves questioning and seeking causes or explanations of what we encounter, thus helping us make sense of what we encounter in our

D. Côté-Arsenault (✉)
St. Louis University, Trudy Busch Valentine School of Nursing, St. Louis, MO, USA
e-mail: denise.cotearsenault@slu.edu

E. M. Denney-Koelsch, D. Côté-Arsenault (eds.), *Perinatal Palliative Care*,
https://doi.org/10.1007/978-3-030-34751-2_2

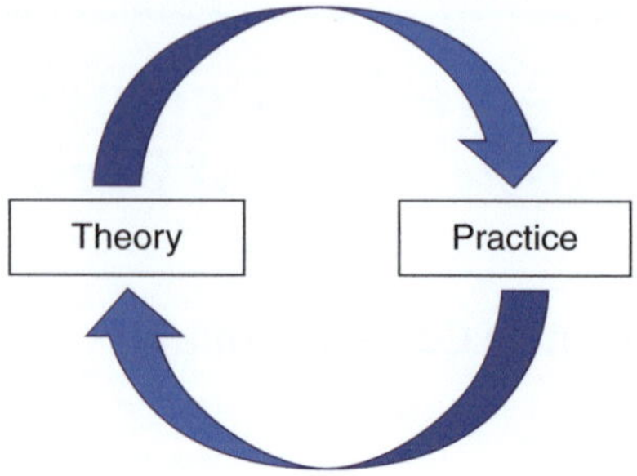

Fig. 2.1 Relationship between theory and practice

practice, providing answers to questions of why, how, when, and what for. Answers include "Because…, Given X, then Y", and "If X intervention is done, Y likely to happen." [3, p. 77].

Theories provide a systematic way to collect data and to describe, explain, or predict what is seen in practice. Theories from other disciplines often broaden and inform our thinking. We provide care to humans, who are psychosocial beings who live within a culture, a community, a family, and who have their own thoughts and feelings. Therefore, theories that inform our practice should be drawn beyond our own discipline in order to meet our patients' needs. Indeed, relevant theories should guide much of our thinking and decision-making, thus guiding our practice. We already think theoretically in practice all the time, often without recognizing it. Understanding more theories will enhance your thinking and improve care practices. Many scholars claim that theory *is* practice.

Once we consider and understand new perspectives and lenses (i.e., new theories) through which to view phenomena and seek to understand human behavior, we broaden our approach to practice. You observe something that triggers your new knowledge and you have, "Eureka!" – "maybe if I do X I might improve Y." Goodson calls this "meaning attribution" (p. 78). This "theorizing" leads practitioners to ask certain questions, question the status quo, seek reasonable explanations, and build a logical sequence of thinking about questions and answers [3].

A commonly known and easy to understand theory is Maslow's Hierarchy of Needs Theory. Abraham Maslow, a psychologist interested in understanding motivation in humans, examined highly successful people such as Einstein and developed his original theory of Hierarchy of Needs in the mid-twentieth century [4]. Maslow found that people are motivated to meet certain needs and that some are more important than others. According to his theory, depicted as a five-level pyramid (see Fig. 2.2), all humans have basic needs including physiological needs such as air, food, and water (bottom level), followed by our need for safety and security. If those basic needs are met, humans seek to meet their psychological needs: belongingness and love, followed by esteem for self and from others. The highest and peak of the pyramid is our need for personal growth and self-fulfillment through self-actualization and achieving our potential. Tay and Diener [5] tested the association of human needs and subjective well-being in 123 countries and generally found support for the universality of these ideas.

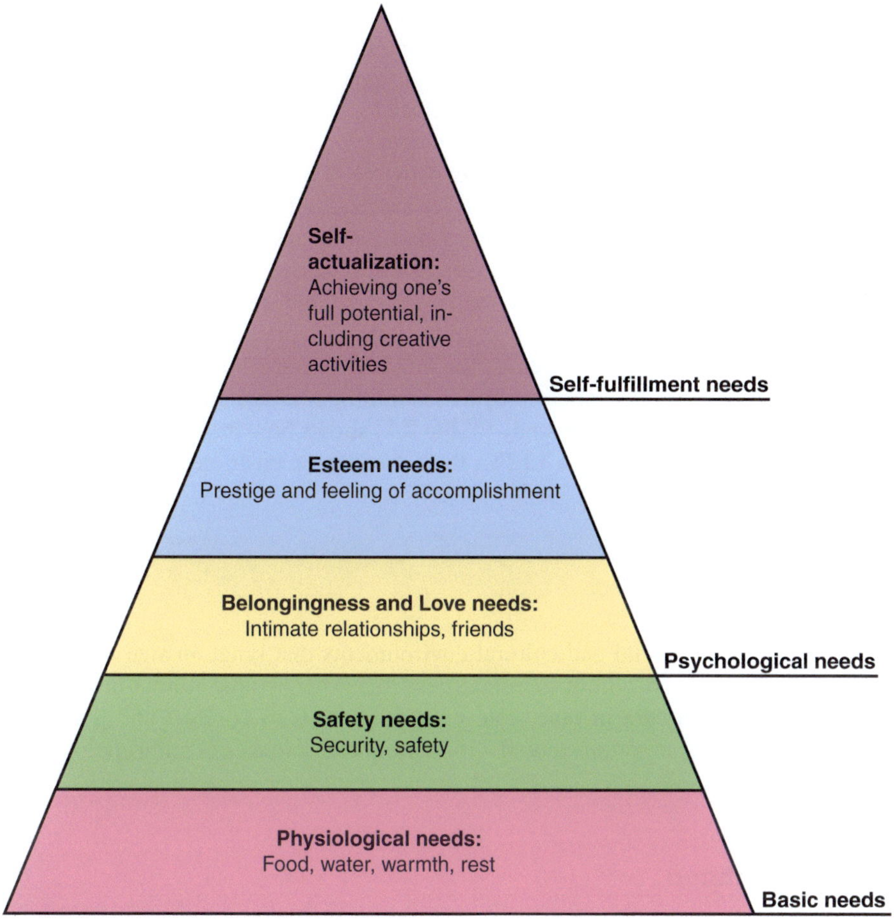

Fig. 2.2 Maslow's Hierarchy of Needs (1962)

Given this brief and incomplete description of Maslow's theory, consider the situation of caring for a parent and their small child who live in very difficult circumstances and never know where their next meal is coming from. As a care provider who sees these clients in clinic, you may identify a concern about a pregnant woman does not come for her prenatal visits, but looking through the lens of Hierarchy of Needs, you first recognize that the primary focus must be on meeting this family's need for food, water, and housing within a safe environment. According to Maslow, the mother may want to come to her prenatal visits but is unable to focus on higher-level needs until her basic ones are met, such as getting enough food to eat. Helping with her basic needs, possibly with a social work consult, may then lead to helping her focus on the issue of transportation to the clinic and facilitate her pursuit of psychological, higher-level ones in the future. Viewing this situation through the lens of Maslow's theory, you can realize that this family's lowest- and most basic-level needs must be met before they will be able to consider psychological needs. Your theory-guided approach will be more effective and less frustrating than simply focusing on your initial concern of getting the woman regular prenatal care. The Hierarchy of Needs is useful in a multitude of settings and circumstances.

Pregnancy is a complicated human experience. There are major physiological changes that occur in the woman's body, of course, but being pregnant has many ramifications for individuals and couples and within society. For many couples, pregnancy is anticipated as a positive event that will lead to a healthy baby and them becoming parents. This scenario is shattered when they receive exceedingly bad news that all is not well with their wished-for baby. Theories from various perspectives provide lenses through which a care provider can see how pregnancy, and in the case of a pregnancy complicated by a life-limiting fetal condition (LLFC), might impact these couples. The case study (Table 2.1) shows how theories are applied to one couple's experience with a LLFC, their pregnancy, birth, death, and bereavement periods.

Sociocultural Theories

Humans are part of social and cultural environments that range in size and scope. Family structures exist within communities; racial and ethnic norms are shared; structures and norms are in place that provide a sense of comfort and guidance. Sociocultural issues are often studied within the social sciences of anthropology and sociology.

Fetal Personhood

The notion of personhood comes out of the social sciences, specifically anthropology and philosophy. Personhood is the condition or state of being a person. Fortes found the universal presence of the category of person in diverse cultures studied in his fieldwork [6]. He claimed that the notion of the person is basic to the structure of human society and human behavior. Personhood is not a single status nor a stagnant one: it is socially and culturally constructed, indicating that it is context dependent. Key transformations of one's personhood occur from pregnancy, life, and death. In the USA, adults are generally accepted as having higher personhood than children, and pregnant women have different capacities than nonpregnant women, thus a change in social status. The question of whether or not a fetus is a person is central to much debate in the USA. Once a baby is born, the majority view the neonate as a person, albeit one with immature personhood due to low socially recognized capacities [7] but with some legal rights.

The notion of fetal personhood is critically important in the field of perinatal palliative care and to the parents whose babies' lives are threatened. Most parents are clear about whether their unborn is or is not a person to them. Naming of the baby is a clear indication of their assignment of personhood to their child [6]. Valuing of and decision-making about the unborn is inherent in the parents' sense of fetal personhood (see Chap. 3, for discussion on changing moral standing from fetus to viability to birth.)

Including fetal personhood in this chapter is intended to illuminate, not obfuscate, key issues. This is not a legal argument but rather a subjective view, i.e., that of a parent. Assignment of fetal personhood has been used as one approach to understanding what a parent feels has been lost with a perinatal loss. Although this notion of fetal personhood is not truly measurable, Côté-Arsenault and Dombeck (2001) developed a brief questionnaire that asked the respondent what they felt they lost: A pregnancy? A baby? A baby with a name? A child who would now be X age? And finally, Did you have a memorial service or funeral? The answers move from "not a person" to increasing degrees of assignment of personhood [8].

Those who work with parents during pregnancy must be aware of their own views of fetal personhood and, more importantly, the views of the parents seeking care and support. If it is clear that parents see their unborn child as a person, through their calling it a baby or a baby with a name, care providers should refer to the fetus as baby or by using the chosen name. This is a clear indication to parents that their perspective is understood, that their baby is seen as a person, and that life is respected. "They treated my baby with respect" has been said by several parents in Côté-Arsenault and Denney-Koelsch studies and is an item in Wool's Parent Satisfaction and Quality Indicators of Perinatal Palliative Care Instrument [8–11].

Personhood, in its broadest definition, refers to the condition or state of being a person as it is understood in any specific context. According to anthropologist scholars, persons are constituted (i.e., made-up or formed), de-constituted (i.e., removed or reversed), maintained, and altered in social practices through life and after death. This process can be described as the ongoing attainment of personhood. Personhood is frequently understood as a condition that involves constant change, and key transformations to the person occur throughout life and death. People may pass from one state or stage of personhood to another. Personhood is attained and maintained through relationships not only with other human beings but with things, places, animals, and the spiritual features of the cosmos [6, 7]. For example, when a formerly productive member of society with high status as a person suffers a massive brain injury and is in a vegetative state with reduced capacities, his personhood very likely diminishes in society.

Of prime concern when thinking of personhood, we need to recognize our own view of fetal and neonatal personhood as well as that of the families we care for. The personhood of the parents can be recognized through respect for their ability to make decisions for themselves and their baby and engaging in person-centered information-giving. As suggested earlier, care providers can acknowledge parental attribution of fetal and neonatal personhood by saying "baby" rather than "fetus" and using the given name.

Rites of Passage

In 1908, anthropologist van Gennep analyzed ceremonies present in all cultures that accompany transitions from one social status to another [12]. He recognized that these *rites de passage* (rites of passage) have a pattern of three phases: separation, transition, and incorporation. Ceremonies, such as baptisms, weddings, and funerals, serve as cultural ways to indicate major life events and bring people together socially to acknowledge the changes in an individual's status in society. Rites of separation indicate the leaving of one's prior status, and rites of incorporation indicate entering a new status; the transition is described as ambiguous, dangerous, and growth producing. These rites or rituals serve as a cushion to ease the passage from one status to another. van Gennep noted that the three subcategories are not equally developed or of equal length in every instance or culture [12]. A common example in our American culture is the rite of announcing an engagement, the intention to be married. This rite of separation indicates that the man and woman are no longer single. An engagement ring is often a sign of this intention and a change in social status of the woman; a verbal announcement or posting on social media publicly notifies family and friends.

The middle transition phase, often referred to as liminality, is the engagement period. This "betwixt and between" phase between two different statuses (term coined by Turner) can be a time of hope for the future but without structure, so it is a time of ambiguity as well [13]. The inherent uncertainty in liminality is uncomfortable. Rituals that might cushion liminality in the engagement example might be wedding showers or bachelorette parties, to indicate support during the transition. Wedding planning, with all of its characteristic decision-making and potential opposing views between families, can be quite stressful for some. The stress might lead some to cancel the engagement and, for others, to seek supportive help to ease the process. The rite of incorporation is clearly the wedding ceremony, often done with many witnesses and partying. The couple is now acknowledged as married by all; expectations, rules, roles, and structures are those of a married couple in that culture. Going away on a honeymoon can serve as another ritual, to allow time away from normal life and to aid in adjustments.

Rites of passage most pertinent to PPC are two: (1) seeing pregnancy as a rite of passage for the woman, from "woman-not-mother" to "woman-mother" and (2) religious or memory-making ceremonies done with babies who are born still or are ill and near the end of life.

Pregnancy When viewed as a rite of passage, pregnancy has distinct rites; the transition phase is by far the longest. Announcement of the pregnancy is the rite of separation; this is often done in stages with close family and friends and social media being the largest audience. The timing of the announcement varies widely, influenced by cultural norms, past experience with perinatal loss, and other concerns.

Pregnancy as a liminal phase The transition or liminal phase is the nine or so months of the woman carrying the baby inside her. This phase of pregnancy is lengthy, with increasing recognition from strangers as the woman's abdominal girth enlarges. The passing weeks may be noted through rituals such as marking off weeks on a calendar, by regular prenatal visits with a provider, or by changes in clothing to accommodate the pregnant woman's "baby bump" [14]. The father's sense of liminality varies widely when he is in his work environment versus at home or at family gatherings. When with his clearly pregnant partner, he is also seen as "in waiting."

Socially shared events such as baby showers, setting up a nursery, and putting a new car seat in one's car are all potential rituals. They serve as milestones and socially acknowledged times that indicate the reality of baby, social support, and the marking of time.

In the Western world, the rite of incorporation generally occurs when the mother emerges with baby in arms (e.g., like what the UK's Duchess Kate Middleton did on the front steps of the hospital where she delivered her newborns; emerging with baby in arms, for all to see) where she is seen as having the status of mother to this baby and baby is introduced to society. This rite of incorporation impacts the personhood of mother, father, and baby; all are elevated.

In the situation of pregnancy loss, stillbirth, or neonatal death, there is no social ceremony, no walking in the neighborhood with the baby that announces the new family member, and new social structure. Parents are left without social recognition and no completion of the rite of passage to parenthood.

Ceremonies with newly born Religious ceremonies such as baptism of infants can be highly valued by parents. When deemed appropriate, baptism can indicate a rite of incorporation into one's faith, communion with God, or as a means of passage to heaven. Baptism is reserved for persons, often only living persons. This is one reason among several that parents hope that their baby is born alive.

Memory-making ceremonies commonly done after birth with an infant death include holding the baby, taking photographs of the baby alone and with family, handprint- and footprint-making, bathing, and dressing the baby. These are things that parents would do with a live infant and/or mark the reality of the baby's existence. Most parents find these ceremonies helpful, but they may be taboo in some cultures and therefore should be offered but not assumed as acceptable [15].

Funerals and memorial services can also be very helpful to those parents who choose to have them. When family, friends, church community members, and others attend, it is a social event as well as a possible religious ceremony. Recognition of the baby as a member of a community and the couple as parents to a baby can be very therapeutic, a rite of incorporation, and may bring a sense of closure for some. Funerals are only done for persons. Babies may also be memorialized through rituals such as a tree planting, flower gardens, balloon lifts, and park benches—all with varying sized gatherings of loved ones.

Grief Theories

When parents learn that there is something gravely wrong with their wished-for child, it is apparent that they are shocked and struggle trying to take in what they have just learned. The response in their head is likely something like, "No, this cannot be so! Our [imagined] baby is perfect. This does not make any sense." Thus, the experience of grief begins, in its many forms. Once seen as pathology, grief is now recognized as a normal, healthy response to loss. Understanding some of the primary grief theories and their roots can provide care providers with knowledge of various forms of grief, such as anticipatory grief and complicated grief. Theories can contribute to one's ability to differentiate normal grief responses from problematic responses. In addition, understanding the perspective from which theories arise can be helpful in distinguishing differences between theories.

The concepts of grief and bereavement were initially recognized by Freud, who founded psychoanalysis and sought to understand human behavior. In his 1917 book, *Mourning and Melancholia*, Freud states that mourning is a normal response to loss, and melancholia is an abnormal state, more like what we now call depression [16]. But our understanding of what this is, what is normal, and how to interpret behaviors has developed immensely through the work of many scholars. Lindemann's study of responses to the Boston Cocoanut Grove fire (1944) focused on the normalcy of grief, its symptomatology, long-term impact, and relationship to trauma [17]. His work lead to a description of common symptoms of grief: (1) somatic distress, (2) preoccupation with images of the deceased, (3) guilt, (4) hostile reactions, and (5) loss of pattern of conduct.

Colin Murray Parkes, a grief psychiatrist, provides foundational understanding of human relationships, i.e., an infant desires to maintain close proximity with its mother and other caregivers [18]. Bowlby introduced attachment theory (1969–1980) and proposed that one's response to loss is dependent on the relationship with that person. He went further in his 1980 book on Loss, likening the death by stillbirth or infant death to the death of a spouse [19]. Bowlby's major contribution is that grief implies loss of someone/thing we are attached to.

Recognized grief theories include the most notable, that of Kübler-Ross, a psychiatrist, who aided in our understanding of what grief looks like from the perspective of the dying patient. While Kübler-Ross opened up this field in 1969 with identified stages of grief in the dying (i.e., denial and isolation, anger, bargaining, depression, acceptance), she also opened the door to conversation and language about death and grief in the USA [20]. While her contributions have been recognized, her stage approach to grief has fallen out of favor (More on Kübler-Ross can be found in Chap. 12).

Current theorists recognize that grief is a process, an adjustment to life without a loved one. Stroebe and Schut see grief as a way of coping with loss. They describe a dual process model of coping in which individuals move from the initial loss orientation to restoration orientation. This flexible oscillation back and forth is dynamic grief work over time resulting in incorporation of life without the loved one but never forgotten [21]. Accordingly, the bereaved cope by moving from confronting the reality of loss at certain times and avoidance of confrontation at other times [22].

Gender differences in response to loss have been noted for a very long time with women known for displaying more reactions such as crying and looking for support from others, whereas men are better known as being stoic, with less display of emotions and a focus on actively doing things. More recent work, notably that of Doka and Martin, indicates that rather than gender-specific types of loss there are various reactions to loss seen as patterns of grieving [23]. The intuitive pattern is seen in individuals who have affective responses to grief; instrumental patterns involve physical responses to grief in the form of restlessness or cognitive responses as often seen in men. These two patterns are the extreme points of a continuum of adaptive approaches to grief with blended patterns or inconsistent patterns across the continuum. Doka and Martin note that patterns are influenced by, but not determined by, gender. They are also influenced by culture and personality style. The scholars espouse that all patterns are effective ways to adapt and respond to grief [23].

This introduction to grief and bereavement theories here is to point out that they are known and referenced by many, and very relevant to all who work in PPC. Their familiarity often renders them invisible; however, the way we view grief greatly impacts our view of variations in grief responses. Providers should consider their own assumptions and experience of grief and then choose a theory they find useful. For example, a theory that sees grief as a way to cope with loss and that it is a healthy process could guide a care provider to encourage parents' grief and suggest resources that might help them cope. A theory that describes grief as a linear process of stages might interpret a parent's return to an earlier stage as concerning, thus instructing her to seek counseling. Much greater detail about bereavement and grief theories can be found in Chap. 12.

Shattered Assumptions

Janoff-Bulman introduced the shattered assumptions' psychology of trauma model [24]. Rape, natural disasters, and the death of a baby are all examples of traumas experienced. Janoff-Bulman's basic premise is that trauma causes psychological disequilibrium because of our basic assumptions of the world, "that the world is benevolent and meaningful and the self is worthy" (p. 6), are shattered. What ensues are attempts at coping with the threats and rebuilding a sense of new normal by revising or creating new assumptions about the world. Within this way of thinking, the death of a baby shatters parents' assumptions that pregnancy leads to a healthy child and that parents outlive their children. The theory states that, through repairing one's worldview, trauma can be overcome. Although this is a brief summary of Janoff-Bulman's model, it does provide a useful way to understand parental trauma and hopefulness for their future [24]. For example, in a subsequent pregnancy after perinatal loss, parents know that pregnancy does not come with guarantees, so they seek more frequent fetal heart tone checks and they strive to enjoy every piece of good news they receive.

Developmental Theories

Developmental theories describe a unidirectional, systematic way that human beings grow or mature over time. Piaget's theory of cognitive development and Freud's stage theory of psychosexual and personality development are two well-known examples. These theories describe, explain, and predict normal, anticipated growth and change within certain contexts. Levels of theory vary from practical to grand and simple to complex, but the movement is generally forward and cumulative. Circumstances can delay or derail development, but professional intervention may assist with achievement of appropriate milestones because current events affect future development [25].

Rubin's Tasks of Pregnancy

Pregnancy is clearly more than a physical-biological experience. While the woman's body undergoes tremendous physical and hormonal changes with conception, implantation, increasing uterine size, and breast changes, there are concurrent tremendous alterations in a woman's psychic world. The woman first recognizes that pregnancy changes her worldview and her responsibility, and her focus now includes her unborn child and her new role as caregiver to that child. Reva Rubin, a nurse researcher and theorist, introduced the notion of the development of maternal identity – the development of viewing self as mother *to this specific child* [26]. This development is evident through maternal undertaking four tasks of pregnancy: (1) to ensure safe passage for self and baby, (2) to ensure social acceptance of self as mother to this baby and acceptance of this baby, (3) binding-in emotionally to this baby, and (4) giving of self to be mother to this baby. These psychosocial tasks are imperatives for mothers and often for fathers. The goal of pregnancy is to have a healthy baby, and parents play a major role in bringing that child into their life, their family, and their community [26].

In the situation of fetal anomalies that may be life-limiting, the mother is keenly aware that she is not able to successfully fulfill the task of safe passage for her child. The fetus is not well, and in some large part, the mother feels responsible. She is supposed to do all that she can to protect her baby and ensure its health. Similarly, her ability to bring her baby into her social sphere is severely hampered by its endangered health. The emotional ties, prenatal attachment, and love are securely there, even though their baby has only been seen through ultrasound. Parents are willing to give a great deal of themselves, to do what they hope is the best for their child. Each task is threatened for couples seen in perinatal palliative care; considering each one brings to light the multiple aspects of becoming a mother and a father and will allow the provider to be more sensitive to their needs.

Revised Tasks of Continued Pregnancy with Fetal Diagnosis

Côté-Arsenault and Denney-Koelsch conducted a longitudinal, phenomenological study of 30 parents who received a life-limiting or lethal fetal diagnosis and chose to continue their pregnancies [27]. In-depth interviews were done individually and jointly with couples, across pregnancy, and through the birth and death of most of the babies (two survived). The purpose of the study was to describe parents' continued pregnancy experiences with a secondary goal to investigate the revised tasks of pregnancy these parents undertook. Five stages or time segments clearly existed for

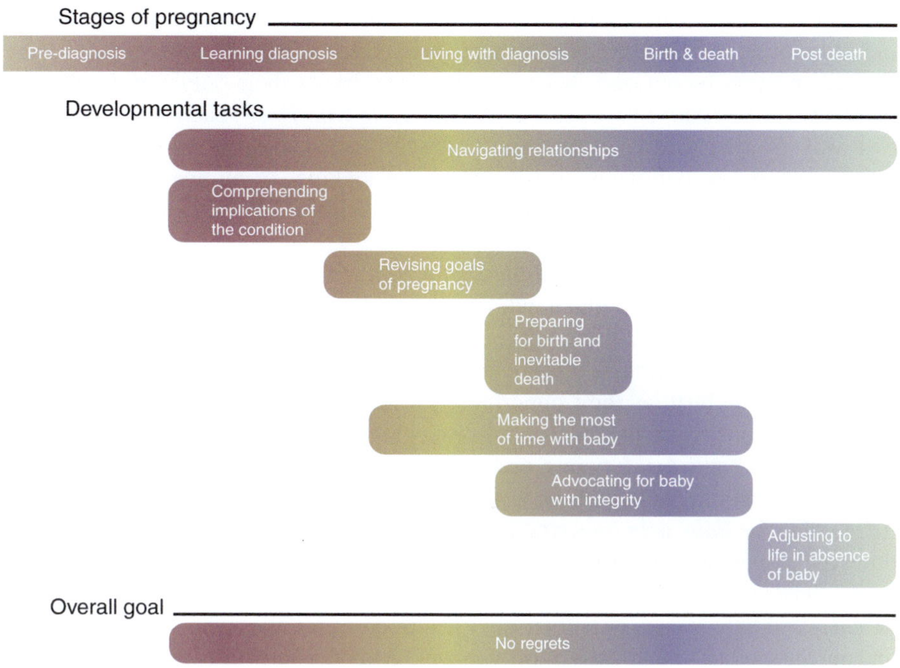

Fig. 2.3 Revised tasks of pregnancy with lethal fetal diagnosis [27]. (Reprinted from Côté-Arsenault and Denney-Koelsch [27], © 2016, with permission from Elsevier)

these parents: (1) pre-diagnosis, (2) learning the diagnosis, (3) living with the diagnosis, (4) birth and death, and (5) post-death (see Fig. 2.3). Additionally, seven tasks of pregnancy were identified through iterative data analysis. The first, *Navigating Relationships*, was ongoing from diagnosis to baby's death and indicates the social aspects of pregnancy in which parents communicate about the new diagnosis and the progress of the pregnancy: who to tell, how much, and in what way to share information. Some parents restricted the number of people they shared with; others spread the news widely. *Comprehending the Implications of the Condition* was the second concurrent task. Parents sought to understand what the diagnosis was and why it meant that their baby's life was in peril. It became clear that unless the parents understood the implications of the diagnosis and accompanying manifestations, they could not psychologically move forward to attend to other tasks. It should be noted that the prognosis was perceived as uncertain for two babies and thus prolonged this task for those parents. Care providers should recognize this task, provide information and time for parents to digest it, and then provide an opportunity to ask further questions. Understanding the fetal circumstances was a turning point for most parents; they were then able to move on emotionally.

Once parents understood why the condition was so serious, they began to *Revise their Goals* of the pregnancy (Task 3). No longer could they look forward to a future with their child, so they grieved what they were going to lose and pondered what they *could* do as they slowly accepted their new reality. Parents changed their expectations and set new goals such as having their baby baptized or to hope that they can look into their baby's eyes at birth, even for a few minutes. As goals were revised, parents recognized that pregnancy was likely their only time with their baby alive. They chose to *Make the Most of Time with Baby*; each did this in their own way. Some found ways to spend time with their baby now by reading books, interacting during ballgames, feeling the baby kicking, or embracing each ultrasound as a way to see the baby moving. This was particularly meaningful for the fathers.

Preparing for Birth and Inevitable Death is the fifth task and one that some parents were reluctant to undertake, while others found the planning as a way to gain some control of the situation. Advancing gestational age forced this shift for all. Location, mode, and timing of delivery were discussed at length. The majority of couples saw the birth as their opportunity to meet their child, and many chose to focus on that positive aspect. All parents recognized that birth also ushered in death; some planned baptisms, funerals, and other family gatherings.

All of the participants took on a parenting role during the pregnancy and began *Advocating for Baby with Integrity*. They saw their baby as a person, with value, who deserved respect and the best care possible. Each decision they made was based on core values, beliefs, and recognition of the gravity of their parenting responsibility. Mothers and fathers were grateful to have health-care providers who valued their baby and put the mother's health as a priority as well. After the baby's death, parents wanted only trustworthy individuals to touch and move the baby's body; they wanted everyone to handle their baby with the same care they would have used if the baby was alive. And lastly, parents began *Adjusting to Life in the Absence of Baby*. Funerals, memorial services, and creating a "shrine" for memorabilia in their home to commemorate their child were done with tears and hugs. Grief and healing took multiple forms and was just beginning as the study came to an end. Parents were grateful for their time with their child, as well as deeply saddened that it was too brief. Adjustments, seeking support, and grief were ongoing. Overall, all parents in the study stated that, above all and after all of their decision-making, they aimed to *Have No Regrets* when all was said and done. Then they could feel that they had made the best choices possible. They were uniformly glad they continued the pregnancy [27].

Recognition of these revised tasks of pregnancy can serve as a guide, a potential timeline, for those caring for these parents who choose to continue their pregnancy. Remember that these tasks are developmental; they build on each other and depend on completion of some tasks before moving to focus on a subsequent one. Task-appropriate interactions with parents during consultations, family meetings, and the birth planning process may contribute to meeting their needs where they are and to help them Have No Regrets.

Prenatal Attachment

Experts agree that feeling an emotional attachment to one's unborn child prenatally is a common and expected psychological aspect of pregnancy, particularly for the mother [28]. For the mother, pregnancy involves the evolution of perceiving the fetus as part of self to recognizing the fetus as separate from self [26, 29]. Concurrent with that shift is an emotional tie and concern for fetal well-being. Rubin referred to this as *binding-in*, but other scholars coined the phrase maternal-fetal attachment to describe the mothers' affiliation with the fetus [30] or prenatal attachment "to know, to be with, to avoid separation or loss, to protect, and to identify and gratify the needs of her fetus" [31, p. 359]. Condon later referred to attachment for both parents [32]. Prenatal attachment is often associated with motivation for healthy behaviors during pregnancy and seems to move individuals psychologically into the role of parent. It is an important theoretical concept to consider when working with parents.

Although prenatal attachment is a difficult concept for researchers and clinicians to measure, it is often apparent when parents demonstrate their connection and love for their child. Mothers may protectively embrace their expanded abdomen and speak tenderly of fetal movements; fathers may refer to their child by a nickname or be entranced watching their baby move during an ultrasound. Expressing concern for their baby's well-being during labor and birth as they struggle to write a birth plan is another indication of their attachment to their child. The absence of attachment would be noticeable if no concern or interest for the fetus is expressed and possibly when parents refer to "the pregnancy" but never to the product of said pregnancy, the "baby."

Studies have indicated that maternal-fetal attachment increases over the course of pregnancy, spiking at quickening when the mother begins to feel fetal movement, and that the level of attachment is greater than that of fathers [33]. This is due, many agree, to the intimate connection a mother has and continual feedback she receives from the fetus inside her as compared with the external and fantasized relationship of the observing father. Findings also indicate that paternal attachment rapidly increases once the baby is born and is held [33].

A word of caution must be given because it is known that some parents withhold their investment and attachment to the unborn baby during pregnancy because of uncertainty of the fetus' health, past losses, and other experiences. Rothman coined the phrase tentative pregnancy in 1986 to describe the emotional stance taken by women at increased risk for genetic abnormalities who sought prenatal diagnosis [34]. These women kept emotional distance from the pregnancy until results from their amniocentesis were known. In the circumstance of pregnancy after prior pregnancy or infant loss, emotional cushioning was identified in the majority of women, in which they attempt to self-protect against another emotional assault if the current pregnancy ends without a live baby, again [35].

The most salient point here is that most parents have an emotional relationship with their fetus during pregnancy. Care providers need to recognize this emotional attachment, assess its degree as best one can, and incorporate this knowledge when speaking to parents and about their potentially highly valued child. Prenatal attachment and fetal personhood are separate concepts; attachment is internal and personal, while personhood is a social construct that is culturally influenced. Both are very important to recognize in working with pregnant mothers, their families, and neonates.

Process of Care

Swanson's Theory of Caring

Fundamental to all of our interactions with patients and families should be a philosophic stance of caring. We all belong to caring professions; we provide *care* to patients and families. But how do we do that? Swanson, a nurse theorist, found that there are several components to a caring process, derived from her inductive analysis of perinatal contexts: mothers in NICU and those who experienced miscarriage. Her Theory of Caring provides a framework for interactions and meeting client needs that guides care. Caring is “a fundamental belief in persons and their capacity to make it through events and transitions and face a future with meaning” [36] (p. 354). Caring is “a nurturing way of relating to a valued other” (p. 165) to be conveyed to others through five caring processes:

1. *Maintaining belief* in another’s ability to make it through events with meaning. Within PPC, this includes offering realistic optimism, helping families to find meaning in their pregnancy with this baby, and standing by the person, not leaving them alone.
2. *Knowing* is accomplished through learning one’s story, understanding what it is like for the one being cared for.
3. *Being with* requires listening and being emotionally present with someone and being available to the family.
4. *Doing for* the other what (s)he would do for self if able. This includes anticipating needs and providing expert knowledge and skill that the one cared for does not have while maintaining their dignity.
5. *Enabling* is facilitating the family’s movement through transitions through informing, explaining, supporting, allowing, and validating.

In PPC, the process of caring means helping parents with the extensive decision-making by getting to know the family story, listen to them as being with, sharing your knowledge that might help them, and giving feedback to the family rather than telling them what to do because you maintain belief in their ability to come through this difficult time. The intended outcome of caring in this theory is *client well-being.*

Côté-Arsenault and Denney-Koelsch found throughout their research that parents want compassionate providers who are caring and nonjudgmental, respect their baby as a person, maintain realistic hope, and use an honest, straightforward manner. Use of the process of caring, as outlined by Swanson, by listening, supporting, and maintaining belief can lead to these desired attributes. Client well-being, as the outcome of caring, would include Having No (Few) Regrets because you made the best decisions you could.

Conclusion

Theories inform the practice of perinatal palliative care in many ways. The concepts of fetal personhood, attachment, grief theories, and shattered assumptions help care providers understand why parents struggle so much with the anticipated loss of their baby. Their whole world has been upended, without the cushioning of the usual rituals to ensure their rites of passage through pregnancy to parenthood. Parents proceed through developmental tasks of pregnancy that are altered because of a life-limiting fetal diagnosis. Perinatal palliative care providers can use their theoretical understanding to help in caring ways for the physical, emotional, psychological, social, and spiritual needs of these families.

Table 2.1 Case study with the application of theories. The story of Michael and Sarah (pseudonyms) and their baby (Joseph) demonstrates many of the theories discussed in this chapter. Their story is outlined in the left column, divided by stages of pregnancy

Case study	Theory and its application to case						
	Fetal personhood	Rites of passage/ liminal phase	Grief	Shattered assumptions	Tasks of pregnancy (revised)	Prenatal attachment/ binding-in	Caring
Pre-diagnosis stage							
Michael and Sarah (M&S) were excited to be pregnant. Family and friends were told about the pregnancy; this was a first grandchild for Sarah's parents so it held extra anticipation. They were eager to learn baby's sex on U/S.	Baby's sex contributes to how the parents and others view baby's personhood. It also allows parents to name their baby.	Announcement of pregnancy is part of the *rite of separation*; excitement from others is part of the sociocultural experience and ritual.		M&S planned this pregnancy, based on the assumption that pregnancy leads to a baby and to them being parents to that baby.	*Rubin* All normal, anticipated responses in a desired and healthy pregnancy. Sought *safe passage* through prenatal care and *social acceptance* through announcing pregnancy to family and friends.	Emotional bonds are to the idea of baby, a fantasized idea.	Prenatal care providers indicate caring by getting *to know* M&S, their story, and their dreams.
At 19 weeks U/S, the sonographer paused and slowed down and finally said that she saw something and went to get their obstetrician. The OB was unable to make a certain diagnosis due to low amniotic fluid, so Michael and Sarah were referred to the closest academic medical center with 3D ultrasound. The earliest appointment was 5 days away, which felt like a lifetime. Sarah continued to work as a therapist, trying to keep busy.	M&S were happy to see their baby on the monitor; learning that it was a boy made him more of a person to them.	The liminal phase was accentuated and made much more difficult when M&S had to wait 5 days for another U/S.	*Anticipatory grief* – M&S knew that something was wrong; their image of a normal pregnancy has been shaken.	Their excitement of seeing baby on U/S was quickly tempered.	*Revised tasks* Family and friends had been so excited to learn the baby's sex that they were eager to come and support Michael and Sarah, but the couple was in shock after their fetal diagnosis; they needed time alone to sort out their feelings.	M&S were becoming emotionally tied to their developing child even though Sarah had not yet felt fetal movement.	The sonographer explained her behavior.

Table 2.1 (continued)

Case study	Theory and its application to case						
	Fetal personhood	Rites of passage/ liminal phase	Grief	Shattered assumptions	Tasks of pregnancy (revised)	Prenatal attachment/ binding-in	Caring
Learning the diagnosis							
At the medical center, the maternal-fetal medicine physician told them that their baby had anomalies consistent with trisomy 13, including a severe heart malformation that could not be repaired. The amount of amniotic fluid was low, suggesting kidney involvement as well. M&S did learn, however, that their fetus was a boy. They struggled with understanding the diagnosis and prognosis, seriously considered terminating the pregnancy, and agonized over what was best for their baby. The sonographer had told them that termination was their only option. They refused to see that person again. After meeting with the genetic counselor a second time and consulting with the cardiologist, they realized they just couldn't terminate. The genetic counselor gave them a copy of the book *The Gift of Time* as a resource.	After learning that they were having a boy, they named him Joseph. A name indicates higher *personhood* assigned to this child.	*Liminality* continues without known rituals that might help this couple.	*Shock and numbness* are often initial feelings after hearing a dire fetal diagnosis. This was in response to the loss of a "normal" pregnancy.	This is not what Michael and Sarah expected in pregnancy. Their view of the world was shattered.	They struggled with *Comprehending the Implications of the Condition* and agonized over what was best for their baby. Once they understood why the condition was so dire, the trajectory of their developmental/ psychological tasks of pregnancy changed dramatically. *Navigating Relationships* was their initial challenge. Sarah continued to work but created information boundaries with others. Her clients could see that she was pregnant but she provided limited information to them; email and social media updates were sent to select individuals. M&S later allowed their parents to come and provide support and comfort.	Anticipated fetal movement did not occur until 30 weeks' gestation because there was so little amniotic fluid. Michael felt the baby move one time. However, M&S still loved their son. They read their favorite children's books to him every evening; they wanted him to know and feel their love.	This sonographer did not demonstrate caring; gave own opinion without *knowing* and *being with* M&S. Genetic counselor came to *know* M&S through listening. *Enabled* them with information and options; provided them a book so that they could be *Doing for self*. Helped them reflect on their own values and priorities as they struggled with decision of whether or not to continue the pregnancy. GC *maintained belief* in their ability to get through this, with support.

Living with the diagnosis							
This mother just wanted to enjoy this pregnancy and time with her baby while she had him. Although family and friends urged Sarah to let them give her a baby shower, she declined. Michael felt that they needed to prepare for birth and death; Sarah was not interested or willing.	This baby was unique and prized by mother.	Family wanted to give Sarah a baby shower because it is a known *ritual* for expectant mothers and a sign of love and support. To this mother, a baby shower would not feel positive. To her, it felt like she was in limbo, with motherhood on hold (*liminal phase*).	Sarah did not want to be grieving so she set it aside. But a baby shower seemed fruitless.		They worked at *Revising Goals* for their pregnancy and themselves. Therefore, *Making the Most of Time with Baby* became their focus, and they were reluctant to *Prepare for the Birth and Inevitable Death* of their son.	Love and attachment were evident. Sarah rubbed her belly and spoke lovingly to Joseph. Michael did not want to feel the baby; he tried to hold back his feelings so that he could take care of others (or so he said).	A caring response would include seeking to understand Sarah's desire to focus on enjoying her baby while alive. Let her know that she has support, no matter how the rest of the pregnancy unfolds.

(continued)

Table 2.1 (continued)

Case study	Theory and its application to case						
	Fetal personhood	Rites of passage/ liminal phase	Grief	Shattered assumptions	Tasks of pregnancy (revised)	Prenatal attachment/ binding-in	Caring
Birth and death							
At 34 weeks, Sarah went for a prenatal visit; no fetal heartbeat was detectable. U/S confirmed fetal death. Sarah went into labor within 24 hours and gave birth at the community hospital. They received excellent supportive care from the bereavement nurse. Every detail was tended to as Michael and Sarah adjusted to Joseph's stillbirth.	After the baby's stillbirth, the grandparents came to meet baby Joseph; he was welcomed as part of the family. He was assigned increased personhood.	After Joseph's stillbirth, holding him, taking photos and footprints, and dressing the baby helped create memories. These were a limited, yet important, *rite of incorporation*. However, the baby did not go home with the parents.	Sarah was hit with the inevitability of Joseph's death. She felt the loss of the anticipated remaining weeks of pregnancy.	Reality came crashing in; time with the baby was over.	Funeral planning was not done and the burden fell on Michael alone. He supported Sarah as she grieved.	M&S were so happy to meet their son. They were happy to hold him.	Care providers listened to M&S, learned, and used Joseph's name. They touched and took care with the baby's body. Michael trusted his son with the bereavement nurse to take him to the morgue.
Post-death							
Michael and Sarah decided to have a very small memorial service for Joseph. His urn and photograph were placed on a special shelf in their bedroom. Sarah decided to pump her breast milk and donate it to the local breast milk bank.	Baby seen as a person whose life has meaning (pumping and donating milk was a way to give meaning to baby's life as well).	A memorial service is a public *rite of passage*, a significant ritual within a family or community. This elevates the baby's personhood.	The reality of Joseph's death hit hard. Michael and Sarah grieved differently; they tried to accept each other's journey.	Struggling to develop a new world view. What is safe?	*Adjusting to life without baby* was ongoing. Pumping her milk was Sarah's way of finding meaning in her son's life.	M&S struggled to move on.	Providing this couple with bereavement counseling, support group information, and other resources will *enable* them to integrate their loss into their lives.

M Michael, *S* Sarah, *U/S* ultrasound, *OB* obstetrician, *GC* genetic counselor

References

1. Young A, Taylor G, Renpenning KM. Connections: nursing research, theory, and practice. St. Louis: Mosby; 2001. p. 11.
2. McEwen M, Will SM. Theoretical basis for Nursing. 4th ed. Philadelphia: Wolters Kluwer; 2014.
3. Goodson P. Theory as practice Ch 4, p. 71–87. In: Butts JB, Rich KL, editors. Philosophies and theories for advanced nursing practice. Sudbury: Jones & Bartlett Learning; 2011, p. 77.
4. Maslow A. Toward a psychology of being. New York: Simon & Schuster; 1962.
5. Tay L, Diener E. Needs and subjective well-being around the world. J Pers Soc Psychol. 2011;101(2):354–65. https://doi.org/10.1037/a0023779.
6. Fortes M. On the concept of the person among the Tallensi. In: Goody J, editor. Religion, morality and the person. Cambridge: Cambridge University Press. p. 247–86. (Original work published 1973) (1973/1987).
7. Harris GG. Concepts of individual, self, and the person in description and analysis. Am Anthropol. 1989;91(3):599–612.
8. Côté-Arsenault D, Dombeck MT. Maternal assignment of fetal personhood to a previous pregnancy loss: relationship to anxiety in the current pregnancy. Health Care Women Int. 2001;22(7):649–65.
9. Côté-Arsenault D, Denney-Koelsch E. "My baby is a person": parents' experiences with life threatening fetal diagnosis. J Palliat Med. 2011;14(12):1302–8. https://doi.org/10.1089/jpm.2011.0165.
10. Wool C, Repke JT, Woods AB. Parent reported outcomes of quality care and satisfaction in the context of a life-limiting fetal diagnosis. J Matern Fetal Neonatal Med. 2017;30(8):894–9. https://doi.org/10.1080/14767058.2016.1195362. Epub 2016 Jun 17.
11. Côté-Arsenault D, Krowchuk H, Jenkins Hall W, Denney-Koelsch E. "We want what's best for our baby": prenatal parenting of babies with lethal conditions. J Prenat Perinat Psychol Health. 2015;29(3):157–76.
12. van Gennep A. The rites of passage. (M.B. Vizedom and G.L Caffee, Trans.) Chicago: The University of Chicago Press; 1960. (Original work published in 1908).
13. Turner V. Betwixt and between: the liminal period in rites of passage. In: Mahdi LC, Foster S, Little M, editors. Betwixt and between: patterns of masculine and feminine initiation. La Dalle: Open Court; 1987. p. 3–19. (Original publication 1967).
14. Côté-Arsenault D, Brody D, Dombeck M-T. Pregnancy as a rite of passage: liminality, rituals & communitas. J Prenat Perinat Psychol Health. 2009;24(2):69–87.
15. Kobler K, Limbo R, Kavanaugh K. Meaningful moments: the use of ritual in perinatal and pediatric death. MCN Am J Matern Child Nurs. 2007;32(5):288–97.
16. Freud S. Mourning and melancholia: the standard edition of the complete psychological works of sigmund freud, Volume XIV (1914–1916): on the history of the psycho-analytic movement, papers on metapsychology and other works; 1917. p. 237–58.
17. Lindemann E. Symptomatology and management of acute grief. In: Parad HJ, editor. Crisis intervention: selected readings. New York: Family Service Association of America; 1965. p. 7–21. (Reprinted from Am J Psychiatry, 1944, September, 101).
18. Parkes CM. Family and relationships. New York: International Universities Press; 1972.
19. Bowlby J. Loss Vol. III. In: Trilogy on attachment and loss. New York: Basic Books; 1980.
20. Kubler-Ross E. On death and dying. New York: Macmillan Publishing; 1969.
21. Stroebe M, Schut H. The dual process model of coping with bereavement: rationale and description. Death Stud. 1999;23(3):197–224.
22. Neimeyer RA, editor. Meaning reconstruction and the experience of loss. Washington, DC: American Psychological Association; 2000.
23. Doka KJ, Martine TL. Grieving beyond gender: understanding the ways men and women mourn. Revised edition. New York: Routledge; Taylor & Francis; 2010.
24. Janoff-Bulman R. Shattered assumptions. New York: The Free Press; 1992.

25. Sage. Overview of developmental theories looking at humans over time. https://us.sagepub.com/sites/default/files/upm-binaries/43318_3.pdf.
26. Rubin R. Maternal identity and the maternal experience. New York: Springer Publishing; 1984.
27. Côté-Arsenault D, Denney-Koelsch E. "Have no regrets:" parents' experiences and developmental tasks in pregnancy with a lethal fetal diagnosis. Soc Sci Med. 2016;154(C):100–9. https://doi.org/10.1016/j.socscimed.2016.02.033.
28. Brandon AR, Pitts S, Denton WH, Stringer CA, Evans HM. A history of the theory of prenatal attachment. J Prenat Perinat Psychol Health. 2009;23(4):201–22.
29. Raphael-Leff J. Pregnancy: the inside story. Northvale: Jason Aronson Inc.; 1995.
30. Cranley MS. Development of a tool for the measurement of maternal attachment during pregnancy. Nurs Res. 1981;30(5):281–4. https://doi.org/10.1097/00006199-198109000-00008.
31. Condon JT, Corkindale C. The correlates of antenatal attachment in pregnant women. Br J Med Psychol. 1997;70:359–72.
32. Condon JT. The parental-fetal relationship: a comparison of male and female expectant parents. J Psychosom Obstet Gynecol. 1985;4(4):271–84.
33. Klaus MH, Kennell JH. Parent-infant bonding. 2nd ed. St. Louis: C.V. Mosby; 1982.
34. Rothman BK. The tentative pregnancy. New York: Viking; 1986.
35. Côté-Arsenault D, Donato K. Emotional cushioning in pregnancy after perinatal loss. Jf Reproductive Infant Psychol. 2011;29(1):81–92. https://doi.org/10.1080/02646838.2010.513115.
36. Swanson KM. Nursing as informed caring for the well-being of others. Image J Nurs Sch. 1993;25(4):352–7.

Perinatal Ethics

3

John W. Wax, Carl T. D'Angio, and Marianne C. Chiafery

Key Points

1. Clinical health-care ethics is a field of applied philosophy that systematically attempts to determine the best action when there are conflicting values and beliefs about the right thing to do for a patient.
2. All health-care providers in the neonatal intensive care unit (NICU) should have a basic understanding of common ethical approaches to dilemmas that occur often, such as neonatal resuscitation at the edge of viability, withholding and withdrawing life support, and using a shared decision-making process to act in the best interest of the infant.
3. Parental authority carries great weight but may be challenged in some circumstances.
4. Moral distress is common among all health-care providers; thus, an understanding of causative and mitigating factors is essential.
5. Hospital ethics committees and consultation services should be available to assist in particularly challenging cases and to provide support for staff via debriefings and ethics education.

J. W. Wax
Department of Family Medicine, Division of Palliative Medicine, Burlington, VT, USA

C. T. D'Angio
Departments of Pediatrics and Medical Humanities & Bioethics, University of Rochester School of Medicine and Dentistry, Rochester, NY, USA

University of Rochester Medical Center, Department of Pediatrics, Rochester, NY, USA

M. C. Chiafery (✉)
University of Rochester School of Nursing, Rochester, NY, USA

University of Rochester Strong Memorial Hospital and Golisano Children's Hospital, Department of Nursing and Bioethics/Humanities, Rochester, NY, USA
e-mail: marianne_chiafery@urmc.rochester.edu

E. M. Denney-Koelsch, D. Côté-Arsenault (eds.), *Perinatal Palliative Care*,
https://doi.org/10.1007/978-3-030-34751-2_3

Introduction and Overview of Ethical Reasoning

The greatest risk of mortality and morbidity for children occurs during the perinatal period, and this is often due to premature delivery or serious genetic, metabolic, or anatomic malformations that present either prenatally or during the first few hours to weeks of life [1]. With more technologically advanced prenatal screening, many potentially lethal conditions are identified weeks to months before delivery; this may create a long period of time during which parents know about the condition and must make complex decisions about the birth and potential death of their baby. Advances in disease directed and life-sustaining therapy have enabled seriously ill children to live longer. However, the cost of increased survival is often invasive medical interventions, surgical procedures, experimental drugs, and prolonged hospitalizations. The neonate is unable to personally weigh the burden of these interventions against a desire for an acceptable quality of life; thus, parents can sometimes struggle with determining what is "the right thing to do." Clinical ethics is a field of applied philosophy which systematically attempts to determine what one ideally should do in individual health-care decisions; in brief, it attempts to answer this fundamental question of what is the "right thing to do." Health-care providers on palliative care teams are often engaged in guiding families through complex medical decisions and should therefore be comfortable using ethical reasoning to help families and their care teams make thoughtful treatment and goals of care decisions in the perinatal period.

In this chapter, we will discuss how to define an ethical dilemma, a broad overview of common ethical approaches, common dilemmas such as neonatal resuscitation at the edges of viability, logical similarities (and emotional differences) between withholding and withdrawing life-sustaining interventions, professional obligations, and moral distress (which can afflict health-care teams when values around health-care decisions conflict).

Types of Conflict

Conflict may be one of the first signs of an ethical dilemma. Ethical dilemmas are generally due to disagreement about values among key family and clinical stakeholders. However, conflicts may be due to factors that are not necessarily ethical in nature. Common factors that can lead to conflict include disagreement about medical facts, confusion or mistakes due to inadequate communication, and/or interpersonal conflict [2]. Each factor will have a different remedy and may not require ethical analysis. Because medical care is technical, involves many professionals and caregivers, and suffers from uncertainty, it is not uncommon for conflict to be due to a combination of factors. Resolution typically involves renewed engagement of families, reevaluation of medical facts, team meetings, family meetings, and conflict mediation.

One example of a dilemma is a parent refusing to permit analgesic medications in a postsurgical, intubated infant with nonverbal evidence of pain. While this may initially appear to be an ethical dilemma, the conflict may resolve with education (if the parents' concern is about causing addiction or misinterpretation of a nonverbal pain cues), building trust (if the parent's refusal is based on a suspicion that the goal of pain medication is to make routine care easier by sedating the infant), or further exploring the emotions and experiences which influence parental preferences. However, this may become an ethical dilemma if the disagreement persists, and the team feels conflict between the duty to prevent avoidable suffering and a desire to respect parent's authority regarding the care of their child.

Introduction to Ethical Frameworks

If an ethical dilemma is the source of conflict, it is important to use a systematic approach to avoid missing salient features that could influence the outcome of deliberation. While most ethical approaches have been generated in the setting of decision-making for adult patients, much of the terminology and principles are applicable to the perinatal and neonatal setting. It is worthwhile to note that there is no "best" ethical approach which will satisfactorily resolve all dilemmas. Instead, multiple approaches are commonly required. Application of different ethical approaches can help the clinician avoid an incomplete analysis of a dilemma and successfully avoid making a premature judgment until all salient factors are considered.

While a detailed review of ethical frameworks is outside the scope of this chapter, we will focus on a few of the most commonly applied frameworks that may have specific importance to perinatal ethics. These can be divided into two types of reasoning: *inductive* (generating general principles based on observations) and *deductive* (applying established principles to a specific situation). (See Fig. 3.1 for common approaches to clinical ethics.) A widely used ethical framework in

Inductive Analyzing a situation to define principles	**Deductive** Application of principles to a situation
Casuistry analysis Applies lessons from similar cases with established and accepted resolutions	Principlism Analyzes a decision based on accepted values such as beneficence, non-maleficence, autonomy, and justice
Relational ethics Explores empathy, compassion, and the importance of relationships present in a dilemma to define ethical goals	Deontological Defines rights and responsibilities (e.g. professional codes of conduct)
Narrative ethics Considers how personal and public stories can examine moral values	Virtue ethics Considers the intention of each actor in a moral dilemma
Consequentialism Defines an ethical act based on the goodness of the outcome	

Fig. 3.1 Common approaches to clinical ethics

Medical indications

Principles of beneficence and nonmaleficence

- How is the problem classified: acute/chronic, reversible/irreversible, emergent/nonemergent
- What is the goal of treatment?
- What is the probability of different outcomes
- based on the proposed treatments?

Parent or guardian preferences

Principle of respect for 'parental' authority

- Is the surrogate capable and legally responsible for making decisions for the patient?
- What are the family's medical values? How do they make complex decisions?

Quality of life

Principles of beneficence, nonmaleficence, best-interests

- What are the short term burdens of therapy? Can these burdens be lessened?
- What is the expected long-term outcomes for the patient? Would parents consider a likely outcome an acceptable quality of life?
- Are there any biases or experiences that may influence clinicians, parents or guardians?
- Should a comfort-directed plan be presented as an alternative to disease-directed therapy?

Contextual features

Principles of justice and fairness

- Are there religious or cultural implications to a decision regarding therapy?
- How will a treatment decision impact other family members?
- Is a decision by a family due to financial concerns?
- Are there scarce medical resources which will be unfairly allocated by a decision?
- Are there professional, inter-professional, research, metric-reporting or business conflicts of interest?

Fig. 3.2 "Four-quadrant" method for ethical decision-making modified for the perinatal period. (Adapted from Jonsen et al. [3])

bioethics is the *four-quadrant approach* to ethical decision-making (Fig. 3.2) [3]. This is a deductive approach that encourages the clinician to consider medical indications, patient preferences, quality of life, and contextual factors as a way of articulating key ethical principles such as *beneficence* (doing good), *non-maleficence* (avoiding harm), *autonomy* (respect for a patient's values and choices), and *justice* (treating people in like situations similarly). Because the four-quadrant model was designed for adult patients, we propose a modified version which may be more readily applied to the perinatal period (see Fig. 3.2). In present-day United States, when there is conflict between these four principles, the principle of autonomy is generally given the greatest weight when making an ethical formulation. The challenges in applying this type of model en bloc to the perinatal setting are evident. Principles of autonomy cannot apply to a neonate who does not have capacity – the neonate cannot define its current quality of life or imagine a future. Thus, responsibility for medical decisions falls to surrogate decision-makers – parents and other caregivers – who will also be impacted by the outcome. Further, traditional concepts of autonomy imagine the patient (or family) as independently able to make an isolated decision if armed with an adequate command of the "medical facts"; this model fails to consider how the messaging a clinician uses to frame each decision can influence the family's process of decision-making [4]. Often, other principles must substitute for autonomy in the perinatal setting: two primary substituted principles are *limited parental authority* (a parent's right to consent or choose between medically reasonable options for their child) and *best-interest standards* (a responsibility to consider the goodness of possible outcomes for the child when making a decision which affects the child). One of the major criticisms of principle-based approaches in the neonatal setting is that there is no universal way to resolve conflicts which inevitably arise between the different principles. The greatest strength of this method may not be in its ability to adjudicate a "right" decision but instead promote a comprehensive discussion about the salient features of an individual case. By allowing decision-makers to actively identify salient principles such as best interest and quality of life using common language, consensus may be more easily reached through shared decision-making [5]. Shared decision-making is discussed at length in Chap. 7.

Deontological ethics is another deductive approach that is based on defining rights and responsibilities for patients and caregivers and applying these principles to a specific situation (Fig. 3.1 outlines this and other common approaches below). For example, if we agree that a child has a right to an upbringing free of violence, then clinicians have a responsibility to report suspicions of non-accidental trauma. This approach is often utilized in legal arguments and provides guidance to clinicians when there are clear rights that are well-defined under professional, organizational, or legal standards.

Virtue ethics analyzes a situation based on the intention of each participant in a dilemma. By choosing aspirational characteristics which seem relevant to a situation, one can ask the following: How would the compassionate nurse share bad news? What would a courageous parent decide when faced with difficult decisions around end-of-life care for an infant? Or, when would an honest physician disclose an error? Virtue ethics is one of the oldest forms of ethical reasoning and complements other ethical reasoning by intuitively analyzing motivation [6]. Key challenges when using this method involve choosing applicable values to a moral dilemma, avoiding oversimplification, and curbing unrealistic expectations of human behavior.

Other accepted models for ethical analysis rely more on inductive reasoning (Fig. 3.1). Examples include *relational ethics* (which emphasize empathy, compassion, and the importance of relationships to define shared ethical goals), *narrative ethics* (considering how personal and public stories can examine moral values), and *consequentialism* (which defines a moral act based on the goodness of an outcome) [7]. These approaches are appealing in the neonatal setting, as they often accommodate the inclusion of the family unit as a part of the ethical formulation rather than just the best interests of the infant.

Finally, case-based moral reasoning, also known as a *casuistry reasoning*, involves defining the ethical dilemma and finding thoughtfully reasoned, established cases which have an accepted resolution [8]. This approach works best if the core components of the ethical dilemma match a well-known test case, and the test case provides an authoritative or instructive answer. This is commonly applied in situations where medicine has a clear legal standard. For example, the moral outcry and subsequent legislative battles following Baby Doe cases in the 1980s led to increased discussion on the rights of a newborns with an expected disability to receive life-sustaining treatment and continue to influence the provision of life-sustaining interventions in the neonatal setting [9]. The specifics of these regulations are reviewed later in the chapter.

Balancing Medical Facts and Surrogate Values

It is critical to attempt to clarify medical facts about a serious diagnosis before attempting any ethical formulation. This can be encapsulated in the need to know (1) what is the precise diagnosis, (2) what is the expected natural history of the disease, and (3) how do we expect interventions to alter the natural history of disease. In the perinatal setting, the answers to these questions may be uncertain. Despite improvements in prenatal screening (such as cell-free DNA testing or improved fetal MRI) and available diagnostics, it may be impossible to have a high degree of certainty about a prenatal diagnosis. Even after delivery, results of genetic or metabolic studies may not be known for several days or weeks. Medical decision-making is further complicated by the fact that it is difficult to prognosticate the course or therapeutic responses to rare diseases or conditions that are extremely heterogeneous (such as some mitochondrial or peroxisomal disorders). Further, there is often a long delay between when a diagnosis is made and an outcome that is meaningful to the patient occurs. For example, a significant intraventricular hemorrhage detected in the neonatal setting may or may not result in a movement disorder or developmental delay in months to years. More common diagnoses, such as prematurity, will have population data available to help guide prognostic decision-making. Database-driven tools like the Neonatal Research Network's Extremely Preterm Birth Outcome Calculator can be used before birth to help guide decision-making but, as will be discussed later, are largely limited to generalities. Over time, each patient's individual prognosis will become more apparent based on clinical response to therapies, and population-based data will become less useful. Diagnostic, prognostic, and therapeutic uncertainties heavily influence decisions about goals of care. Specifically, in the setting of uncertainty, clinicians and parents may be most comfortable with trials of indicated therapies with a plan to reevaluate, rather than choosing a comfort-oriented approach early in the clinical course of a serious illness.

Based on the medical facts available, parents must make decisions based on their core values and the acceptability of different probable outcomes. This is a challenging task for several reasons: (1) It requires considering a future where one likely has little experience (as would be the case for healthy parents caring for a child with a chronic medical condition); (2) decisions are often coupled with medical uncertainty; (3) decision-making can be complicated by active grief (as in the loss of a twin or mother) or the anticipatory grief for a future that is no longer possible for the child. Therefore, we should anticipate that parents or guardians of seriously ill neonates need significant emotional support and additional time to make well-reasoned decisions. Clinicians can help reduce this cognitive load and angst by attempting to understand the family's values and making clear recommendations that are consistent with these values. Further, it is important to only present options when the input from the decision-maker will change the care plan and not burden families with options which are generally accepted as unreasonable or obligatory.

Limitations to Parental Authority

As previously noted, autonomy is the ethical principle which authorizes capacitated adults to make broad medical decisions – this principle allows individuals to embark on experimental or cosmetic procedures which carry risk with little expected medical benefit (such as stage I clinical trials) or avoid therapeutics which have unquestionable benefit and manageable risk (such as insulin for diabetes mellitus). Autonomy is bounded by the principle of futility. Futility has been extensively debated and typically can be understood as either quantitative (e.g., meeting the intended goal less than 1% of the time) or qualitative (e.g., an "unacceptable likelihood of achieving an effect that the patient has the capacity to appreciate as a benefit") [10]. The term futility is problematic in that it is particularly value-laden, and alternative terms (such as "potentially inappropriate") have been recommended as a replacement in the ICU setting [11].

In the pediatric setting, parental authority is the corollary to patient autonomy. Parental authority is more limited than autonomy such that while it is reasonable to expect that children will develop similar value systems as their parents, it is unreasonable to assume that children will always develop value systems that precisely match the values of their parents (Fig. 3.3). We define the limits of parental authority by the bounds of the following: (1) *obligatory interventions*, which occur when anticipated benefits *greatly* outweigh harms (right side of Fig. 3.3), and (2) *unreasonable interventions*, which are withheld when anticipated harms *greatly* outweigh benefits (left side of Fig. 3.3). The classic example of an obligatory intervention is to administer a blood transfusion after a blood loss due to a significant trauma; the benefits of transfusion can be life-saving and medical risks are few. Therefore, while individuals may refuse a blood transfusion based on personal or religious beliefs, we do not allow parents to refuse a life-saving blood transfusion for a minor child [12]. Aggressive resuscitation attempts for a newly delivered anencephalic infant are an example of a potentially unreasonable or inappropriate intervention based on near certainty regarding early death [13].

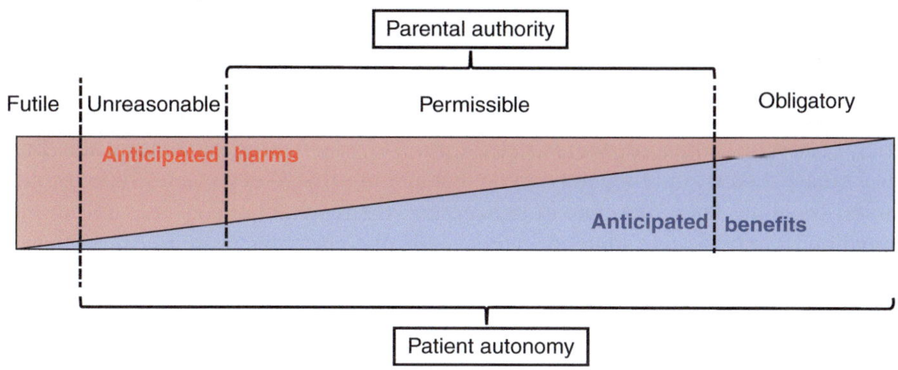

Fig. 3.3 Limits of parental authority and patient autonomy

The borders of parental authority are a potential cause of conflict between a medical team and families. Therefore, it is important to proactively identify which interventions are beyond the scope of parental authority, ensure consensus among medical providers, and present a medical care plan to a family that does not suggest a false choice that is not subject to parental authority (see more on this in Case 3.2). In other words, clearly defined "obligatory" interventions should be presented to parents as the standard of care, and "unreasonable" or "impermissible" interventions may be explained but clearly identified as inappropriate. The interventions defined as obligatory or unreasonable will be institution-specific; therefore, it is important to develop and understand local standards to ensure that similar patients are treated similarly. Parental authority may also be limited if there is clear evidence that the parent is making decisions that are not in the best interest of the infant or if the parent is incapacitated. Examples of an incapacitated surrogate include someone who has a cognitive disability which impairs their ability to make informed decisions, someone under the influence of mind-altering substances, or someone delirious secondary to serious illness. If a surrogate is unable or unwilling to participate in decision-making, involvement of a hospital ethics committee and risk management team is essential – appropriate emergent interventions should be initiated and efforts should be made to identify and appoint a guardian. Often, this will be a grandparent or other involved adult relative.

Principle of Moral Standing

Moral standing, or moral status, is a principle which attempts to weigh how much an entity's interests should be considered when making an ethical decision (Fig. 3.4) [14]. This is an important concept in perinatal ethics because there are clinical circumstances where the best interests of a mother and the best interests of a fetus may come into conflict (such as continuing potentially teratogenic, mood-stabilizing medications during a pregnancy or early induction of labor so that a mother can start chemotherapy for a newly identified cancer) (see Chap. 16, Case 16.4). The concept of moral standing is useful but can lead to controversy. While elective abortion is not within the scope of perinatal palliative care, conflict surrounding abortion rights provides a practical example of disagreements about moral standing. Someone who is strictly pro-life would interpret a moral standing as a binary distinction; they may argue that an unfertilized egg carries little (or no) moral standing, but at the time of conception, the resultant embryo has full moral standing. Alternatively, someone who is strictly pro-choice would argue that a fetus has lesser moral standing than the mother, so the mother has rights to terminate a pregnancy based solely on her own interests. The concept of partial moral standing can be used as a justification for maintaining the liberty rights of a pregnant mother who actively exposes her fetus to the harms of alcohol or tobacco. In general, in the United States, two significant thresholds in the perinatal period result in a dramatic increase in the moral standing of a fetus – the age of viability

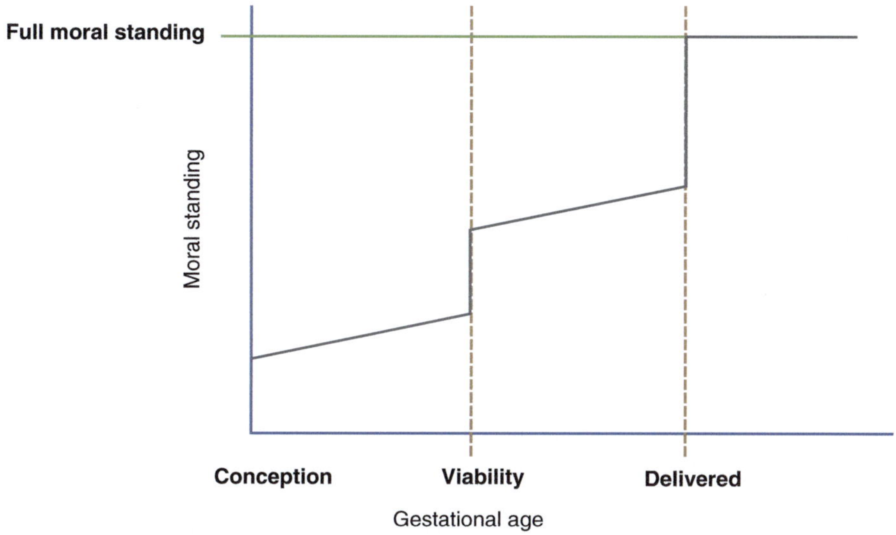

Fig. 3.4 Stepwise development of moral standing

(when a fetus could reasonably be expected to survive outside of the uterus) and immediately after delivery, when the fetus is no longer subject to the mother's interest in bodily integrity (Fig. 3.4) [15].

Perinatal Resuscitation Decisions

Case 3.1
Two families, each with a woman carrying a 23-week-gestation fetus at risk for delivery in the next several hours, have made differing decisions about neonatal resuscitation. The fetuses are similar in all known respects. One family has opted for full resuscitation, while the other, no resuscitation. The neonatologists plan to honor both decisions. Why?

Discussion

While the discussion of this case will focus on resuscitation and treatment decisions for periviable premature infants, the approach to other infants with high risks for morbidity and mortality, e.g., major prenatal anomalies, trisomies 13 or 18, is similar in concept to what will be described here. Regardless of the circumstance that makes survival unlikely, morbidity significant, and/or the burden of therapy high, similar principles and reasoning apply.

Decision-making for fetuses and newborn infants differs from the typical American biomedical ethical construct that elevates the importance of autonomy above other principles. While a woman is pregnant, she is generally felt to have a near-absolute right to refuse interventions (e.g., Cesarean section) that might be necessary to save the life of her fetus. Once an infant is born, deference is often given to the parental authority, which is more limited than an individual's autonomy to make decisions regarding her or his own health care (Fig. 3.3). Decision-making regarding resuscitation of a medically tenuous newborn often takes place while a mother is still pregnant – in the space between a mother's autonomy and the parents' authority over decisions for their child.

The most common circumstance in which prenatal discussion of resuscitation occurs is in the setting of impending delivery of an infant on the cusp of viability, defined in 2015 by some experts as 22–24 weeks' gestation, where the prognosis for survival is guarded and the likelihood of significant health sequelae, including neurodevelopmental impairment, is high [16]. It is important to note that this range has varied over time, as medical care has improved and outcome data have changed. Discussions in the early 2000s often described the periviable period as 23–25 weeks [17, 18]. The American Academy of Pediatrics' Committee on Fetus and Newborn recommends that "the approach [to periviable infants] should be shared decision-making with the family, guided by considering both the likelihood of death or morbidity and the parents' desires for their unborn child" [16]. However, others have argued that there are situations within this range where the risks are so high and the benefits so uncertain that treatment could be considered "unreasonable" or even "inhumane" and parental decision-making authority limited (such as resuscitation under 22 weeks' gestation) [19–22]. It should be noted that this conception is broader than the ethical definition of futility (where the chances of achieving the stated goal of therapy are extremely low) [23]. As infant maturity advances and/or prognosis improves, treatment eventually crosses into being considered "obligatory," and parental authority is again limited [20, 21, 24]. In the current era, many neonatologists would consider resuscitation to be obligatory for uncomplicated deliveries of otherwise healthy fetuses above 25–26 weeks' gestation, where survival may approach 80–90% [16]. Once again, the most difficult and complex decision-making occurs at an intersection – between "unreasonable" and "obligatory" treatments – an area often referred to as the "gray zone" [16–18, 25, 26].

Evidence-Based Ethics

While the concepts of perinatal decision-making apply to many situations beyond extreme prematurity, the wealth of data surrounding outcomes of extreme prematurity have made it particularly amenable to discussions of using data to determine best approaches, a concept termed "evidence-based ethics" [21]. It should be stressed, however, that the same data are viewed differently by different participants in conversations and that treatment approaches are shaped by societal consensus [27].

The most straightforward approach both to prenatal decision-making and to attempting to define the borders of the gray zone for shared decision-making is to use easily ascertained parameters, e.g., an estimate of gestational age, often combined with an estimate of fetal weight (or, similarly, a specific chromosomal or anatomic anomaly). These rules of thumb, however, encompass a wide range of outcomes and do not take into account other prenatally available factors known to influence outcome [28–31]. In 2008, Tyson and colleagues published an outcomes prediction model for infants born at 22–25 weeks' gestation that incorporated, in addition to estimated fetal weight and gestational age, exposure to antenatal corticosteroids, fetal sex, and singleton vs. multiple birth [31]. This was subsequently made available as an online calculator (https://www1.nichd.nih.gov/epbo-calculator/Pages/epbo_case.aspx) that produces estimates of survival and survival with various levels of neurodevelopmental impairment at 18–22 months of age. However, these data were drawn from infants born between 1998 and 2003 at a limited number of perinatal centers, making applicability many years later and/or in other settings unclear. Work is underway to update this estimator. In addition, prenatal estimates of survival are based on sometimes imprecise values (for instance, estimations of fetal weight), making the estimates themselves imprecise. Since the ultimate consequence for an infant is either to experience a particular outcome or not (100% or 0%), percentage likelihoods of outcomes are also, by nature, unable to be accurate for an individual infant. Further factors not considered in such a calculator, such as coexisting congenital anomalies, perinatal infection, or route of delivery, may also alter its prognostic validity [32, 33].

In an attempt to refine estimates of survival, some have suggested using immediate delivery room impression and course [34]. However, among extremely preterm infants, physical estimates of gestational age correlate poorly with (often reliable) antenatal ultrasound estimates [35, 36], and initial response to resuscitation also poorly predicts eventual outcome [25].

Rare conditions, for which extensive natural history information is often unavailable, are notoriously harder to prognosticate than prematurity. This can make clear delineation of what is obligatory vs. unreasonable more variable, based on the individual center or physician. For example, some centers will not offer complex congenital heart surgery for infants with severe chromosomal disorders, feeling that this would be an unreasonable level of intervention. On the other hand, some centers will permit this if parents desire.

Trials of Therapy

Another reasonable approach to resuscitation at the borderline of viability (or any condition with uncertain prognosis) is a trial of therapy, incorporating an initial attempt at resuscitation and continuous reassessment of prognosis based on early postnatal course. Some have found that such an approach allows clearer delineation of infants extremely unlikely to survive or survive without major impairments, based either on objective data (e.g., intraventricular hemorrhage, inability to maintain oxygenation despite respiratory support), subjective impression, or both [37–39]. This approach has the advantage of delaying decision-making until more data have accrued and the precision of outcome estimates have improved. Potential disadvantages include suffering among infants unlikely to survive and the possibility that parents will not accept recommendations that therapy be limited in the face of evidence of poor prognosis, leading to further suffering of infants who will ultimately die or suffer severe impairments. In addition, trials of therapy do not directly address the question of the lower limit below which it is unreasonable to provide resuscitation, which would leave the ever-moving target of futility as the only setting in which resuscitation would not be attempted.

A similar approach is also often chosen by parents of infants with prenatally diagnosed anomalies with expected poor or uncertain prognosis. Allowing infants to "declare themselves" can provide parents and clinicians with reassurance that reasonable attempts were made to save or prolong life and only abandoned when the prognosis was clear. The approach has the same potential risk (for instance, in accepting extremely risky surgery) of inflicting suffering upon infants not destined to survive.

Withholding and Withdrawing

Adult palliative care providers will likely be comfortable with the ethical equivalency of withholding and withdrawing life-sustaining treatments, as explored in the literature [24, 40]. However, for many parents and some direct care providers in the NICU, these ethically equivalent decisions carry a different emotional weight. In the setting of neonatal resuscitation decisions, withholding and withdrawing place primacy on different concerns. Prenatal decision-making (withholding treatment) focuses on minimizing suffering. It aims to limit the number of infants who will have poor outcomes (death or significant disability) by accepting the possibility that some non-resuscitated infants would have gone on to have good outcomes. This approach highly values non-maleficence (avoiding harm). Postnatal decision-making (that can result in withdrawing treatment) focuses on minimizing the number of infants with eventually good outcomes who would be harmed (die) by nontreatment, an approach valuing beneficence (avoiding death) highly. While either of these approaches is ethically valid, they emphasize different values (avoiding suffering vs. maximizing survival). The preferred approach for an individual family will depend, in part, on the weights they place on these values.

Guidance for Decision-Making

A potentially reasonable approach to shared decision-making regarding neonatal resuscitation is for the decision-making to be collaborative when an infant's best interests are unclear (the "gray zone," middle of Fig. 3.3), but to be more heavily provider-led when an infant's best interests are relatively clear, i.e., where treatment appears either "unreasonable" or "obligatory." Although some variation on this model is commonly used to guide neonatal resuscitation throughout high-income countries, perinatal decision-making models with differing emphases on provider and family input are used in various settings [41–43]. Some centers operate largely on clinician-led decision-making, with tacit or expected parental assent to the decisions. In other centers, decisions are likely to be family-led in nearly all situations outside of "obligatory" treatment. This often results in more trials of therapy, as families are more likely than providers to emphasize positive aspects of an infant's prognosis [41, 44]. Arguably, a balanced approach that defines the zone for shared decision-making as broadly as possible, but leaves room for provider direction outside this zone, is the best of imperfect systems – maximizing parental authority but keeping infants' best interests paramount when they are clear [45]. One way that palliative care clinicians can support this process is by creating space to acknowledge emotions, eliciting hopes, fears, goals, and values and then reflecting these key values – by exploring these topics, one can help parents better understand the meaning of the choices in a clinical situation and promote shared decision-making [46].

Several additional complexities regarding perinatal decision-making bear mention. The first is that ethicists disagree on whether factors other than an individual infant's best interests (e.g., the family's broader interests, other societal interests) should be considered when discussing decisions [47]. For instance, some ethicists would insist that considering the effect on a family's other children of embarking on arduous and risky treatment regimen for one child would not be a legitimate concern, as it was not directly related to the index child's best interests. Secondly, the available data suggest that, if a resuscitation plan has been agreed upon by family and physicians prenatally, unilateral departure from the plan by a physician based on delivery room characteristics or course (short of some substantial, unexpected alteration of circumstance) may not be warranted. Although the courts have sided with physicians in cases where such departures have been made [48], the ethical ground for the departures is shaky. Finally, it should be acknowledged that the width of the gray zone and the limits of "unreasonable" and "obligatory" care vary from institution to institution and, sometimes, from provider to provider within an institution. This is particularly true for infants of 22 and 23 weeks' gestation, for whom resuscitation might not be offered as an option in one institution, while it is offered in another. While this appears to contravene the ethical principle of justice (treating persons in like situations similarly), it may often reflect differences in local institutional experience with survival, disability, and suffering in those infants, as well as the relative values the institution and surrounding community place on survival and suffering [19, 20, 24, 49].

To provide appropriate guidance to parents regarding the choices they face, compassionate and complete prenatal consultation is required. Ideally, the neonatal and perinatal care providers would help parents, where appropriate, arrive at a plan for delivery room and immediate postnatal management. Where time and circumstances allow or require (e.g., the expected delivery of an infant with a prenatally diagnosed major anomaly), prenatal consultation with other relevant services, including palliative care, is encouraged. The reader is referred to Chaps. 5, 6, and 7 for a comprehensive discussion of the conduct of prenatal consultations.

The effects of perinatal decisions have also been studied longitudinally. Parents are generally comfortable with their decisions, even in the face of significant disability among their children, as are their children when they are old enough to speak for themselves [41, 50, 51]. There are two main caveats to these conclusions, however. The available data focus mainly on parents who have decided in favor of resuscitation, and there is a minority of parents who are extremely distressed by the survival of an infant who goes on to have significant, lifelong disability. Effects on medical care providers are more mixed. Providers, particularly nurses, may experience significant moral distress caring for infants undergoing trials of therapy or who are otherwise gravely ill, where there is perceived suffering and the expected outcome is poor [52].

Case 3.1: Conclusion

To return to Case 3.1, infants born at the cusp of viability, or who have other conditions that make survival uncertain and the risk of sequelae high, present particular challenges. It may be possible to avoid needless, prolonged suffering by forgoing the provision of life-saving resuscitative measures at birth, but applying even the best prognostic estimates will result in the deaths of some infants who would have survived with good function. Making the best decisions for these soon-to-be born infants requires high-quality evidence, careful exploration of a family's wishes and values, and compassionate, shared decision-making [45]. Qualitative evidence from family interviews confirms that families expect a mixture of expert advice and latitude for the family's values [41]. Although, in some cases, an infant's best interests will make provision of resuscitation either unreasonable or obligatory, in most cases, respect for parental authority to define those best interests is the most reasonable approach. The differing parental decisions in the case, based on their own interpretations of the best interests of their children, are justified.

Case 3.2

A couple has been informed that their 36-week-gestation fetus has a cardiac defect. The severity of the lesion is unclear, but they remain optimistic that it can be surgically corrected. At birth, it is apparent that the infant has a genetic defect as evidenced by facial deformity, cryptorchidism, low-set ears, and swallowing difficulties that require nasogastric feeding to prevent aspiration. Further investigation leads to a diagnosis of CHARGE syndrome. The family learns about the high prevalence of developmental and intellectual disabilities for children with CHARGE syndrome, ranging on a continuum from mild disability to those who will require full custodial care all their life. The parents ask that the nasogastric feeding tube be removed and feedings stopped because they are concerned about the poor quality of life that they anticipate as the child grows. The infant enjoys his pacifier, is comforted when held, cries when hungry, and calms after being fed. The ethical question to consider is as follows: Is it ethically justifiable to forego life-sustaining treatments, specifically to stop nutrition, in this infant with a disability of unknown eventual severity?

Discussion

Generally, parents are given authority to make health-care decisions on behalf of their minor children. This authority is partially based in the belief that parents have a profound bond with their child that compels a parent to do that which is ethically just. Since young children have never had capacity, and cannot make rational, thoughtful decisions about their care, parents are asked to make decisions that are in the child's best interest. Such decisions are not made in isolation. Decisions are made with information about medical facts from health-care providers, as well as factors such as perception of the future challenges the child will face including pain and suffering; fear of social ostracization; impact of the child's needs on other family members, especially siblings; and financial concerns. Thus, some could argue that parental decisions made are not always purely in the best interest of the affected infant. Often, poor decisions are a result of poor communication and high emotions.

Neonatologists may find it difficult to predict the severity of disability that will persist among some infants. The infant brain is plastic, yet some children will not achieve the hoped-for gains. The parents of a child born with congenital anomalies are often asked to make decisions in settings where prognosis is uncertain. Thus, parents may find that goals of care conversations with the physician and care team are overwhelming due to prognostic uncertainty [53].

Goals of care conversations often include a discussion of quality of life, and such concerns are not uncommon among parents who have an infant with disabilities. The perception of the disability is critical. It is often the case that parents are more optimistic than health-care providers about a child's potential future, and parents are generally more accepting of possible severe disability than nurses or physicians [54]. However, in the case at hand, the staff and ethics team are concerned that the parents are not acting in the best interest of the child, based on negative perception of a children with developmental disabilities – they imagine a future without friends, perpetual suffering, and a detrimental effect on the siblings' lives. While there is sympathy for the parents, it is important to recognize there are boundaries to parental decisions regarding foregoing life support.

Precedents

A series of legal cases in the 1970s and 1980s brought government and public attention to the rights of infants born with disabilities and defined limits to withdrawal of life support [55]. The initial case occurred in Indiana in 1982, when an infant was born with Trisomy 21 and esophageal atresia. The parents refused to give consent for surgical repair of the atresia based on the child's high likelihood of intellectual disability, and the baby died within days due to lack of fluid and nutrition. Other similar cases followed. Alerted and concerned, President Ronald Reagan asked the US Department of Health and Human Services (DHHS) to investigate. DHHS responded to the cases with rules that became known as the Baby Doe Regulations. The rules stipulated that fluid and nutrition and medical treatment could not be withheld from infants based on a handicap or disability. Ultimately, after several legal challenges, the rules were changed and incorporated as amendments to the 1988 Child Abuse and Protection and Treatment Act [56]. The current law states that treatment may be withheld if (1) the infant is irreversibly comatose or (2) treatment is futile (with regard to survival) or (3) the treatment is likely futile (with regard to survival) *and* is inhumane. Critics argue that the law is vague (particularly regarding lack of agreement on the definition of futility), has no associated professional or criminal sanctions, and has never been tested in the court. Therefore, there is room for interpretation that allows for thoughtful discussion between the medical team and infant's parents to develop the best plan for their infant. It is critical to the process that parents are provided with the necessary information to make informed and ethically justifiable decisions. As part of information gathering, the clinician should elicit information about the parents' perceptions of their infant's current and future situation, as well as their values and goals for their infant.

Obligations of Health-Care Providers

It is rare for health-care providers to question parent decisions to have an infant forgo live-saving care, yet there are times when it is appropriate to do so. Health-care providers have an ethical duty to advocate for the infant's best interests when parental decisions are dangerous, precipitous, or ill-conceived [57].

In the case at hand, the infant's prognosis is unclear. He has no known medical conditions that pose imminent death or cause suffering. He demonstrates normal infant developmental needs for food and comfort as evidenced by crying when hungry and satiety after feedings and calms when held.

The parents, struggling with the discovery of multiple new problems nearly daily, believe that their infant's life is not worth living based on a perhaps premature assessment of the child's future quality of life. Limits to parental authority to refuse medical treatment should be considered when the proposed treatment has clear benefit and minimal harm or risk to the patient. Such is the case with continuing to provide nutrition to this infant: the burden of hunger and starvation is greater than the burden of continued feedings, which carry low risk and are not highly invasive. In the situation where the burden of treatment rises to the level that there is greater harm than perceived benefit, and as the amount of technological support and severity of illness and future disability increases (moving to the right in Fig. 3.3), reasons for interference in parental decisions to forego life-sustaining treatments diminish. Conversely, when the burden is viewed as less than the perceived benefits (moving to the left on Fig. 3.3), then there is a greater moral justification for health-care providers to question the parents' decision, and as noted previously, care could be considered "obligatory." The American Academy of Pediatrics stated that "medical care that is clearly beneficial should always be provided" and that "anticipated limited potential of an individual and present or future lack of available community resources are irrelevant and must not determine care decisions" [58]. The facts about the medical condition and assessment of the benefits and burdens of treatment should be integral to decision-making.

The parents may be upset to have their choice denied. A gentle explanation of the rationale for the decision is critical. Additionally, the family should be reminded that the child's progress, or lack thereof, should continue to be monitored by the family and medical team. Future medical decisions should be made based upon evolving and continuing assessment of the child's prognosis.

Moral Distress

The nature of the neonatal intensive care unit (NICU) requires that ethical decisions are made and enacted daily. Advances in technology and ability to save babies in the gray zone of viability continue to push the boundaries of treatment. Additionally, members of the health-care team may have differing values, beliefs, and obligations in a given situation. Moreover, the values and beliefs of the infant's parents/caregivers are often paramount. With so many stakeholders, conflict about what is the right course of action is not uncommon. Ultimately, the staff may not agree with a decision made by others, usually the infant's parents, yet must enact the decision, thus creating a personal ethical dilemma, often termed "moral distress" [59]. Moral distress has recently been defined by Fourie as the "psychological response to morally challenging situations such as those of moral constraint, moral conflict, or both" [60, p. 92]. All health-care providers can be affected by moral distress, but the burden is highest among direct care providers [52].

Moral distress is often confused with burnout, stress, or grief responses. In the latter situations, measures such as rest, temporary reassignment, attention to self-care, and working through the grieving process bring relief of these stressors, which are generally temporary in nature. Moral distress differs, however, in that it creates a state of moral dissonance within the affected person and a belief that personal integrity has been violated. The effect of moral distress is profound and can last a lifetime [61].

The impact of moral distress on staff can be significant, including physical and emotional responses such as anger, sleeplessness, and guilt [62, 63]. Nurses report a statistically significant direct inverse relationship between poor communication among care providers and patient outcomes as well as moral distress and patient outcomes [64]. Epstein and Hamric note that unresolved moral distress may result in moral residue, defined as an accumulation of moral distress that continues to build or "crescendo" to high levels [65]. Unmitigated or unresolved moral distress may result in nurses leaving the environment and, ultimately, the profession [66].

Causes of moral distress include (1) poor interprofessional communication [66, 67], (2) actions that prolong the patient's death [68–70], (3) treatment that is perceived as being overly burdensome and not in the child's best interest [71], and (4) medical interventions that are viewed by the staff as "futile" [72]. Nurses in the NICU report the situations that cause the most moral distress are as follows: (1) following the family's wishes to continue life support or perform CPR when the actions prolong dying and are not in the child's best interest, (2) carrying out orders for unnecessary treatments in a dying child, and (3) poor pain control and burden of suffering because of physician fear that increased medication will hasten death [72]. Thorne et al. (2018) undertook a qualitative study to explore moral distress among NICU physicians, nurses, and respiratory therapists and found moral distress could be attributed to clinical situations and organizational factors [73]. Clinical factors include health-care provider perception of wanting to do more to support families, difficulty delivering bad news, feeling that actions violated the best interest of the child, and disagreement with parental decisions. Organizational factors that caused moral distress included lack of access to resources including supportive care for stressed families and the complexity of being part of a large practice team. This was evident by disagreements among physicians about the treatment plan and having to act upon a plan decided by a physician-colleague with whom one disagrees [73].

Those who suffer from moral distress are often emotionally upset, sometimes making reasoned, calm discussion difficult [74]. The first step to address moral distress is to create a safe environment where staff are comfortable broaching and discussing ethical concerns. Factors that contribute to a collegial interprofessional environment and may help to diminish moral distress include respectful communication, open sharing of perspectives and beliefs, and emotional support among team members. An ethical work environment is fostered when workers perceive that team members look out for each other, are involved in a process for decision-making to the fullest extent possible, and believe that all are working for the best interest of the patient [75].

Measuring moral distress is somewhat subjective; thus, reports of effectiveness of attempts to mitigate moral distress are often anecdotal. Interventions that may be helpful to decrease moral distress include structured ethical decision-making meetings, formal ethics debriefings, and case discussions in a supportive and caring environment [76]. Staff members who have had more exposure to ethics education and ethical reasoning demonstrate lower levels of moral distress than peers who have not had this benefit [77]. Ongoing ethics education should be a goal in NICUs, and can be achieved via planned in-service programs, and case discussions in a supportive environment, often with the assistance of a clinical ethicist. Additionally, it is helpful to encourage providers to explore and attempt to understand the parents' values and perspectives that influence their decisions. Such information can be valuable in working toward a shared decision.

Structured interprofessional ethics discussions can provide a framework to guide team conversations about how to proceed in ethically challenging cases. A shared decision-making model is most helpful, and many NICUs embrace this model. Decision-making frameworks incorporate steps such as (1) identify the nature of the ethical question, (2) explore viewpoints of all stakeholders, (3) explore and weigh suggestions for how to proceed, (4) develop consensus on a decision, and (5) make a plan for action/implementation [78]. Evaluation of the process and/or outcome is an important step and can be accomplished via ethics debriefings.

Ethics Committee Consultation

Despite the best intentions or clinical experience of a palliative care consultant, complex ethical issues may not be able to be resolved through shared decision-making. With this in mind, a team approach to ethical decision-making provides greater authority and validity to the outcomes of any deliberation. After the Joint Commission on Accreditation of Healthcare Organizations (JCAHO) mandated the availability of ethics committees in the 1990s in hospitals, there has been near-universal availability of hospital-based ethics committees. Despite universal acceptance, there is no universally accepted composition or function of ethics committees [79, 80]. However, despite the heterogeneity of ethics consult services, there should be a clear mechanism for requesting formal ethics consultation if the invested parties are unable to come to a mutually satisfying conclusion. All staff should have access to clinical ethics consultation, without fear of reprisal or fracturing team communication or workflow. Ethics consultation can provide assistance in difficult situations by providing clarity about the ethical question, improve communication among stakeholders, mediate conflict, and provide education about ethical boundaries based on historical cases and the legal basis for decisions. Additionally, ethics consultants can provide staff with a venue to address moral distress via planned interdisciplinary ethics rounds and debriefings about difficult cases.

Conclusion

Clinical decision-making in the neonatal setting is often complicated by unique and challenging ethical dilemmas. Neonates are a vulnerable population, and surrogate decision-makers may have conflicting values and perspectives regarding which clinical actions are in an infant's best interests. More commonly than in other populations, medical care providers may perceive limits to parental decision-making authority, either to provide or withhold interventions. As this chapter illustrates, negotiating good decisions requires many skills. By applying principles of ethical reasoning, the palliative care clinician can help ensure a fair and thoughtful process. Engaging parents and caregivers in honest and empathic shared decision-making process can minimize conflict and angst. Finally, identifying and addressing signs of moral distress among colleagues in an open and supportive way can maintain collective resilience and cohesion among team members. If disagreements around ethical dilemmas persist despite the best efforts of a multidisciplinary team, hospital ethics team consultation should be sought. Ultimately, health-care systems should promote a fair, transparent, and systematic approach to ethics consultation and conflict resolution.

References

1. Kochanek KD, Murphy SL, Xu J, Tejada-Vera B. Deaths: final data for 2014. Natl Vital Stat Rep. 2016;65(4):1–122.
2. Lo B. Resolving ethical dilemmas: a guide for clinicians. 5th ed. Piladelphia: Lippincott Williams & Wilkins; 2013.
3. Jonsen AR, Siegler M, Winslade WJ. Clinical ethics: a practical approach to ethical decisions in clinical medicine. New York: McGraw-Hill; 2010.
4. Walter JK, Ross LF. Relational autonomy: moving beyond the limits of isolated individualism. Pediatrics. 2014;133(Suppl 1):S16–23.
5. Macauley R. Ethics in palliative care: a complete guide. 1st ed. New York: Oxford University Press; 2018.
6. Pellegrino ET, Thomasma DC. Virtues in medical practice. New York: Oxford University Press; 1993.
7. Marty CM, Carter BS. Ethics and palliative care in the perinatal world. Semin Fetal Neonatal Med. 2018;23:35–8.
8. Jonsen AR, Toulmin S. The abuse of casuistry: a history of moral reasoning. Philos Rhetor. 1988;24(1):76–80.
9. Kopelman LM. Are the 21-year-old Baby Doe rules misunderstood or mistaken? Pediatrics. 2005;115(3):797–802.
10. Schneiderman LJ. Defining medical futility and improving medical care. J Bioeth Inq. 2011;8(2):123–31.
11. Bosslet GT, Pope TM, Rubenfeld GD, Lo B, Truog RD, Rushton CH, et al. An official ATS/AACN/ACCP/ESICM/SCCM policy statement: responding to requests for potentially inappropriate treatments in intensive care units. Am J Respir Crit Care Med. 2015;191(11):1318–30.
12. Black L. Limiting parents' rights in medical decision making. Virtual Mentor. 2006;8(10):676–80.
13. Ethical aspects of CPR and ECC (Part 2). Circulation. 2018;102(Supp 1). https://www.ahajournals.org/doi/full/10.1161/circ.102.suppl_1.i-12. Accessed 20 Feb 2019.
14. Jaworska A, Tannenbaum J. The grounds of moral status. Metaphysics Research Lab, Stanford University. 2018. Available from: https://plato.stanford.edu/archives/spr2018/entries/grounds-moral-status/.
15. Dickenson D, editor. Ethical issues in maternal-fetal medicine. Cambridge, UK: Cambridge University Press; 2002.
16. Cummings J, Committee on the Fetus and Newborn. Antenatal counseling regarding resuscitation and intensive care before 25 weeks of gestation. Pediatrics. 2015;136(3):588–95.
17. Lui K, Bajuk B, Foster K, Gaston A, Kent A, Sinn J, et al. Perinatal care at the borderlines of viability: a consensus statement based on a NSW and ACT consensus workshop. Med J Aust. 2006;185(9):495–500.
18. Condie J, Caldarelli L, Tarr L, Gray C, Rodriquez T, Lantos J, et al. Have the boundaries of the 'grey zone' of perinatal resuscitation changed for extremely preterm infants over 20 years? Acta Paediatr. 2013;102(3):258–62.
19. Mercurio MR. Physicians' refusal to resuscitate at borderline gestational age. J Perinatol. 2005;25(11):685–9.
20. Mercurio MR. Parental authority, patient's best interest and refusal of resuscitation at borderline gestational age. J Perinatol. 2006;26(8):452–7.
21. Tyson J. Evidence-based ethics and the care of premature infants. Future Child. 1995;5(1):197–213.
22. Ahluwalia JS, Lees C, Paris JJ. Decisions for life made in the perinatal period who decides; on which standards? Arch Dis Child Fetal Neonatal Ed. 2008;93(5):F332–5.
23. Bernat JL. Medical futility: definition, determination, and disputes in critical care. Neurocrit Care. 2005;2(2):198–205.

24. Beauchamp TL, Childress JF. Principles of biomedical ethics. New York: Oxford University Press; 2009. p. 417.
25. Singh J, Fanaroff J, Andrews B, Caldarelli L, Lagatta J, Plesha-Troyke S, et al. Resuscitation in the "gray zone" of viability: determining physician preferences and predicting infant outcomes. Pediatrics. 2007;120(3):519–26.
26. D'Angio CT, Mercurio MR. Evidence-based ethics in the "gray zone" of neonatal viability: promises and limitations. Pediatr Health. 2008;2(6):777–86.
27. Pignotti MS, Donzelli G. Perinatal care at the threshold of viability: an international comparison of practical guidelines for the treatment of extremely preterm births. Pediatrics. 2008;121(1):e193–8.
28. Garite TJ, Clark RH, Elliott JP, Thorp JA. Twins and triplets: the effect of plurality and growth on neonatal outcome compared with singleton infants. Am J Obstet Gynecol. 2004;191(3):700–7.
29. Liggins GC, Howie RN. A controlled trial of antepartum glucocorticoid treatment for prevention of the respiratory distress syndrome in premature infants. Pediatrics. 1972;50(4):515–25.
30. Shinwell ES, Reichman B, Lerner-Geva L, Boyko V, Blickstein I. "Masculinizing" effect on respiratory morbidity in girls from unlike-sex preterm twins: a possible transchorionic paracrine effect. Pediatrics. 2007;120(3):e447–53.
31. Tyson JE, Parikh NA, Langer J, Green C, Higgins RD. Intensive care for extreme prematurity--moving beyond gestational age. N Engl J Med. 2008;358(16):1672–81.
32. Batton DG, DeWitte DB, Espinosa R, Swails TL. The impact of fetal compromise on outcome at the border of viability. Am J Obstet Gynecol. 1998;178(5):909–15.
33. Wylie BJ, Davidson LL, Batra M, Reed SD. Method of delivery and neonatal outcome in very low-birthweight vertex-presenting fetuses. Am J Obstet Gynecol. 2008;198(6):640.e1–7; discussion e1–4.
34. Seri I, Evans J. Limits of viability: definition of the gray zone. J Perinatol. 2008;28(Suppl 1):S4–8.
35. Ballard JL, Khoury JC, Wedig K, Wang L, Eilers-Walsman BL, Lipp R. New Ballard Score, expanded to include extremely premature infants. J Pediatr. 1991;119(3):417–23.
36. Donovan EF, Tyson JE, Ehrenkranz RA, Verter J, Wright LL, Korones SB, et al. Inaccuracy of Ballard scores before 28 weeks' gestation. National Institute of Child Health and Human Development Neonatal Research Network. J Pediatr. 1999;135(2 Pt 1):147–52.
37. Lagatta J, Andrews B, Caldarelli L, Schreiber M, Plesha-Troyke S, Meadow W. Early neonatal intensive care unit therapy improves predictive power for the outcomes of ventilated extremely low birth weight infants. J Pediatr. 2011;159(3):384–91.e1.
38. Meadow W, Lagatta J, Andrews B, Lantos J. The mathematics of morality for neonatal resuscitation. Clin Perinatol. 2012;39(4):941–56.
39. Andrews B, Myers P, Lagatta J, Meadow W. A comparison of prenatal and postnatal models to predict outcomes at the border of viability. J Pediatr. 2016;173:96–100.
40. Reichlin M. On the ethics of withholding and withdrawing medical treatment. Multidiscip Respir Med. 2014;9(1):9–39.
41. Partridge JC, Martinez AM, Nishida H, Boo NY, Tan KW, Yeung CY, et al. International comparison of care for very low birth weight infants: parents' perceptions of counseling and decision-making. Pediatrics. 2005;116(2):e263–71.
42. Arzuaga BH, Meadow W. National variability in neonatal resuscitation practices at the limit of viability. Am J Perinatol. 2014;31(6):521–8.
43. Laventhal N, Verhagen AA, Hansen TW, Dempsey E, Davis PG, Musante GA, et al. International variations in application of the best-interest standard across the age spectrum. J Perinatol. 2017;37(2):208–13.
44. Arnolds M, Xu L, Hughes P, McCoy J, Meadow W. Worth a try? Describing the experiences of families during the course of care in the neonatal intensive care unit when the prognosis is poor. J Pediatr. 2018;196:116–22.e3.
45. Leuthner SR. Decisions regarding resuscitation of the extremely premature infant and models of best interest. J Perinatol. 2001;21(3):193–8.

46. Lantos JD. Ethical problems in decision making in the neonatal ICU. N Engl J Med. 2018;379(19):1851–60.
47. Leuthner SR. Borderline viability: controversies in caring for the extremely premature infant. Clin Perinatol. 2014;41(4):799–814.
48. Annas GJ. Extremely preterm birth and parental authority to refuse treatment--the case of Sidney Miller. N Engl J Med. 2004;351(20):2118–23.
49. Sayeed SA. Legal challenges at the limits of viability. Lahey Clin Med Ethics. 2007;14(2):6–8.
50. Saigal S, Lambert M, Russ C, Hoult L. Self-esteem of adolescents who were born prematurely. Pediatrics. 2002;109(3):429–33.
51. Tideman E, Ley D, Bjerre I, Forslund M. Longitudinal follow-up of children born preterm: somatic and mental health, self-esteem and quality of life at age 19. Early Hum Dev. 2001;61(2):97–110.
52. Whitehead PB, Herbertson RK, Hamric AB, Epstein EG, Fisher JM. Moral distress among healthcare professionals: report of an institution-wide survey. J Nurs Scholarsh. 2015;47(2):117–25.
53. Rempel GR, Blythe C, Rogers LG, Ravindran V. The process of family management when a baby is diagnosed with a lethal congenital condition. J Fam Nurs. 2012;18(1):35–64.
54. Saigal S, Stoskopf BL, Feeny D, Furlong W, Burrows E, Rosenbaum PL, et al. Differences in preferences for neonatal outcomes among health care professionals, parents, and adolescents. JAMA. 1999;281(21):1991–7.
55. Menikoff J. Law and Bioethics: an introduction. Washington DC: Georgetown University Press; 2002.
56. US Government Printing Office (2010). CAPTA Reauthorization Act of 2010. PL 111-320 111th Congress 12/20/2010. Retreived from: https://www.congress.gov/bill/111th-congress/senate-bill/3817/text.
57. Diekema DS. Parental decision making. Available from: https://depts.washington.edu/bioethx/topics/parent.html.
58. Principles of treatment of disabled infants. Pediatrics. 1984;73(4):559.
59. Epstein E, Delgado S. Understanding and addressing moral distress. OJIN. 2010;15(3):Ms 1. https://doi.org/10.3912/OJIN.Vol15No03Man01.
60. Fourie C. Moral distress and moral conflict in clinical ethics. Bioethics. 2015;29(2):91–7.
61. Nathaniel A. Theroy of moral reckoning. New York: Springer Publishing; 2008.
62. Meltzer LS, Huckabay LM. Critical care nurses' perceptions of futile care and its effect on burnout. Am J Crit Care. 2004;13(3):202–8.
63. Walsh A. Pulling the heartstrings, arguing the case: a narrative response to the issue of moral agency in moral distress. J Med Ethics. 2010;36(12):746–9.
64. Baggs JG, Schmitt MH, Mushlin AI, Mitchell PH, Eldredge DH, Oakes D, et al. Association between nurse-physician collaboration and patient outcomes in three intensive care units. Crit Care Med. 1999;27(9):1991–8.
65. Epstein EG, Hamric AB. Moral distress, moral residue, and the crescendo effect. J Clin Ethics. 2009;20(4):330–42.
66. Karanikola MN, Papathanassoglou ED, Kalafati M, Stathopoulou H. Exploration of the association between professional interactions and emotional distress of intensive care unit nursing personnel. Dimens Crit Care Nurs. 2012;31(1):37–45.
67. Baggs JG, Schmitt MH. Nurses' and resident physicians' perceptions of the process of collaboration in an MICU. Res Nurs Health. 1997;20(1):71–80.
68. Varcoe C, Pauly B, Storch J, Newton L, Makaroff K. Nurses' perceptions of and responses to morally distressing situations. Nurs Ethics. 2012;19(4):488–500.
69. Zuzelo PR. Exploring the moral distress of registered nurses. Nurs Ethics. 2007;14(3):344–59.
70. Pavlish C, Brown-Saltzman K, Hersh M, Shirk M, Rounkle AM. Nursing priorities, actions, and regrets for ethical situations in clinical practice. J Nurs Scholarsh. 2011;43(4):385–95.
71. Prentice T, Janvier A, Gillam L, Davis PG. Moral distress within neonatal and paediatric intensive care units: a systematic review. Arch Dis Child. 2016;101(8):701–8.

72. Cavaliere TA, Daly B, Dowling D, Montgomery K. Moral distress in neonatal intensive care unit RNs. Adv Neonatal Care. 2010;10(3):145–56.
73. Thorne S, Konikoff L, Brown H, Albersheim S. Navigating the dangerous terrain of moral distress: understanding response patterns in the NICU. Qual Health Res. 2018;28(5):683–701.
74. Howe EG. Fourteen important concepts regarding moral distress. J Clin Ethics. 2017;28(1):3–14.
75. Rathert C, Fleming DA. Hospital ethical climate and teamwork in acute care: the moderating role of leaders. Health Care Manage Rev. 2008;33(4):323–31.
76. Chiafery MC, Hopkins P, Norton SA, Shaw MH. Nursing ethics huddles to decrease moral distress among nurses in the intensive care unit. J Clin Ethics. 2018;29(3):217–26.
77. Allen R, Butler E. Addressing moral distress in critical care nurses: a pilot study. Int J Crit Care Emerg Med. 2016;2(1):1–6.
78. de Boer JC, van Blijderveen G, van Dijk G, Duivenvoorden HJ, Williams M. Implementing structured, multiprofessional medical ethical decision-making in a neonatal intensive care unit. J Med Ethics. 2012;38(10):596–601.
79. Annas G, Grodin M. Hospital ethics committees, consultants, and courts. AMA J Ethics. 2016;18(5):554–9.
80. Aulisio MP. Why did hospital ethics committees emerge in the US? AMA J Ethics. 2016;18(5):546–53.

Parental Experiences and Needs After Life-Limiting Fetal Diagnosis

4

Amy Kuebelbeck and Erin M. Denney-Koelsch

> "People often use physical terms to try to describe what it feels like to hear devastating news—that it's like being punched in the stomach, like being hit by a truck, or like the world is crashing in on them. To me it felt like falling backward, as though the tiled concrete floor, the clay underground, all the subterranean layers of rock were simply and soundlessly parting to let me through to some other dimension. What followed was an extraordinary journey of grief, joy and love as we waited with Gabriel, simultaneously preparing for our son's birth and for his death. Despite some wrenchingly aggressive surgical options, no one could give our son a good heart. So we set out to give him a good life [1]."

Introduction

Any situation in which a family is faced with unexpected news about their baby, born or unborn, is challenging. Sudden premature birth or an unexpected post-birth diagnosis (such as hypoxic brain injury or undiagnosed congenital anomalies) causes significant shock and rapid need for decision-making. These situations can be highly traumatic, and there is little time to prepare. When parents receive a prenatal diagnosis of a life-limiting condition in their baby, they experience the shock at the time of the diagnosis and then are faced with many weeks or months to prepare and make decisions. While there are differences in their experiences, many of the recommendations described in this chapter apply to both populations. In this chapter, names will be pseudonyms unless parents have given specific permission to use their real names.

A. Kuebelbeck (✉)
Editor, perinatalhospice.org, St. Paul, MN, USA

E. M. Denney-Koelsch
University of Rochester Medical Center/Strong Memorial Hospital, Department of Medicine, Division of Palliative Care, Rochester, NY, USA

E. M. Denney-Koelsch, D. Côté-Arsenault (eds.), *Perinatal Palliative Care*,
https://doi.org/10.1007/978-3-030-34751-2_4

Parental Experiences After Life-Limiting Fetal Diagnosis

The description at the beginning of this chapter obviously cannot represent every family's experience. Diagnoses, personalities, values, and countless other factors may differ. Even so, parents often do share similarities in their experiences, including emotions of shock, grief, anger, and disbelief; the need to make decisions and the need for up-to-date information and appropriate support from their health-care providers; questions about the impact on their relationships with their partners; and questions about the impact on extended family and siblings.

Case Part 4.1

Susan and Jack had difficulty getting pregnant. They had one early miscarriage at 10 weeks and one stillbirth at 20 weeks of pregnancy for unclear causes. They have one living biological child, a 5-year-old boy. They had been wanting another child, especially a girl, and now were pregnant for the fourth time. They were cautiously optimistic when everything seemed to be going well. At their 19-week ultrasound, they could sense that the sonographer was pleasant enough but a little quiet. When the exam was completed, they were told to wait for the doctor. The doctor explained that there were some abnormalities on the ultrasound: calcifications in the brain, an abnormal appearance to the hands, an "echogenic bowel," and what appeared to be a hole in the heart. It was not clear what the cause was, but the doctor was concerned that it may be a genetic or chromosomal problem. The doctor recommended an amniocentesis to clarify if the problem was genetic while also explaining that the amniocentesis can – rarely – cause labor to begin prematurely. Very worried, the couple went home to try to figure out what to do, and they ultimately decided to undergo the test.

Emotions

Although in hindsight some parents say they had a foreboding sense that something was wrong, most parents are blindsided by the news that their baby has a problem. Shock and disbelief are common initial reactions, making it difficult to process the news on the spot and perhaps clouding decisions that are made quickly. Said one parent, who later opted to continue her pregnancy:

> For a minute or two, sitting in the genetic counselor's office, I was crying a lot, and there was definitely a piece of me that thought, you know, maybe termination is the answer. Let's just end this nightmare right now [2].

As in any death or major life crisis, parents may experience a swirl of emotions including denial, anger, and eventually acceptance. This emotional journey is not a linear one, and not all parents experience the same emotions. Importantly, for caregivers, parents' initial emotions upon receiving the diagnosis may not be the same emotions they may feel after having had some time to process the news, and many parents have reported that being allowed some time before making irrevocable decisions was valuable in their emotional journey (normal and complicated grief and theories of grief and mourning are covered in Chap. 12).

Navigating Social Relationships

Parents often talk about the challenges of being pregnant and still having to appear in social situations, knowing that their baby may not survive. They are often approached by well-meaning people who express excitement about the coming baby or ask questions that they may or may not want to answer [3]. Providers can help parents by providing anticipatory guidance of what is to come, and helping them prepare scripts for certain common situations (such as the stranger in public or colleagues at work).

Process of Obtaining a Diagnosis

Some conditions, such as anencephaly, are able to be identified quickly. Other parents describe agonizing waits for a definitive diagnosis. One parent described it this way:

> It seemed like we were being dropped from the top of the stairs by stages. First, at my Level 2 ultrasound, they found that Katherine had a diaphragmatic hernia. Then I had an amnio test, then that same day our doctor sent us to an infant cardiologist, who found Katherine's heart condition. Then three days later, we were hit with the Trisomy 13 [2].

The waiting for a clear diagnosis, through multiple tests and visits with specialists, was described by other parents as "torture" [4]. There also can be time pressure for parents to consider the option of termination vs. continuing the pregnancy. Parents cannot begin to accept and prepare for the future without clarity about the diagnosis and prognosis; therefore, any delay causes stress and anxiety.

Case Part 4.2

Three weeks later, the amniocentesis results confirmed that the baby was a girl, but she had a rare chromosomal abnormality for which there were only a few case reports available as guidance. In those cases, most of the newborns died within hours to a few days of life, and the longest-surviving child had severe developmental delays and died at the age of 4 of pneumonia and respiratory failure. The parents returned to discuss the diagnosis with the doctor, who explained what she knew about the condition and its prognosis, which was uncertain, but not good. The parents were extremely sad, worried, and in shock. The doctor assured them that this condition was nothing they caused or could have prevented and was not their fault. The parents volunteered that terminating the pregnancy was not an option for them, and they asked, "What do we do now?"

Relationship with Partner

It goes without saying that being confronted with the death of their baby is a major life event and stressor in a couple's relationship. A common assumption is that bereaved parents have a higher divorce rate than other couples. While statistics vary, two studies from The Compassionate Friends, an international support group for bereaved parents of children of any age, found that the divorce rate was actually *lower* than that of the general public [5, 6]. In contrast, another study found that couples experiencing perinatal loss, especially unmarried couples, were more likely to break up than those without a loss [7]. A study specifically about parents who had chosen to continue a pregnancy after a lethal fetal condition found that the experiences of the pregnant parent and the nonpregnant parent are inherently different [8]. They each had individual responses to adversity that impacted their individual experiences. The strength of the couple's relationship prior to the diagnosis clearly impacted how both parents coped with the diagnosis, and like other relationship stressors, the impending death of a baby can break relationships that are already frayed [8].

On the other hand, those who offered mutual support, shared in decision-making, and understood each other's coping behaviors usually found that they were closer after the experience, and it strengthened the bonds of couples whose relationships already were strong [8].

Said one mother:

> My husband and I have a great marriage, and I didn't want to lose that on top of losing our baby. I later found out that those divorce statistics are usually overstated, and my husband and I are closer than ever. I don't see how you can look into the depths of absolute heartache and despair with someone and not come out with a more intimate understanding and appreciation for each other. I love my husband now more than ever [2].

Impact on Extended Family and Siblings

Many parents are concerned about the potential impact on their baby's siblings. Some parents avoid talking about the fetal diagnosis with their children, because of young age and developmental level or because of a sense of protection. It is generally recommended to include siblings in the experience at a developmentally appropriate level. In a survey of 411 parents who had a baby who was stillborn, the parents overwhelmingly recommended taking steps to include older siblings in the experience to "make the stillborn baby and the loss real for the siblings" [9]. Younger children might not understand the permanence of death and will need sensitive explanations that avoid euphemisms such as "sleep" or "pass away," so children don't interpret those words literally. Children also may benefit from hearing that mommy and daddy are sad because of the baby, not because anything an older child may have done or not done, and that it is OK for everyone to be sad, and it is also OK for everyone to be happy about other things.

Some hospitals and home-based programs have child life specialists who can provide valuable support for children. Parents also can follow their older children's lead and gently guide them toward understanding that something is very wrong with their baby brother or baby sister's body and that the baby might not live for very long but that the baby will be loved and protected. (See also Chap. 14, which covers the role of child life in working with siblings.)

Extended family is affected by a severe fetal diagnosis, too. Grandparents bear a double grief: grief over their grandchild's condition and impending death, as well as grief over seeing their adult children in emotional pain. Like most parents, even parents of adult children can have a deep drive to try to fix a situation, even one that is unfixable. Extended family and friends often are intensely concerned about the parents' emotional health, which may translate into what some parents report as pressure to terminate the pregnancy and "get it over with" in an attempt to spare parents from pain. Conversely, some extended family and friends might maintain an unrealistically hopeful attitude that does not align with medical information. Parents may find it more helpful when their family accompanies them on their journey with a heartfelt acknowledgment of the baby's life, rather than offering advice or pressure to take a particular course of action. Wrote one mother:

> My entire family wanted me to terminate (I still can't bring myself to write "abort"). They thought it would be easier on me. In the end everyone was so glad that I decided to continue. We all fell in love with her [2].

One study found that, in some families, parents and grandparents found ways to share their grief in a constructive manner, while in other families the intergenerational relationships were strained. "Bereaved parents found comfort and healing in grandparents' simple behaviors such as seeing and holding the deceased baby, attending the funeral, understanding the significance of the baby's loss to the parents, and keeping in close contact after the funeral" [10].

Health-care providers should consider the impact of the experience on the entire family, offering information where desired by the parents, emotional support always, and referrals for specialized counseling when needed.

"Treat My Baby as a Person"

Many parents talk about wanting their baby, regardless of the serious condition or diagnosis, to be treated as a person [11]. In most cases, they want providers to ask permission to use their baby's name. They talk about wanting everyone to treat the baby (even after death) with gentleness and dignity. Some parents talk about wanting the body to be kept warm, to not be harmed, or to be loved [11, 12]. This overarching theme should pervade all care provided.

Case Part 4.3

The parents decided to meet with a palliative care team in a prenatal meeting with the doctor, nurse, and social worker. The parents announced that they decided to name the baby "Hope." They had been considering the options presented to them by their obstetrician: comfort care, attempted resuscitation, and NICU care. "Do we do everything we can to keep our baby alive, or do we let her go?" they asked. "We don't want her to suffer, but we also want her to have a chance." At the end of the visit, the parents agreed to the suggestion of preparing a birth plan document.

Process of Parental Decision-Making

After a life-limiting fetal diagnosis (LLFD), parents are faced with many challenging decisions, both medical and personal. Working through all these decisions takes both time and effort. From interviews with couples who were faced with life-limiting fetal diagnosis, decision-making was a major part of their overall experience, for which they consulted each other as well as their health-care team. The process involves a three-step risk-benefit analysis in which they identify the decision to be made, weigh subjective (personal) and objective (medical facts) factors, and come to a decision (Fig. 4.1). All parents have differences in how they process

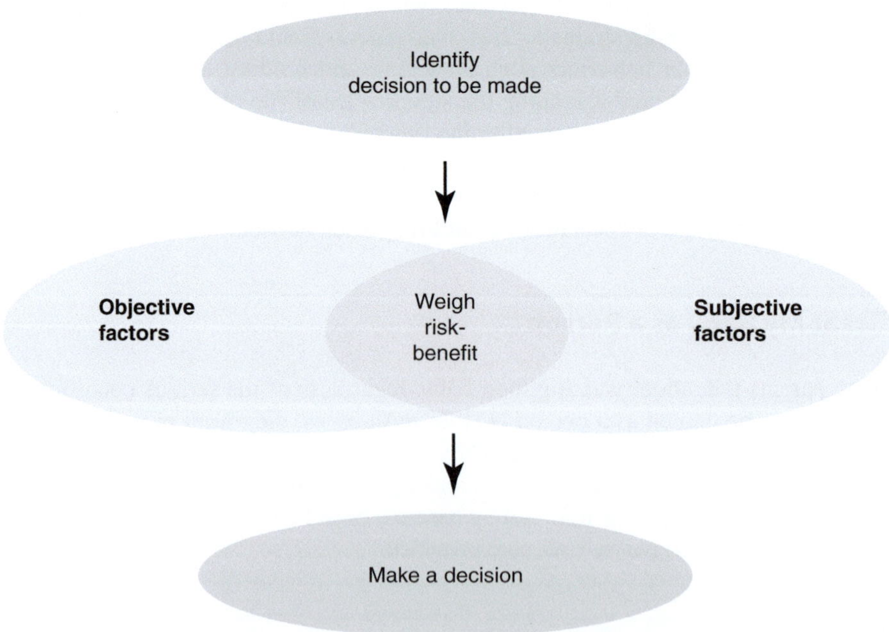

Fig. 4.1 Process of parental decision-making in lethal fetal diagnoses

medical information and receive guidance from their health-care providers. They have varied personal beliefs, spiritual and religious backgrounds, family structures, and values. Commonalities in the objective and subjective factors primarily considered for the most common decisions are listed in Table 4.1.

Table 4.1 Objective and subjective factors considered by parents when making decisions in life-limiting fetal conditions

	Primary considerations	
Decision to be made	Objective factors	Subjective factors
Continue pregnancy vs. termination	Diagnostic certainty Prognostic certainty Treatment options	Personal values and spirituality Impact on maternal health Avoidance of suffering Desire to have no regrets Sense of control
Additional testing Amniocentesis Cell-free DNA testing Specialist consultations	Diagnostic certainty Prognostic certainty Treatment options Expertise of the health-care team	Impact on baby Impact on maternal health
Choosing care team Team members Obstetrical/MFM Neonatal Specialists Location of care	Expertise of health-care team Treatment options Clinical implications of choice	Impact on family
Prenatal care plan Frequency of visits Fetal monitoring (ultrasound, Doppler)	Treatment options	Impact on maternal health Sense of control
Labor and delivery plan Fetal monitoring Mode of delivery Vaginal (induction vs. expectant) C-section (scheduled vs. for fetal distress)	Clinical implications of choice	Impact on maternal health Impact on baby Impact on other children/family Sense of control
Care for baby after birth Overall goals of care Comfort Life-prolonging Middle-ground approach Neonatal resuscitation preferences Location of care NICU Newborn nursery In mother's room Home when able Feeding options	Diagnostic certainty Prognostic certainty Fetal health status Treatment options	Avoidance of suffering Likelihood of a good outcome Sense of control Impact on other children No regrets
Memory-making Rituals (baptism, funeral planning) Bathing Dressing in special clothing Photography Locks of hair, foot-/handprints How, and how much, to include other family members	Baby's health status	Values and spirituality Impact on self Impact on partner Impact on other children

Case Part 4.4

Three weeks later, the parents again met with the team to discuss the birth plan. In the meantime, they had pregnancy photos taken with their son at one of their favorite parks and started a baby album with the baby's ultrasound photos. The parents had many questions about the various labor and delivery options and what to do for the baby after birth. They wanted to know what would happen if she's "a little bit stronger than they think she will be" and they don't intervene to support her breathing. They said they don't want to do anything that would "make her suffer just for us," but they wanted her to "have a chance" and for the doctors "not to just leave her there to die." The parents, together with the obstetrical and neonatal teams, agreed upon a birth plan. The family's overall goal was to have the baby born alive and be baptized and to "give her a chance at life" if possible, but not to undertake any "heroic measures." They chose natural delivery but with monitoring in labor with a backup plan for a C-section for fetal distress only if the mom could be awake for the delivery, because she didn't want to miss any potential time with the baby. The parents opted for a time-limited trial of medical interventions, including resuscitation and intubation in the delivery room with a possibility of NICU transfer for further testing and monitoring. They were aware that they could transition to comfort care at any time if things were not going well.

Understanding Their Choices: A Spectrum of Care

After a life-limiting fetal diagnosis, most families are told of the option to terminate the pregnancy. Families who choose termination often say their main concern is whether the baby will suffer from his or her terminal condition and that they feel this is the best choice for them under the circumstances. Those who terminate a desired pregnancy for a LLFD often experience intense grief that may have some similarities to those who carry to term. Some desire memory-making rituals similar those who carry to term [13]. Whatever the reasons, these families deserve compassionate care throughout their experience, opportunities for memory-making, and expert bereavement support. For the purpose of this book and the rest of this chapter, however, we will focus on the decisions of those who choose *not* to terminate, as they are eligible for palliative care services. In a survey of 405 bereaved parents looking at their perceptions of palliative care, 97.5% reported that they did not regret their decision to continue the pregnancy as it provided opportunities to cherish their time with the baby [14].

Choosing to continue a pregnancy with a life-limiting anomaly opens up a number of further decisions for the approach to care for the pregnant mother and the baby. When considering the type of care parents may want for the pregnancy, birth, and neonatal period, there exists a *spectrum* of care options from *life-sustaining*

Comfort approach		Life-sustaining approach
Holding Swaddling Warming Stimulating Blow-by oxygen Morphine	Stimulating blow-by oxygen Positive-pressure ventilation NICU admission Noninvasive testing Palliative procedures	Intubation Chest compressions Resuscitation Medications NICU admission Long-term ventilation Invasive testing Surgery

Fig. 4.2 Spectrum of care options for baby at birth with life-limiting fetal diagnosis

approach to a *comfort approach to care* with middle-ground approaches in between (Fig. 4.2). It is important that both providers and parents understand this as a spectrum and not a black-and-white choice.

Choosing a Care Team

When parents are considering all of their options, one major consideration is the care team. Once learning of a LLFD, some parents prefer to continue care with their known obstetrician or midwife and stay as close as possible to home in a hospital or clinic that they are familiar with, perhaps close to support such as extended family and friends. On the other hand, some parents feel that the unexpected diagnosis and poor or uncertain prognosis warrant a higher level of care, such as at a tertiary-care center where the providers have more experience with complex pregnancies and newborns or there are specialists in the area of their baby's condition. These decisions require education about their options, referrals from local providers, and often travel for families. The decision to stay closer to home often stems from the proximity to support of family and friends as well as concerns for their other children's welfare if they deliver far from home. There is no right or wrong decision, and parents should be supported in their decision.

Prenatal Care

Prenatal care in the context of a LLFD must be sensitive to the needs of the mother and her goals for the pregnancy and baby. Typical assessment for maternal health must of course continue. Some providers may feel that monitoring fetal status through growth monitoring, heart rate checks, and ultrasounds is less essential when the outcome is expected to be poor. However, most parents want to continue to know what is happening, to be up-to-date on the status of the developing baby, and to be able to enjoy the time they have through the pregnancy. Ultrasounds for the purpose of bonding can be extremely valuable to parents, especially to fathers who bond more through visual and direct contact with the baby [4]. The frequency of prenatal visits and the nature of these visits should be discussed with parents to ensure it is meeting their medical and psychological needs. Mothers may find sitting in waiting rooms with other pregnant mothers to be too difficult. They also find it extremely burdensome when office staff are not aware that their situation is different from the norm and request that their charts be marked in some way to add additional sensitivity to their care [3].

Labor and Delivery

Parents want to know the range of options they have for labor and delivery. In a normal pregnancy, the standard care is naturally tailored to maximize the chances of a healthy mother and a healthy, live baby. Careful monitoring for fetal distress is a standard part of hospital labor and delivery, with the usual recommendation of an urgent delivery (either through augmented delivery (e.g., vacuum or forceps) or cesarean section (C-section) when there are signs of fetal distress. This typical plan may be altered in the case of a LLFD. While labor and delivery happens chronologically before care of the baby, the parent's goals and wishes for overall approach to care for the baby should inform the delivery plan.

Parents should be offered some choice in labor management, timing, mode, and location of delivery, which can allow some degree of control in an otherwise largely uncontrollable situation. A scheduled delivery (either by induction or C-section) can allow the location and timing to be aligned with parent preferences. On the other hand, some parents with likely lethal conditions feel that choosing the day of delivery is akin to choosing the day their baby will die. In some conditions, especially chromosomal anomalies, the baby may die during labor or birth, and some parents would prefer to have a C-section in hopes of a live birth and some meaningful time with the baby alive [3]. In this case, parents must be informed that there is still a potential for fetal demise in utero, resulting in stillbirth, and that C-sections carry risks to maternal health and future fertility. Some hospitals permit a scheduled induction earlier than full term, depending on state laws, and some parents who are otherwise continuing their pregnancy as long as possible choose to induce a few weeks before their due date if their baby's condition is deteriorating and they wish to have the chance to meet their baby alive.

Fetal heart rate (FHR) monitoring during labor should also be discussed. Typically, FHR monitoring is intended to alert the medical team to fetal distress, allowing either augmented delivery or an urgent C-section. Some parents with LLFDs still want an urgent C-section for fetal distress if the plan for neonatal care includes resuscitation and life-sustaining therapies. However, others who choose a more comfort-oriented approach to neonatal care may not want to put the mother through a C-section for fetal distress, knowing that it would not improve the baby's poor prognosis. Some parents may want to know what is happening with the baby, even if they don't intend to change their plans based on the information. For example, one mother in Côté-Arsenault and Denney-Koelsch's study whose baby did not have monitoring during labor and was stillborn wished she had known at what point the baby had died [3]. All of these decisions are linked to the overall parental goals and approach to care for the baby (discussed below).

Care for the Baby After Birth

After a normal birth if the infant does not have adequate respiratory effort, heart rate, or color, neonatal resuscitation including augmented respiratory support (e.g., positive-pressure ventilation (PPV), intubation), chest compressions, and administration of emergency medications is the standard of care. If these interventions are required, the newborn would be taken to a higher level of care (special care nursery or neonatal ICU). However, it may be reasonable to consider some alterations to this standard plan in the setting of a life-limiting condition, particularly when the likely prognosis is extremely short (minutes to hours). For example, some families may choose not to resuscitate in the case of inadequate breathing or heart rate to sustain life, feeling that this would be too much to put the baby through if there is little or no chance of survival. In this case, they are likely to also choose not to have an urgent C-section for low fetal heart rate during labor. Therefore, fetal heart rate monitoring during labor could be intermittent or not checked at all. If the parents' overall goal is for comfort care, they may want the baby to be kept with them and not transferred to another unit (e.g., NICU). Again, the approach to care for the baby should inform the labor and delivery planning as discussed above.

Middle-Ground Approaches

There are also middle-ground approaches to care that are neither fully life-sustaining nor fully comfort-focused. Many families find it difficult to make no attempt to facilitate the infant's transition from in utero to the external world, which even in normal circumstances can take a few minutes. They may feel that a limited resuscitation or a time-limited trial of aggressive care may be appropriate, with a plan to transition to comfort measures only if these fail to improve the baby's condition.

Limited Resuscitation

Between full resuscitation and no resuscitation, parents may choose to have a limited resuscitation, in which some early efforts are made by the neonatal team to stimulate the baby's breathing and circulation, but not go so far as to start chest compressions or intubate. This is sometimes enough to "buy some time" for the infant to transition and be able to spend more time with the family while alive.

Time-Limited Trial of Aggressive Care

Another option can be a time-limited trial, in which a life-sustaining treatment such as intubation and mechanical ventilation can be attempted for a few hours or days to allow time to assess the baby's condition, run some tests, or confirm the diagnosis. This option can also "buy time" for parental certainty of the right course of action as well as bonding and memory-making.

When a Time-Limited Trial Goes Well

In the event that a baby does better than expected, parents have more time to make decisions about future care, including potential discharge home. Discharge planning may include a plan for comfort measures at home (hospice), palliative care (which can include life-sustaining medical interventions as well as measures intended to improve the baby's quality of life), and/or ongoing life-sustaining care including medical equipment (feeding tubes, respiratory support, etc.), specialist follow-up, and home nursing needs.

Importance of Understanding Diagnosis and Prognosis

Despite the improvements in prenatal diagnosis through high-tech ultrasounds and genetic testing (both via amniocentesis and cell-free DNA testing on mother's peripheral blood), there are many situations in which the diagnosis and/or prognosis are still unclear. Sometimes, the imaging is difficult due to fetal positioning or lack of amniotic fluid. Sometimes, genetic testing comes back normal despite a clear constellation of findings that imply a syndrome or genetic abnormality. Genetic testing may yield abnormal results of uncertain significance without a clear prognosis. Sometimes, parents decline further testing, feeling that additional results would not change their plans or decisions. (See also Chap. 6) Often, parents are told that "there is something wrong, but we're not sure what it is." Some parents find it so emotionally difficult to hear their baby's poor prognosis that they avoid medical interactions in which they have to hear more details. Lastly, a small minority of parents do not believe – or actively deny – the medical information they are presented. In the authors' experiences, in any case of diagnostic or prognostic uncertainty, parents are much less likely to modify standard prenatal or neonatal care because of the condition.

Case Part 4.5

At 36 weeks of pregnancy, Susan came to the hospital after her water broke at home. The baby's heart rate was fine, so Susan was moved to a labor room. Eventually, she was fully dilated and had been pushing for about 10 minutes when the baby began to show decelerated heart rates, some deep. Together with her caregivers, she and her husband decided to proceed with a vacuum-assisted delivery, which was successful. Hope was born floppy, blue, and with no respiratory effort. She had a full head of hair, and while her face showed indications of anomalies, consistent with what was seen on ultrasound, her parents thought she was beautiful. The NICU team brought Hope over to the resuscitation area, where positive-pressure ventilation (PPV) yielded a good response in Hope's heart rate, but whenever the ventilation was stopped, her heart rate dropped again. The team asked the parents if they'd like to intubate, and Susan and Jack both nodded yes and said, "Please try." The team attempted to intubate three times but were unsuccessful, so they continued PPV. After 10 minutes, Hope's heart rate began to fall again, even with PPV. The team asked the parents if they would like Hope to receive chest compressions. Susan and Jack look at each other and again nodded yes. After about 2 minutes of chest compressions, the parents tearfully agreed that this was "too much." Susan said, "I just want to hold her." The team respectfully carried Hope to her parents, who swaddled her and held her in her final moments.

Personal Factors that Affect Parental Decision-Making

While parents need to understand the medical diagnosis, prognosis, treatment options, and implications of their choices, parents use many factors in making decisions that are not fact-based, objective, or data-driven (subjective factors in Fig. 4.1). Their personal "gut feeling," values, religious or spiritual beliefs, their perception of how the decision will impact themselves personally, their other children or family, a sense of control, and a desire to have no regrets all play a major role in decision-making.

Religion and spiritual beliefs are extremely important for some families, especially in the decision to continue vs. terminate the pregnancy. Many families talk about the decision being less about religion than just a sense of what is the right thing to do for them as parents. Other decisions for care of the baby may have religious implications, such as the desire for a live birth in order to have a baptism as soon as possible. Regardless of religious affiliation, all parents have spiritual and existential questions, such as "Why did this happen to us?" and "What meaning does this have in our lives? "Spiritual care is extremely important through this highly life-changing experience. (See Chap. 11, for more information.)

The *impact of their decisions on other children* is considered carefully by many parents, in particular with choosing a care team and the location of delivery. Some parents also consider the impact on their other children of having a child with a significant disability who may require extensive care for years to come.

Parents also consider carefully what decision is likely to produce a "good" outcome, whatever this means for them. For some parents, a good outcome may be a living child regardless of disability; for others, a good outcome is a life free of pain and suffering even if it is short; for others, it is knowing that they tried everything they could for their baby. Whatever a good outcome is for them, they want to make the right decisions that will ultimately lead to a feeling of having done the right thing and having "no regrets" [3]. In the end, it is the parents' lives who go on after this experience, and this lack of regret may be the best possible outcome.

Memory-Making

Many parents find deep meaning in making thoughtful plans for creating memories with their baby, implementing those plans, and later cherishing the memories of the time with their baby. Which memories and keepsakes each family may desire will vary, but options should be offered. Many families don't realize the range of possibilities. Memory-making experiences can include the following:

- Rituals of birth, such as a baby shower (tailored to the circumstances with keepsake gifts such as photo frames).
- Rituals such as baptism, blessing, or a naming ceremony.
- Caring physically for the baby in life and after death, including bathing, diapering, feeding (if possible), kangaroo care, and dressing and swaddling the baby.
- Inviting extended family and friends to participate in various ways during the pregnancy and the baby's life and death, in person or virtually via online sites such as Caring Bridge [15].
- Creating intentional experiences with the baby even before birth, such as visiting a special location, having a pregnancy photography session, or listening to special music.
- Collecting tangible keepsakes such as footprints, photographs, hospital bracelets, clothing worn by the baby, blankets, and even the fragrant soap used for bathing the baby.
- Caring physically for the baby in death, including bathing and dressing the baby and making plans for a respectful disposition of the body. Some families choose to transport their baby's body to a funeral home themselves, and some choose to host a vigil in their home [16]. Limbo and Lathrop [17] describe afterdeath care as "final acts of caregiving" that express love for the child as well as validate the roles of the parents.
- Funerals, memorial services, and other rituals of death.

Research has confirmed the importance of memory-making and ritual for parents experiencing perinatal loss. "Rituals provide an opportunity for adding new meaning or reconstructing a prior meaning to profound life events" [18]. Tangible keepsakes promote healthy grieving and give concrete memories and meaning to their baby's life [19] and make it easier for parents to visualize the baby as a missing member of their family [20]. Memory-making helps parents to weave the baby's story into the fabric of their lives [21, 22]. Conversely, not having the opportunity to perform memory-making tasks can have a detrimental effect on parental grieving [20, 22].

Ritual can also be meaningful for caregivers. Limbo and Kobler use the term "co-creating ritual" to describe caregivers and parents working together to add ritual and meaning to the experience [22]. (See "Memory-Making" also in Chaps. 5, 13, and 15)

Parental Needs from the Health-Care Team

Though most of parents' time coping with a life-limiting fetal diagnosis occurs outside of health-care settings, care providers interact with families in numerous and varied encounters from the moment of detection of an abnormality, through the diagnostic process, the rest of pregnancy, the labor, birth and delivery, the care of the baby after birth, the hospital stay, postpartum care, neonatal care, and bereavement in some cases. Care can be provided by numerous types of providers, with an interdisciplinary team model being the ideal. Nearly always, initial detection of an abnormality comes from the obstetrician and/or ultrasonographer. These professionals may give the initial information about the abnormal test result but not know the cause of the problem. For example, an abnormal prenatal screen may show higher risk for a trisomy, but not which type. Then, parents typically have subsequent visits with specialists, including higher-resolution ultrasounds, specialist high-risk obstetricians (maternal-fetal medicine (MFM) physicians), genetics counselors, palliative care team members, neonatologists, and other specialists depending on the fetal condition (e.g., cardiology, surgery, and neurology). All of these specialties have physicians, nurses, social workers, office staff, and other care team members who interact with the patients and families.

The study of 405 bereaved parents whose babies died following prenatal diagnosis of a life-limiting condition, referenced earlier, showed that most were satisfied with their prenatal care (75.6%), and they were more likely to be satisfied with their care when they received compassionate care and help coping with their emotions [23]. Quality care can significantly improve parents' experience, whereas poor care can make the experience more difficult than it already is [12]. Parents report that while many did not mind being given the option of terminating the pregnancy, they resented providers who pressured them to abort. They also were frustrated when they felt providers were not sharing full information or were "sugarcoating," but parents wanted balanced information that was not entirely negative at all times. They craved a bit of positive news, and hope was essential – even hope that was reframed, such as hope that the baby would be born alive and live for a few minutes, not necessarily hope that the diagnosis was wrong. Families want honest, straightforward information about the current clinical situation as it is known, with updates as more information becomes available. They also need expert guidance about diagnostic testing and treatment options and the implications of those choices. In addition to sharing information, it is essential that providers seek to understand what the parents are going through, their goals and values, and their reasoning for making the decisions they do. This can reduce conflict and improve overall family satisfaction [12] (Table 4.2).

Table 4.2 Tips for health-care teams for increasing parent satisfaction [11, 12]

Tips for health-care teams	Examples
Treat baby as a person	Ask about baby's name and whether you can use it Note: Some parents strongly dislike the medical term "fetus" and prefer to use the word "baby"
Encourage parenting and memory-making	*Before birth:* Involve parents in decision-making Offer bonding ultrasounds Assist with prenatal memory-making (e.g., family photos) *After birth:* Care for baby in typical ways such as bathing, clothing, and feeding Invite family and friends to meet the baby Document their time with the baby through video and photographs Collect keepsakes such as handprints and footprints Use existing rituals such as baptism or a naming ceremony, adapting rituals, or creating new ones
Allow time for parents to make decisions	Assess where they are in their thinking Give them a timeline for when decision must be made "We realize this is a lot to take in. Would you like to talk more about the next steps today?"
Be a supportive presence	"This must be so difficult. What is the hardest part?" "What are you worried about?" "Is there anything we can do to make this a little easier for you?"
Assess parental understanding of condition prior to sharing information	"What is your understanding of your baby's condition? What have the doctors told you so far?"
Provide medical information in a frank, honest, straightforward, and compassionate manner Diagnosis and prognosis Treatment options and their implications	"This is what we know so far about your baby's condition…" "What questions do you have?"
Maintain some hope	May help to reframe hope, what is realistic to hope for Hoping for the best and preparing for the worst at the same time Make note of what is going well and what is normal "While this looks very serious, it's hard to know for sure what will happen. We will keep you informed at all times about what is going on, good or bad" "What information would you like to hear more about?"
Attempt to understand parents' goals and values	"What are some of the things you are thinking about as you make this decision?" "What is most important to you as you think about how we should care for your baby?"

Table 4.2 (continued)

Tips for health-care teams	Examples
Offer nonjudgmental guidance: once goals and values are understood, help guide the treatment options that fit	"From what I know about you, your baby's condition and what is important to you, may I make a suggestion for how we might proceed?"
Increase continuity of care	Avoid rotating visits with team members
Minimize waiting times to see specialists	
Things to avoid	
Be mindful of "never say" phrases that parents report as being unhelpful or even hurtful	"Withdraw care" (palliative care is still care, albeit a different kind of care) "You can have another baby" (maybe not, and even if they do have another baby, human beings aren't replaceable) "I understand what you're going through" "Closure" or "moving on" (grief isn't so neatly resolved)

Resources for Families

Books

Thanks to the pioneering perinatal bereavement work of professionals and caregivers through organizations such as Resolve Through Sharing Bereavement Education [24], Share Pregnancy and Infant Loss Support [25], and others, resources have gradually become available for parents experiencing miscarriage, stillbirth, and infant death. But as recently as the 1990s, parents who wished to pursue a palliative care approach during their pregnancy and for their baby after birth – whether the parents had terminology for this type of care or not – could find virtually no resources available specifically for them. In 1999, for example, one of the authors of this chapter could find only a single bare-bones website with a small number of parent stories [26]. In response to the need, she subsequently wrote a memoir that was the first mainstream book describing this experience [1] and later coauthored a more extensive guidebook for parents that included quotes and stories from well over 100 parents whose babies were diagnosed with a wide range of life-limiting conditions [2]. Other books have followed, including a children's book for siblings [27], and perinatal hospice even was highlighted in a sidebar in the 2016 revised edition of what many parents consider to be the pregnancy bible, *What to Expect When You're Expecting*, under the heading "If a problem is found" [28].

Support Groups

Although a growing number of parents are choosing to continue their pregnancies following prenatal diagnosis of a life-limiting condition, the total numbers are small when compared not only with parents experiencing healthy pregnancies but also with the subset of parents experiencing pregnancy loss or infant death. It is possible that there may not be more than one perinatal palliative care patient in the same OB practice or even in the same city at the same time. Therefore, as much as these patients are desperate for support, offering an in-person support group for perinatal palliative care patients and their partners may be impractical. Some parents have tried attending regular pregnancy and infant loss support groups, and they have been welcomed by group facilitators and other group members, but some parents have reported finding these general groups less than helpful. Parents often are most in need of support while they are still pregnant, because anticipating the loss over many weeks and months can be extremely stressful. Attending a typical pregnancy and infant loss support group while pregnant can cause awkwardness all around. Some parents and group facilitators have reported tension and unhelpful dynamics if a support group also includes parents who have chosen termination. Even when all involved have good intentions, grief and judgment and second-guessing of one's own or another's choices can complicate the group and make the goal of offering and receiving support difficult to reach.

Websites and Online Forums

Consequently, many parents have turned to seek support online. Parents have established websites specific to certain conditions, such as the Trisomy 18 Foundation [29], a site begun by a mother in the USA, or Anencephaly.info [30], a site begun by a mother in Switzerland and now available in 11 languages including English. Conditions such as these are relatively rare in pregnancies overall (anencephaly is estimated to occur in approximately 1 in 1000 pregnancies; T-18 in approximately 1 of 3000 girls and 1 in 8000 boys), so health care providers might not have had experience with a particular diagnosis before or might not have the most current information about the condition. But within moments at a computer, parents can find extensive information at their fingertips.

Also within a few keystrokes, parents can be connected with a large community of other parents dealing with a similar condition. For example, the Facebook support groups for Anencephaly.info [31] and for the Trisomy 18 Foundation [32] each have more than 1000 members. Some more targeted groups are much smaller but can also offer great consolation to affected parents, such as a private Facebook group for parents who have chosen to continue their pregnancies with babies diagnosed with hypoplastic left heart syndrome and also chose to decline surgical intervention and provide palliative care instead [33]. Other message boards and support sites, some public and some private, are not condition-specific but offer general peer-to-peer support to parents who are choosing to continue their pregnancies in the face of a wide range of life-limiting prenatal diagnoses. For example, the Carrying/Carried Pregnancy Despite Poor or Fatal Prenatal Diagnosis message board at BabyCenter.com was begun in 2009 and has more than 1500 members [34]. While these resources can be extremely valuable, care providers should advise parents to be cautious about online sources and to seek high-quality information.

Parents may also feel strong pressure from other parents to make a particular decision. They should be encouraged to consider all the reliable information they have and make the right decision for themselves.

An extensive list of websites, online forums, and other resources for parents has been compiled on the Resources for Parents page at perinatalhospice.org [35].

References

1. Kuebelbeck A. Waiting with Gabriel: a story of cherishing a baby's brief life. Chicago: Loyola Press; 2003.
2. Kuebelbeck A, Davis DL. A gift of time: continuing your pregnancy when your baby's life is expected to be brief. Baltimore: Johns Hopkins University Press; 2011. 408 p.
3. Côté-Arsenault D, Denney-Koelsch E. "Have no regrets": parents' experiences and developmental tasks in pregnancy with a lethal fetal diagnosis. Soc Sci Med. 2016;154:100–9.
4. Denney-Koelsch EM, Côté-Arsenault D, Lemcke-Berno E. Parents' experiences with ultrasound during pregnancy with a lethal fetal diagnosis. Glob Qual Nurs Res. 2015;2:2333393615587888.
5. The Compassionate Friends, NFO Research Inc. When a child dies: a survey of bereaved parents [Internet]. 1999. Available from: https://docplayer.net/21487803-When-a-child-dies-a-survey-of-bereaved-parents-conducted-by-nfo-research-inc-on-behalf-of-the-compassionate-friends-inc.html.
6. The Compassionate Friends. Only 16 percent of bereaved parents divorce, new study reveals [Internet]. 2006. Available from: www.compassionatefriends.org/CMSFiles/X101206Press_Release_Survey,_Divorce-National.pdf.
7. Gold KJ, Sen A, Hayward RA. Marriage and cohabitation outcomes after pregnancy loss. Pediatrics. 2010;125(4):1202–7.
8. Côté-Arsenault D, Denney-Koelsch E. Love is a choice: couple responses to continuing pregnancy with a lethal fetal diagnosis. Illn Cris Loss. 2018;26(1):5–22.
9. Avelin P, Erlandsson K, Hildingsson I, Bremborg AD, Rådestad I. Make the stillborn baby and the loss real for the siblings: parents' advice on how the siblings of a stillborn baby can be supported. J Perinat Educ. 2012;21(2):90–8.
10. O'Leary J, Warland J, Parker L. Bereaved parents' perception of the grandparents' reactions to perinatal loss and the pregnancy that follows. J Fam Nurs. 2011;17(3):330–56.
11. Côté-Arsenault D, Denney-Koelsch E. "My baby is a person": parents' experiences with life-threatening fetal diagnosis. J Palliat Med. 2011;14(12):1302–8.
12. Denney-Koelsch E, Côté-Arsenault D, Jenkins Hall W. Feeling cared for versus experiencing added burden: parents' needs from health care providers in pregnancy with a lethal fetal diagnosis. Illness, Cris Loss [Internet]. 2016:293–315. Available from: https://doi.org/10.1177/1054137316665817.
13. Sandelowski M, Barroso J. The travesty of choosing after positive prenatal diagnosis. JOGNN – J Obstet Gynecol Neonatal Nurs. 2005;34(3):307–18.
14. Wool C, Limbo R, Denney-Koelsch EM. "I would do it all over again": cherishing time and the absence of regret in continuing a pregnancy after a life-limiting diagnosis. J Clin Ethics. 2018;29(3):227–36.
15. Caring Bridge [Internet]. Available from: www.caringbridge.org.
16. When your baby dies: information and resources for bereaved parents about the option to bring your stillborn or deceased baby home.
17. Limbo R, Lathrop A. Caregiving in mothers' narratives of perinatal hospice. Illn Cris Loss. 2014;22(1):43–65.
18. Kobler K, Limbo R, Kavanaugh K. Meaningful moments: the use of ritual in perinatal and pediatric death. MCN Am J Matern Nurs. 2007;32(5):288–95.

19. Limbo R. Caring for families experiencing stillbirth: a unified position statement on contact with the baby. Illn Cris Loss. 2012;20(3):295–8.
20. Leon IG. Helping families cope with perinatal loss. Glob Libr Women's Med [Internet]. 2008. Available from: https://doi.org/10.3843/GLOWM.10418.
21. Côté-Arsenault D. Weaving babies lost in pregnancy into the fabric of the family. J Fam Nurs. 2003;9(1):23–37.
22. Limbo R, Kobler K. The tie that binds: relationships in perinatal bereavement. MCN Am J Matern Nurs. 2010;35(6):316–21.
23. Wool C, Repke JT, Woods AB. Parent reported outcomes of quality care and satisfaction in the context of a life-limiting fetal diagnosis. J Matern Neonatal Med. 2017;30(8):894–9.
24. Resolve Through Sharing Bereavement Education [Internet]. Available from: http://www.gundersenhealth.org/resolve-through-sharing/.
25. Share Pregnancy & Infant Loss Support [Internet]. Available from: http://nationalshare.org.
26. Waiting with love [Internet]. Available from: http://www.erichad.com/wwl.
27. Tioleco-Cheng M. Special delivery. Rise-and-Shine Studio; 2013.
28. Murkoff H, Mazel S. If a problem is found. In: What to expect when you're expecting. 5th ed. New York City: Workman Publishing Company; 2016. p. 60–1.
29. Trisomy 18 Foundation [Internet]. Available from: www.trisomy18.org.
30. Anencephaly.info [Internet]. Available from: www.anencephaly.info.
31. Anencephaly.info Facebook group [Internet]. Available from: www.facebook.com/groups/anencephaly.info.
32. Trisomy 18 Foundation. Expecting Trisomy 18 Facebook group [Internet]. Available from: www.facebook.com/groups/ExpectingTrisomy18.
33. HLHS Comfort Care, private Facebook group for parents of babies with hypoplastic left heart syndrome [Internet]. Available from: www.facebook.com/groups/1597312227239884.
34. BabyCenter. Carrying/carried pregnancy despite poor or fatal prenatal diagnosis message board [Internet]. Available from: https://community.babycenter.com/groups/a6711405/carrying_pregnancy_to_term_despite_fatal_prenatal_diagnosis.
35. Kuebelbeck A. Resources for parents, perinatalhospice.org [Internet]. Available from: www.perinatalhospice.org/resources-for-parents.

Part II

Clinical Care for Families Facing Life-Limiting Fetal Conditions

5 Obstetric Management in Life-Limiting Fetal Conditions

Stefanie J. Hollenbach, Elizabeth A. Westen, and Loralei L. Thornburg

Introduction

Each year in the United States, approximately 15,000 infants are born with conditions incompatible with prolonged life [1]. As technology – including prenatal ultrasound and antenatal genetic testing – continues to improve, prenatal diagnosis of life-limiting conditions is becoming more common. It is important to note that while some life-limiting fetal conditions (LLFC) are diagnosed antenatally (genetic syndromes, structural anomalies), others are not identified until the time of delivery. Additionally, each year, thousands of infants face imminent demise secondary to extreme prematurity or sudden preterm birth. Regardless of the cause of the fetal or neonatal life-limiting condition, it is prudent to consider the antenatal period as a time for planning and discussion of goals of care. The role of the antenatal care provider is to empower patients to identify their preferences and values for their pregnancy in light of the life-limiting fetal condition. These values can help guide the creation of a plan to optimize the attainment of their preferences throughout pregnancy and their birth experience.

S. J. Hollenbach · E. A. Westen · L. L. Thornburg (✉)
Department of Obstetrics and Gynecology, Division of Maternal-Fetal Medicine, University of Rochester Medical Center, Rochester, NY, USA
e-mail: loralei_thornburg@urmc.rochester.edu

E. M. Denney-Koelsch, D. Côté-Arsenault (eds.), *Perinatal Palliative Care*,
https://doi.org/10.1007/978-3-030-34751-2_5

Antepartum Diagnosis and Prenatal Care

Key Points

1. Prenatal diagnosis of LLFC is increasing and having an antepartum plan of care and an interdisciplinary care network providing support for families is essential.
2. Encouraging families to have autonomy to make plans for their infant in utero allows them to be involved in all aspects of decision-making about their infant's care.
3. Creating a birth plan provides a framework and helps guide families through the delivery process in order to make the experience with their infant what they want it to be.

Prenatal Diagnosis

In most developed and many developing countries, 2D prenatal ultrasound has become the established standard of care for accurate dating and viability confirmation as well as for screening and identification of structural and chromosomal anomalies [2]. The Internal Society of Ultrasound in Obstetrics and Gynecology (ISUOG) provides guidelines on conducting a screening and more targeted fetal anatomic survey examination. A majority of lethal structural abnormalities can be detected at 18–22 weeks (during the now routine anatomic survey); however, some abnormalities such as acrania or anencephaly can be reliably diagnosed earlier by 11–12 weeks of gestation. In addition, first trimester screening and cell-free DNA screening identify a large proportion of chromosomal abnormalities in the first trimester. Approximately 90% of lethal abnormalities are identified following either first or second trimester serum or ultrasound screening [2]. However, some diagnoses, such as lissencephaly, have a very poor prognosis but cannot be diagnosed until later third trimester. Clinicians and parents often seek further reassurance from a second imaging modality (such as specialized ultrasound or CT/MRI) or follow-up confirmatory imaging study before making irrevocable decisions about the pregnancy. Fetal MRI has increasingly been used to corroborate ultrasound findings [3]. Confirmation of prenatal diagnoses of fetal chromosomal anomalies is achieved by invasive diagnostic procedures including amniocentesis or chorionic villus sampling (CVS), which are discussed further in Chap. 6.

When prenatal testing reveals that an unborn infant has a life-limiting condition that is expected to result in a high risk of death before or shortly after birth, many parents find themselves in an extremely challenging and emotional situation. The conversation during which healthcare providers reveal a life-limiting fetal diagnosis to parents is an important one which will undoubtedly leave a lasting impression. The provider task of breaking bad news of a LLFC to parents can be improved by approaching it as a stepwise procedure and applying well-established principles of communication and counseling [4]. In 2000, The Oncologist published the SPIKES

Table 5.1 SPIKES protocol for delivering bad news adapted for life-limiting fetal diagnoses

SPIKES
Step 1: *S – Setting up* the interview
Arrange for privacy (quiet room, limit disturbances). Have tissues available.
Involve significant others (offer to put partner on speakerphone if not present in person).
Sit down (limit barrier between you and the patient, allow patient to use bathroom first).
Make connections (eye contact, holding the patient's hand if they are comfortable with this).
Limit interruptions (set phone/pager on silent, inform office staff of need to use the room).
Step 2: *P* – Assessing the patient's *perception*
Open-ended questions – "What have you been told about your infant's condition so far?"
"What is your understanding of why you have been sent to see our high-risk practice today?"
Step 3: *I* – Obtaining the patient's *invitation*
Some patients will want to know every detail of their fetus's diagnosis, while others will not.
If patients do not want to know details, offer to answer any questions they may have.
Step 4: *K* – Giving *knowledge* and information to the patient
Try to use nontechnical words such as "brain" rather than "calvarium" or "side of the heart" rather than "ventricle."
Avoid excessive bluntness such as "the baby has a bad problem and is going to die."
Give information in small chunks and check periodically for the patient's understanding.
Step 5: *E* – Addressing the patient's *emotions* with emphatic responses
Show support for the patient's emotion – touching their arm or handing them a tissue.
Empathetic responses such as "I wish I did not have to give you this news."
Step 6: *S* – Strategy and *summary*
Patients who have a clear plan for the next step are less likely to feel anxious and uncertain
Before making a follow-up plan, ask the patient if they are ready for such a discussion
Some patients may need to go home and process the information they have just received

Adapted from the SPIKES protocol [4]

protocol for giving bad news to cancer patients. In many ways, this protocol is suitable for relaying a LLFC to parents (see Table 5.1). As mentioned in the SPIKES protocol (see also Chap. 17), having a follow-up visit arranged or defining a next step in the care plan is often comforting for some patients. It is important to note however that other patients will need to leave the office and process this diagnosis alone or with family before they are ready to address further decisions. This conversation is the starting line of an emotional marathon which has a certain end but a variety of paths. The path that parents take can be a self-directed journey.

Once parents are aware of a LLFC and ready to pursue further discussions regarding goals of care, building the individualized foundation for caring for their infant can begin. Best practice models focus on advance care birth planning in which prenatal and palliative teams offer guidance and support to parents who are faced with their infant's death [1]. Palliative care in the perinatal period is distinct in that typically this is a time of joy and anticipation of welcoming a newborn into the family. The concept of a baby with a life-limiting condition or fetal/neonatal death is in abrupt contrast to the "normal" pregnancy and natural labor families anticipate [2]. Emphasis during care planning for LLFC should surround treating families with respect, including them in all decisions, and making them a part of the care team. When parents feel they have a critical role in their infant's care, they retain a sense of control in the midst of an out-of-control situation. Because there is an increased risk for in utero fetal demise (IUFD), early delivery, and pregnancy complications, it is ideal to have care planning discussions relatively soon after a LLFC has been discovered.

Prenatal Care

Different women and families will have varied emotions surrounding their obstetric visits during a pregnancy complicated by a life-limiting prognosis. For some women, these prenatal care visits may feel like a piece of "normal" where the focus on the pregnancy (which friends and family may be avoiding) gives them space and time to discuss their baby, listen to the fetal heartbeat, watch the baby on ultrasound, and have the opportunity to bond. For others, the office may be extremely stressful and may represent continued confrontation of the abnormal findings, the poor prognosis, and the forced reality that things are not progressing normally.

Further complicating prenatal care are the different pay structures related to antenatal testing and visits by different health insurance plans. Most insurances cover prenatal care, labor, and delivery under a single global fee. For some families, avoiding fees outside the routine pregnancy care and delivery charge may be imperative. This can be especially true in patients that participate in community-based cost-sharing (e.g., the Mennonite and Amish communities) and those where a delivery and pregnancy will fall across two calendar years (resulting in the need to meet two deductibles, one in each year). For these reasons, there is not a "one-size-fits-all" approach to the prenatal period for these families. Therefore, after a LLFC has been made and before follow-up testing is ordered, it is necessary to have a frank discussion about the value of this testing and if the family desires to have it. In a scenario of extreme growth restriction, for example, if performing an ultrasound to confirm that the fetal weight is not in a viable range is helpful to providers and families, then it should be offered. However, if interval scans for fluid volume and Doppler which occur between growth ultrasounds (growth scans are typically spaced at least 2–4 weeks) are unlikely to yield actionable results, the family may wish to forgo this interval testing.

The decision of whether to continue or end a pregnancy when a LLFC has been made prior to the age of viability is a personal and complicated one for many families. Families should be informed of all of their options as regards to the pregnancy. State limitations regarding pregnancy termination and accessibility to local resources for abortion care should be discussed. If a certain region does not have pregnancy termination services, patients should be informed of other centers in the country where these services are available. When faced with a LLFC, some families view pregnancy termination as a palliative process – limiting both fetal suffering and emotional suffering to the mother and family of continuing the pregnancy. Autopsy and confirmation of fetal diagnoses should be offered following termination. In addition, baptism or religious services as well as photos and footprints should be offered if appropriate based on the clinical scenario. Options and considerations for medical and surgical pregnancy termination are included in the intrapartum section of this chapter.

Maternal Prenatal Complications

When pregnancy continues, discussions regarding care during pregnancies affected by LLFC are further complicated if there is ongoing maternal disease. There are a number of maternal diseases that can lead to poor fetal outcomes, and there are genetic disorders that either worsen through generations or have variable expressivity – which makes it possible for the mother or father to have the disease but the disease in the fetus to be far more serious. Therefore, it is possible that even if the family chooses to decline fetal evaluation, visits may still be needed to evaluate and monitor maternal disease. In addition, many fetuses with LLFC are at risk for hydrops and polyhydramnios. Both of these conditions can develop suddenly, and both can be associated with maternal health compromise (see the intrapartum special considerations section). In the case of polyhydramnios, some women may need amnioreduction (removal of some of the excess amniotic fluid via amniocentesis-type procedure) due to maternal respiratory or vascular compromise. Prenatal exam monitoring for sudden increase in fundal height or serial ultrasounds to screen for hydrops and/or polyhydramnios in the at-risk fetus may be of value to prevent maternal compromise. In other scenarios, delivery is recommended for the health of the mother. For example, if a woman develops severe preeclampsia and HELLP (hemolysis, elevated liver enzymes, low platelet syndrome) syndrome at 21 weeks, delivery is recommended for her well-being. Although delivery is needed imminently for maternal health, this also implies delivery of a fetus that is previable and will not survive. The balance of maternal and fetal well-being is a complicated one which occasionally requires making impossible choices to let one go in order to save the other. Monitoring for development of maternal disease (e.g., preeclampsia) is an important part of routine prenatal care and should not be overlooked in cases affected by LLFC. For the family that finds weekly visits stressful, costly, or distant from home, this can be an added stressor. The clinician should explore what stressors in the visit can be eliminated and discuss the value of the testing and what is being monitored for with the family. Some proposed strategies for limiting family anxiety and optimally supporting maternal care are listed in Table 5.2.

Table 5.2 Family-centered prenatal care in life-limiting fetal diagnosis

Prenatal visit suggestions
Early/late appointments to not disrupt the family's work schedule.
Exiting the office through a back door (avoid the waiting room).
Schedule visits during time frames when less pregnant women are likely to be in the office (lunch hour, early morning, late afternoon).
Allow for extra time during visits – especially when relaying an initial diagnosis
Have tissues available in patient care rooms.
Co-manage care with providers located closer to the mother's home if possible so the patient does not have to travel hours for every prenatal visit.
During ultrasounds – offer to print photos or to have the family record the baby's heart beat
Electronic records should clearly display LLFC upon opening the chart.

(continued)

Table 5.2 (continued)

Charts of infants who have passed should be flagged (e.g., Epic™ uses a carriage with broken wheel icon).
Refer to the infant by name (if chosen) or with usual epithet baby/infant.
Plan multidisciplinary meetings when possible so the obstetricians and pediatric providers are both available during discussions and on the same page with the parents regarding the care plan.
Have social work or therapists available if possible to provide additional support to these women and their families (spouse/partner, grandparents, and other children at home).
Creation of a birth plan early in the process to provide families a vehicle through which to consider all options and what is important to them.
When a comfort care plan is chosen
Let the pregnant mother/family know they will have support in this process; offer frequent visits/contact for support.
Discuss how to get in touch with the care team if questions/concerns arise.
Attempt to have one or two points of contact to maintain consistency – a care coordinator or one provider in particular.
Hold conversations in a private, quiet place. Avoid interruptions (turn off pager/cell phone ringer).
Offer to write down details, including diagnosis, or tape-record conversations for later use.
At delivery
Provide time to create memories – offer for parents to dress/bathe/feed their infant.
Offer relocation to a back hallway or private room if desired for comfort and space for family.
Be supportive of parents holding their infant, and allow the family to stay with the infant as long as they need – including after death occurs.
Offer to take photos and make footprints or memory boxes.
Limit the number of providers assigned to care for the patient/infant to further provide continuity of care.
Provide assistance in making memorial/burial plans. Discuss options for autopsy and baptism/blessing.
Postpartum period
Establish contact with a social worker, chaplain, or grief counselor prior to discharge.
Discuss possibility of lactation and methods of treating breast engorgement. In general, medication therapies to reduce lactation are not recommended. Some mothers may be interested in breast milk donation.
Provide a pamphlet on community resources, support groups, and spiritual centers.
Consider a home visit by a staff member, care coordinator, or public health nurse within a few days.
Two-week follow-up physician visit (rather than the typical six-week postpartum visit).
Consider not billing for this visit or having a no-charge appointment for families with LLFC.
Phone calls scheduled on significant days (Mother's Day, infant's due date, anniversary of death).
Schedule a future post-loss consult to review diagnoses, pathology results, and preconception counseling prior to considering a future pregnancy attempt.
Consider desires for family planning. Discussion of pregnancy spacing.
Review pregnancy course, delivery complications, and impact on future pregnancy implications.
Optimize method of family planning to prevent recurrent pregnancy until emotionally and physically ready.

Sensitivity to Parent's Needs in Prenatal Care

Importantly, the infant's name and prognosis should be clearly visible to all staff that open the medical chart, and staff should refer to the infant as much as possible by name (if known) or by usual epitaphs (baby, little one) instead of by diagnosis ("the woman with the Downs baby," "the baby with the brain anomaly") when rooming or discussing patient. If an infant has died, the mother's chart should be marked (e.g., Epic places a carriage with broken wheel adjacent to the mother's name in the banner of her chart for the year following the event) so that staff taking calls, reviewing results, making appointments, and rooming patient will not inadvertently ask insensitive questions or make an inappropriate comment. This may require adjusting routine forms at check-in (e.g., questionnaire about breastfeeding and pediatric care at the postpartum visit). It is important to facilitate prenatal bonding during pregnancy (as well during intrapartum), and it is crucial to treat the baby as a person (particularly when the parents say "baby" or use a specific name) [5].

Birth Plan

Developing a birth plan is pivotal to helping the family determine their goals of care for the pregnancy and for assuring that families understand and are prepared for challenges likely to occur at delivery. Further, this can help to provide a "road map" for the labor and delivery team (which in many cases may be different than the outpatient care team), and as such, the development of the birth plan needs to include values clarifications so that the entire team knows what is important to the family. It also may help families create a framework upon which they can make decisions if/when they encounter any unexpected events or questions that come up urgently. Birth plans can also be helpful to interconnect the entire care team including obstetric care providers, neonatologists/pediatricians, and palliative care specialists so that all involved are aware of parents' wishes and goals of care.

One common misconception with families in developing a birth plan is that it is an "a la carte" menu where each decision is independent and equal. Unfortunately, delivery planning is a bit more of a "fractal" layout in which each decision opens one pathway for intervention and care and closes another. A common example of this is the scenario where a woman who wants "every intervention including cesarean" if her fetus is in distress also wants no monitoring in the office or during the labor process. Unfortunately, monitoring is the only way to assess if there is a need for fetal intervention. Another common example is the woman who wants no interventions for fetal distress but prioritizes seeing and holding the baby alive above all other outcomes. These discussions can be extremely difficult, and starting with "key goals" or "primary objectives" to care and infant evaluation of "what is your goal for your infant's birth" instead of with individual events such as "do you want a cesarean" can help develop a framework where events can be seen as "congruous" or "incongruous" to their goals.

In addition to consideration for route of delivery and antenatal monitoring, birth plans should also include plans for the infant once delivered. Parents should be encouraged to clarify their goals of care for the infant. Understanding a family's primary objectives can help providers to ensure directed care towards family goals. MOLST (Medical Orders for Life-Sustaining Treatment) forms can be reviewed prior to birth of the infant to discuss which interventions the family would consider. The individual context in which palliative care is applied is different for every family. Some families may find an active NICU with a lot of staff around comforting – knowing they are not alone when their infant dies. Other families may wish to take their infant home to die. What is right for one family may not be what is best for another family with the LLFC. Exploring these wishes and understanding a family's needs and goals prior to delivery of the infant help to make the process smoother for all those involved (see also Chaps. 4 and 7). In a medical world driven by aggressive therapies and a fix-it approach, it is important to revise treatment goals for these infants who cannot benefit from intensive intervention and shift focus in a palliative direction [6]. Parents need to be aware of options for comfort care and interventions focused on easing of suffering rather than "curing." Parents should be informed regarding what to expect and encouraged to participate in the dying process of their infant in a manner and environment they find meaningful. A few suggestions for family-focused palliative care are included in Table 5.2.

Intrapartum Care of Women and Their Families

Key Points

1. Personalized goals for delivery should inform discussions regarding intrapartum plan of care and should be initiated as early as possible in the antenatal setting.
2. For patients bringing pregnancies to a close in the second trimester, most will be appropriate candidates for either medical or surgical options.
3. Prior uterine surgery with subsequent uterine scar is not a contraindication to attempted vaginal birth prior to 28 weeks or even at term when fetal interventions are not desired.
4. Decisions on utilization of intrapartum obstetric interventions should be guided by individualized patient- and family-centered discussions.
5. Family-neonatal bonding can be facilitated through supported interactions in the peripartum period and collection of physical remembrances.

The planning for peripartum care of women and their families with pregnancies affected by life-limiting conditions begins in the antepartum setting with a particular focus on the evolving plans regarding mode and timing of delivery [2, 7]. The acuity of presentation in labor, the higher incidence of issues such as malpresentation and fetal distress, and the lack of time to clarify family goals intrapartally make pre-labor planning of the utmost importance [2]. Because there is an increased risk for early delivery and pregnancy complications, it is important to have discussions to begin clarifying goals and birth plans as early as possible with a goal to establish a framework by 24 weeks. The execution of these delivery plans can be facilitated by comprehensive documentation so that all members of the care team understand the family's goals for delivery.

Depending on the types of anomalies or conditions present in the fetus, both early labor and medically indicated deliveries may be increased. The focus in planning for delivery should be on the "big picture" of the family's goals for the pregnancy and the expected postnatal course for the neonate [8]. Some families may modify their goals for the pregnancy and birth from the typical expectation of a healthy infant and mother to having more time with their infant alive. Specifically, there is value to patients in determining delivery planning goals that empower them to feel some control through an experience that is otherwise very much out of their control [9]. However, it is important not to lose sight of the variations in risk-benefit profile from healthy pregnancies to inform the individual patient's delivery planning. It is further important to help families understand that with a medically complicated pregnancy a birth plan cannot be viewed as an absolute delineation of the course of events, as evolution of planning will be needed as findings and medical conditions change.

Making Decisions for Mode of Delivery in the Mid-trimester

Shared decision-making with the patient and her family begins with the discussion of mode of delivery [10]. A primary goal in the decisions regarding mode of delivery should be in providing family-centered care with the aim of alleviating a range of suffering – physical, emotional, and spiritual – by guiding families through their treatment choices [11].

For some patients, even if the goal is term delivery, this may not be possible due to a variety of maternal and fetal complications or issues. Pregnancies with a fetus with life-limiting conditions are at higher risk for presenting with mid-trimester labor, cervical dilation/threated abortion, bleeding, or early rupture of membranes. Further, maternal complications are more common, including mirror syndrome and HELLP, which may necessitate delivery or bringing a pregnancy to a close in the mid-trimester. For patients in which there is a need for the pregnancy to come to a close in the previable period – either by choice or due to pregnancy complications or in the setting of extreme growth restriction rendering the baby less than 24-week size – it is generally appropriate for patients to choose between medical and surgical options. The medical route of delivery is accomplished through labor induction. The surgical route of delivery is performed as a dilation and evacuation (D&E) or an intact surgical extraction. This choice is based on maternal, fetal, and cervical characteristics, as well as access to these services in the region of the country where the patient is being cared for, as most states offer limited access to D&E services outside of major cities, and laws have restricted access even within major centers that have trained providers. The National Abortion Federation can help patients and providers locate these services (1-877-257-0012) and can even help with financial assistance in some cases (1-800-772-9100).

Specifically, for infants with a biparietal diameter (head size) less than about 24-week size, it is appropriate to consider D&E for surgical completion of pregnancy versus labor induction. For mothers experiencing medical complications in mid-trimester, this method allows for more rapid delivery and resolution of some pregnancy complications (such as bleeding, maternal mirror syndrome, preeclampsia, infection). Performing this procedure at advanced gestational ages requires operators skilled in the safe performance of this procedure, which may limit availability. Mid-trimester procedures are generally safer with cervical preparation, which may include prostaglandins, antiprogesterones, and osmotic dilators based on gestational age, fetal size, and regional practice patterns [12, 13].

For viable pregnancies at advancing gestational ages, some practice patterns frequently include performing feticide prior to mid-trimester medical or surgical termination of pregnancy. Feticide may decrease the time from induction to completion of delivery of baby and placenta when medical termination (induction of labor) is performed in the second trimester and has the ancillary benefits for emotional, ethical, and legal sequelae that come with avoiding signs of life at the time of birth. However, there is no evidence that feticide prior to surgical procedures in the second trimester improves procedural safety and therefore should only be performed if local laws dictate its use, such as times when intact extraction is anticipated or at times to "stop the clock" when gestational age is approaching legal limits within the state while performing cervical preparation or induction, which can take several days [14].

For medically complex patients, decision-making should be individualized for each patient's particular risk profile. While the benefits of D&E include less blood loss and the ability to coordinate the timing with availability of a comprehensive anesthesia and obstetric team, it does generally require a higher burden of anesthesia than even neuraxial anesthesia (e.g., epidural) for labor induction. Timing is also a concern for an acutely decompensating patient such as those who experience very preterm preeclampsia and/or HELLP syndrome. In these circumstances, the need to place cervical dilators for safe cervical preparation prior to surgical procedures must be weighed against the unpredictable timing of labor induction.

Medical Induction of Labor for Fetal Loss or Nonviable Fetus

While it is beyond the scope of this book to provide complete medical details on pregnancy termination procedures and care for patients undergoing labor induction, a general outline of best practices and medications is included to familiarize all members of team with these strategies. Protocols are similar, but there is variation in typical dosing by weeks of gestation.

Protocols for Labor Induction in the Mid-trimester: 13–24 Weeks

The ideal treatment strategy for induction of labor prior to 24 weeks includes mifepristone and misoprostol in combination. Misoprostol is a prostaglandin analog which facilitates uterine emptying and is especially valuable in the setting of retained placenta, a common complication in early delivery. Mifepristone is an antiprogesterone which prepares the cervix, uterus, and placenta for delivery and therefore is proposed to decrease time to completion of delivery and lower rates of retained placentae.

Typical dosing includes mifepristone 24–48 hours prior to initiating high-dose misoprostol 400 mcg vaginally or sublingually every 3 hours. If there is an inability to administer mifepristone for logistical or legal reasons, misoprostol alone can be used but is likely to incur prolonged time to completion. If using misoprostol as a single agent, it may be appropriate to consider a loading dose of 600–800 mcg vaginally followed by the high-dose misoprostol dosing strategy described above [15].

Protocols for Labor Induction in the Mid-trimester: 24–28 Weeks

The ideal treatment strategy for induction of labor from 24 to 28 weeks gestational age includes mifepristone 200 mg or 600 mg administered 36–48 hours prior to initiating high-dose misoprostol 200 mcg–400 mcg every 4 hours. If there is an inability to administer mifepristone, misoprostol alone can be utilized. If undelivered following 24–48 hours of misoprostol administration, there can be consideration of a rest period, continuation of the misoprostol protocol, or transition to an oxytocin protocol; however, there is limited evidence regarding the optimal completion strategy for patients experiencing prolonged induction [16].

Mid-trimester Labor Induction for Women with Prior Uterine Surgery

Some patients and providers may offer questions regarding the safety of trial of labor after cesarean (TOLAC) to attempt vaginal birth after cesarean section (VBAC) or after other forms of uterine surgery such as prior transmural myomectomies. Although limited data exist, uterine scar of any type does not appear to be a contraindication to labor prior to 28 weeks. For these patients, it may be appropriate to consider using a lower dosing strategy for misoprostol administration; however, there are no data to suggest this changes risk profile and may prolong time to completion of delivery [16].

For the most updated, evidenced-based guidelines for surgical and medical completion of pregnancies in the second trimester, see the Society of Family Planning Clinical Guidelines webpage at https://www.societyfp.org/Resources/Clinical-guidelines.aspx [17].

Making Decisions for Mode of Delivery as Pregnancy Advances

With advancing gestational age, many patients may inquire about appropriate indications for cesarean delivery versus a planned attempt for vaginal birth. For pregnancies affected by life-limiting conditions, standard obstetric indications for cesarean may be considered, but special attention should be paid to the balance of risks and benefits when prolonged neonatal survival is not expected [7]. Because of the imbalance of risk, most obstetricians do not recommend cesarean delivery unless necessary for maternal safety [2].

Even absent a recommendation for cesarean delivery, patients may specifically request this type of delivery. Absent a medical indication for cesarean, this practice is referred to as cesarean delivery on maternal request. In the case of pregnancies affected by complex fetal anomalies, this request usually arises from a desire to see/hold an infant alive prior to its death [2]. These circumstances require extensive pre-labor counseling which includes the key points that (1) there are additional maternal risks, (2) surgical delivery will not change the ultimate fetal/neonatal outcome, and (3) the medical recommendation is for attempted vaginal delivery [2]. Further, the discussion of risk must include the risks in subsequent pregnancies, including the ability to access TOLAC services, increased risk of pregnancy complications, and increased risk for bleeding and morbid placentation (such as placenta accreta). Therefore, the "risk" cannot be simply viewed within the single maternal-fetal dyad, but within the entire life course of the patient, their/her plans for further reproduction, risks to other children (of maternal death/complications in future pregnancies), and risks to the "future" fetus as well. If patients are able to exhibit good understanding of these key points, then the choice for delivery mode must include the patient's considerations on "best" approach, and supporting mothers through a surgical delivery where they sustain additional risks in exchange for psychosocial benefit can be appropriate in the model of beneficence-based care [9].

Labor Management in the Setting of a Comfort-Oriented Approach to Care for the Fetus/Neonate

A critical component of labor management decision-making for the delivery of fetuses with life-limiting illnesses revolves around the strategy for fetal monitoring. While some patients and providers may find the application of continuous electronic fetal monitoring generally comforting, the ability to reveal non-reassuring fetal status when a patient has elected to forgo aggressive intrapartum or neonatal interventions may simply generate family distress without leading to a change in management. There is therefore a strong role for clear and thorough discussions about the risks and unindicated downstream consequences of performing fetal monitoring. Choosing no interventions and accepting that a child may die during the labor course is markedly different than listening to the slowing and stopping of the heart rate over many minutes or hours as a child dies during labor. Therefore, for families that do not wish to undergo cesarean section for fetal indications, the strong preference should be for tocodynamometer alone (to assess contraction strength and frequency without monitoring fetal heart rate) to assist with medication titration. Breech presentation is not a contraindication to vaginal delivery in these infants.

Some patients will elect to proceed with no monitoring throughout the labor process, while others may elect to utilize intermittent auscultation in order to facilitate knowledge of the viability status of the neonate at the time of delivery. Although data exist that intermittent monitoring is equal to continuous monitoring in the low-risk setting, this cannot be extrapolated to the fetus with life-limiting condition. In fetuses that are strongly anticipated to exhibit abnormal rhythms absent a family's desire for aggressive intrapartum interventions, many families will specifically forgo continuous monitoring [7]. In contrast, some patients would accept the maternal risks of cesarean in order to deliver a baby prior to onset of intrapartum demise, and in these circumstances, continuous fetal monitoring could be considered after full discussion of risks and benefits with family [2].

The medical management of induction and labor for a pregnancy affected by a life-limiting condition does not generally differ from standard obstetric practices. This includes the application of standard analgesic approaches [7]. This should include comprehensive pain relief including for patients undergoing second trimester inductions as the pain experienced requires a full complement of analgesia services including nitrous oxide or neuraxial anesthesia, if desired [9].

The role of emotional support throughout the labor process is of the utmost importance for these patients and their families. Extensive emotional support can be provided to the patient and family by the provider team as well as by specialized nurses with additional training in perinatal bereavement or palliative care providers [7]. Perinatal support counseling before and after delivery, and planned follow-up after discharge home (not "as needed" but scheduled for short interval after discharge), is key to assuring the team is able to check in on the family at regular intervals, perform screening for postpartum depression, and assure timely referrals for ongoing psychiatric care if needed.

It is also noteworthy that delivery of infants with life-limiting illnesses can cause secondary trauma for the care team as well. It is important to be aware of the emotional effects of caring for these families with complex infant needs and provide appropriate support to the care team so that they may continue to provide empathic care [18]. Appropriate planning should assure that all team members are aware of staff options for support, counseling, and stress relief offered to prevent emotional burnout and detachment.

Special Considerations

Some deliveries for the fetus with life-limiting prognosis may require additional planning beyond the planning for fetal intervention and postdelivery support, evaluation, and care. Although the number of fetal syndromes and combinations of findings cannot possibly be covered in this chapter, many fetal syndromes will lead to one or more of a common cluster of physical manifestations – hydrops, growth restriction, fetal disproportional growth, malpresentation, and polyhydramnios. Further, after delivery, hemorrhage and incidence of retained placenta can be increased due to early delivery or increased uterine distension.

Special Delivery Circumstances: Extremely Low Birth Weight

When delivering fetuses of extremely low birth weight, there are a variety of issues that can be encountered due to both the fetal size and fetal proportions. Due to the much larger proportion of fetal weight distributed to the head in extremely small infants, especially at early gestational ages and in the setting of extreme growth restriction, there can be significant complications with non-vertex presentation (any position other than head down). Moreover, these presentations are more likely to occur or even develop during labor with a previously vertex presentation due to the small fetal size allowing the physical space to transition positions, even at advanced stages of labor. While it may feel tempting to artificially rupture the fetal membranes to either augment the labor process or decrease the chance of variable lie for vertex fetuses, this is not usually the correct intervention. Whenever possible, keeping the membranes intact even to the point of delivery en caul (intact delivery of the amniotic fluid sack and baby) can decrease the incidence of birth injury, especially for non-vertex presentations, as well as reduce the risk of head entrapment behind the cervix and the risk of retained placenta.

When attempting non-vertex delivery of extremely low-birth-weight infants (either viable infants or following intrauterine fetal demise), it is of particular importance to remember that the large head size in relation to body size strongly contributes to increased risk for head entrapment. This occurs because the small fetal body is able to slip through the cervix with restriction of the cervix at the level of the fetal neck and the fetal head remaining within the uterus. Avoidance of early rupture and en caul delivery can help prevent this, but if delivery after membrane rupture occurs, then, as with breech deliveries at more advanced gestational ages, predominant reliance on maternal expulsive efforts increases the safety of breech vaginal delivery. If head entrapment is encountered regardless of reliance on maternal expulsive efforts, it should be managed with standard obstetric interventions with one exception. If the fetus is nonviable or the family has elected for nonaggressive care, then maneuvers do not need to be attempted immediately. Instead, the fetus should be allowed to remain in place (head inside the cervix, body out) while uterine contractions continue to allow for further dilatation of the cervix. If maneuvers are done, the significant disproportion between head and body size can contribute to risk for unintentional disarticulation of the fetal head (this is especially a risk in the infant with hydrops or in one that has been demised for a period of time); therefore, maneuvers should be performed with much less force than on term infants, and a much lower threshold should be considered for the placement of cervical incisions (Dührssen incisions) to attempt to release the entrapment atraumatically.

Special Delivery Circumstances: Polyhydramnios

Many fetal conditions that limit prognosis can be accompanied by or predispose to polyhydramnios, which can subsequently precipitate early delivery, impinging on the maternal diaphragm or venous system leading to respiratory or vascular compromise, and markedly increase risk for malpresentation, protracted labor, and postpartum hemorrhage. Most of the disorders at risk for polyhydramnios relate to abnormal fetal swallowing seen with certain gastrointestinal and central nervous system disorders as well as obstructive disorders within the chest – either due primarily from a chest mass or from displacement of contents into chest, like in a diaphragmatic hernia [2]. In some cases, women may need amnioreduction serially for comfort. Evaluating for sudden increase in fundal height or performing serial ultrasound are strategies to monitor the at-risk fetus for this complication. Alternatively, evaluation can be prompted by maternal symptoms of rapid abdominal distention, discomfort, or shortness of breath. Typically in these cases, polyhydramnios occurs suddenly after 28 weeks and worsens from there. A type and screen and hematocrit on admission should be ordered on all these women, and the team and family should be aware of this potential risk. Active management of the second stage with oxytocin immediately following delivery of the infant may help to decrease the risk of hemorrhage arising from polyhydramnios.

Special Delivery Circumstances: Delayed Initiation of Labor in Anencephaly

Anencephaly (congenital absence of a major portion of the brain, skull, and scalp) is the most severe and most common neural tube defect [19]. The incidence of other congenital malformations is 13–41%, and approximately 65% of fetuses with anencephaly die in utero. Those who survive tend to have polyhydramnios due to dysfunctional swallowing mechanisms. Labor and delivery is often complicated by unstable fetal lie, malpresentation, dysfunctional labor (poor dilation or dystocia), and postpartum hemorrhage. Given that there is often no firm presenting part pushing on the cervix, initiation of labor may be delayed in pregnancies with an anencephalic fetus. Parents should be counseled on these findings as well as what to anticipate as regards to appearance of their newborn. Care can be taken to place a hat on the infant following delivery if the parents would find this comforting or if the appearance of the exposed cranial tissue is daunting. Most of these infants will pass away within hours to days after birth; however, survival has been confirmed out to 2 months of life, although this would be rare. Breech presentation is not a contraindication to vaginal delivery in these infants and in fact may be preferable to allow for better pressure from a presenting part. Head entrapment is rarely if ever a concern.

Case 5.1: Anencephaly

MF is a 30-year-old G4P2012 who presents for first trimester screening. At the time of her screening ultrasound, anencephaly was identified. She was extensively counseled regarding the uniformly lethal nature of this finding and the availability of all pregnancy management options including the availability of resources for termination of pregnancy within this institution. After extensive discussion with her partner, family, and care team, she made the decision to continue the pregnancy expectantly. She met with the palliative care team on three occasions throughout the remainder of the pregnancy to discuss comfort care measures for the infant following delivery. The plan was made to perform monthly ultrasound assessments for viability and amniotic fluid volume, but no antenatal fetal surveillance was planned. Polyhydramnios was identified late in the second trimester and continued to increase in the third trimester.

At 35 weeks, MF presented to the labor and delivery unit in preterm labor at 4 cm. Amniotic fluid index at the time of presentation was 41 cm and the fetus was in breech presentation. As per her antenatal plan of care outlined in her medical record, a vaginal delivery was pursued even in the setting of non-vertex presentation, and no fetal monitoring was performed. Following spontaneous rupture of membranes at 6 cm, there was slow progression in labor over the next 7 hours to full dilation.

Preparations were made for delivery in the standard labor room with the palliative care team readily available for assessment and initiation of comfort care measures. Maternal pushing was only partially successful in delivering the infant to the level of the shoulder blades requiring the provider to assist with delivery of the arms using Loveset maneuvers. The fetal head delivered without additional maneuvers.

The infant was passed to the mother and her family who was supported through their goal of bonding with their infant throughout his first day of life. Compassionate comfort care measures were provided to the infant, and the family was supported through holding, bathing, and dressing their infant. He subsequently passed away at hour of life 18 and remained with the family for an additional day of bonding and memory-making with the assistance of a cooled bassinet. MF was discharged home from the hospital on postpartum day #2 with a collection of physical remembrances of her infant.

Special Delivery Circumstances: Anhydramnios

Anhydramnios is defined as the absence of amniotic fluid. Pregnancies can be affected by anhydramnios for a variety of reasons – for example, no amniotic fluid may be produced (bilateral fetal renal agenesis) or fluid may be leaking (premature rupture of membranes). Regardless of the inciting cause, anhydramnios complicates labor. Without the normal amniotic fluid cushion around the fetus and umbilical cord, uterine contractions in the setting of anhydramnios put pressure directly on the umbilical cord. Given the umbilical cord compression, variable decelerations and non-reassuring fetal status during labor are more common. In one retrospective review of low-risk pregnancies at term affected by anhydramnios, the cesarean section rate was 56.6% in primigravidas [20]. Women should be counseled about the increased risk of cesarean delivery due to fetal distress during labor or induction in the setting of anhydramnios. This may influence decisions regarding fetal monitoring during labor/induction in this setting, especially considering concerns for lung hypoplasia in these fetuses.

Special Delivery Circumstances: Delayed Third Stage and Retained Placenta

Delivery of fetuses with life-limiting conditions may be more likely to be affected by delayed third stage (increased length of time to deliver the placenta) and retained placentae due to contributions from abnormal placental development and increased incidence of mid-trimester delivery. For pregnancies delivering preterm, and in particular before 28 weeks, there is an increased incidence of prolonged third stage of labor and retained placenta. When undergoing mid-trimester induction of labor, it is appropriate to continue high-dose misoprostol following delivery of the infant with otherwise expectant management of the placenta. Continuing misoprostol administration for 4–6 hours following delivery of the infant can be appropriate to attempt augmentation of spontaneous placental delivery if maternal bleeding is unremarkable with otherwise stable maternal status.

For patients in whom the decision is made that manual or instrumented placental delivery is required, this can cause particular challenges in the palliative maternal-neonatal dyad. The need to augment delivery of the placenta may be occurring during the neonate's final hours of life or during a time when critical decisions may need to be made based on evaluation of the neonate's condition or confirmation of suspected diagnoses. The management of the placenta can be completed in standard obstetric fashion; however, anything that can be done to decrease the need for operative anesthesia, transfer to an operative suite, or separation of mother from neonate is ideal. There are a variety of methods to elicit delivery of the placenta without extensive anesthesia or transfer of the mother requiring separation of the maternal-neonatal dyad. Paracervical blocks and/or pudendal blocks can be placed to facilitate maternal comfort with the required instrumentation in the delivery room. Bierer forceps (ideal if available) or ring forceps can be utilized under ultrasound guidance to surgically evacuate the placenta with much greater maternal tolerance than manual extraction. Manual vacuum aspirators (MVAs) can also be utilized at the bedside for evacuation of very small placentae or clearance of retained placental fragments, again with better maternal tolerance than manual exploration. All of these allow the family to remain together in room with the infant, during this important and limited time. If there is heavy bleeding, inability to completely assess, and maternal intolerance/need for pain control, then evaluation and care in the OR suite due to maternal risks should NOT be delayed to allow for bonding.

Case 5.2: The Unexpected Palliative Care Patient

MR is a 41-year-old G1 with a medical history of systemic lupus erythematous (SLE) and chronic hypertension. She presented to establish prenatal care in the first trimester with stable SLE symptoms and labs and a mild range blood pressure on a stable dose of a beta-blocker. Baseline laboratory evaluation revealed no protein in the urine as well as normal kidney and liver function.

At 24w3d, she presented to labor and delivery with a headache. Physical exam revealed clonus (rhythmic beating of the feet indicating hyperreflexia) but an otherwise normal neurologic exam and severe range hypertension (220/115). Acute management of blood pressure required multiple doses of IV medications to decrease blood pressure to the mild range. Laboratory evaluation revealed profound abnormality including liver transaminases (AST/ALT

540/490), elevated creatinine (3.1), and thrombocytopenia (platelet count 32). Lupus blood work revealed no evidence of increased disease activity. Formal ultrasound revealed a fetus in complete breech presentation with significant intrauterine growth restriction (estimated fetal weight 405 g). All of these findings are consistent with the diagnosis of HELLP syndrome (hemolysis, elevated liver enzymes, and low platelet count), which can cause seizures, stroke, disseminated intravascular coagulation (DIC), and risk for maternal death. Magnesium was started for seizure prophylaxis. The recommendation was made to proceed with delivery due to the significant risk of maternal health compromise and anticipated further decompensation if she remains pregnant.

The intrauterine growth restriction was discussed with the patient as was the anticipated poor prognosis for an infant affected by such profound growth restriction in the peri-viable period. Following extensive discussion with the obstetrics and neonatal teams, the patient decided to proceed with delivery and forgo any resuscitative efforts for her infant given the significance of the growth restriction. She was offered surgical and medical options to move towards delivery and elected to proceed with induction of labor as she had a strong desire to hold her infant following delivery. Only intermittent fetal auscultation was performed as MR voiced a concern she wanted to be emotionally prepared for whether her infant would be born alive.

Mifepristone and misoprostol were administered for labor induction, and a transfer to the MICU was eventually required for a continuous antihypertensive infusion to control severe range blood pressures. Following 24 hours of medical induction, she called out with pelvic pressure, and fetal parts were noted to be palpable just past the vaginal introitus. She rapidly delivered the baby, who had some respiratory effort. The infant was wrapped and handed to MR to hold as per her previously discussed preference. Within minutes of delivery of the infant, heavy bleeding developed. She was uncomfortable with attempt at manual removal of the placenta. MR strongly desired to avoid a surgical placental removal as she understood this time with her living infant would be limited and, in fact, her infant may pass away during the time she was in the operating room. She also valued the presence of her partner at bedside and did not want to be separated during this time so they could both participate in bonding with their infant. Given this, placental removal was performed at the bedside under ultrasound guidance using Bierer forceps. The patient was able to tolerate the procedure without additional analgesics and held her infant throughout the procedure. Her infant was noted to be without cardiac activity 15 minutes following her bedside placental extraction.

HW remained in the MICU for an additional day of aggressive antihypertensive support with her partner at bedside throughout. Her infant remained at her bedside as well with the support of a cooled bassinet. During this time, her family came to her bedside to provide emotional support to MR and her partner and to experience holding their infant. Once stabilized, she was transferred to the high-risk labor and delivery unit for four additional days of postpartum stabilization. She was discharged home on postpartum day #5 with a box of physical remembrances of her infant and arrangements made for a private cremation with plans for close outpatient follow-up of blood pressure and bereavement support.

Special Delivery Circumstances: Destructive Procedures

There are some delivery circumstances where decompression of the fetus is required to facilitate vaginal delivery of an infant that otherwise would require surgical delivery. Due to the destructive nature of these procedures, they are generally reserved for nonviable infants or those with profoundly devastating prognoses. Procedures that may be required include cephalocentesis during which the fetal CSF is drained to decompress the calvarium and cleidotomy where surgical division of the clavicles is performed to decompress the thorax [9]. While these procedures are generally utilized to facilitate vaginal delivery, they can also be employed at the time of hysterotomy to facilitate delivery through a smaller uterine (i.e., low transverse) incision.

Special Delivery Circumstances: Microcephaly and Fetal Disproportions

Typically in a vertex birth, the head is of the largest width, allowing the remainder of the fetus to delivery easily. For the fetus with a small head (microcephaly) or enlarged abdomen (for a variety of reasons), the proportions are off. This is no different than the disproportionate infant proportions seen in the fetus of a diabetic mother where the abdominal growth is ahead of the gestational age, leading to an increased risk of shoulder dystocia. Therefore, the team should look not just at fetal size, but at fetal proportions as well when preparing for delivery. This does not mean that a cesarean is necessarily warranted in these circumstances but that the team should be aware and prepared. Fetuses with profoundly small head circumferences are at increased risk for complications during delivery. Although it would seem at first glance that the delivery would be "easier," care must be taken as the head may slip through the incompletely dilated cervix with a relatively larger abdomen still needing to pass through. Therefore, shoulder dystocia can occur with the profoundly microcephalic infant as the abdomen attempts to follow the small head. Similarly, in a fetus delivering with enlarged polycystic kidneys (like in Beckwith-Wiedemann or a variety of other conditions) or with profound fetal ascites (prune belly) where the abdomen is far ahead of the head circumference, the team should be prepared for shoulder dystocia.

Special Delivery Circumstances: Mirror Syndrome

Pregnancies affected by significant fetal hydrops can be complicated by maternal mirror syndrome in which profound maternal edema develops. The condition is frequently difficult to differentiate from preeclampsia and may, in fact, be part of the preeclampsia spectrum of pathologic processes. Regardless of the etiology, the maternal presentation includes hypertension, hemodilution, hepatic lab aberrations, and pulmonary edema [21]. These maternal hemodynamic changes may present challenges to optimizing maternal safety and placental perfusion during delivery. The progression and severity of mirror syndrome can be fulminant and severe; therefore, delivery should not be delayed in the patient with this condition for steroids or other fetal interventions, especially given the poor fetal prognosis of severe hydrops in early gestational ages. In addition, the fetal hydrops itself can precipitate difficulty with delivery – shoulder dystocia can be a significant problem for fetuses affected by hydrops, especially at advancing gestational age.

Case 5.3: Fetal Hydrops and Maternal Mirror Syndrome

JR is a 25-year-old G1P0 with a fetus known to be affected by monosomy X (a single copy of the X chromosome) following CVS sampling performed at the time a cystic hygroma (swelling of the neck often found in chromosomal disorders) was noted on first trimester screening. The patient underwent comprehensive counseling and elected to proceed with the pregnancy expectantly (continuation of pregnancy rather than termination). The cystic hygroma resolved, but congenital abnormalities of the aorta were noted at the time of the anatomic survey. The pregnancy continued without significant issues into the third trimester when, at 36 weeks, an ultrasound was obtained for fundal height measuring larger than expected for gestational age with significant maternal edema. Ultrasound revealed massive polyhydramnios (AFI 40) with fetal findings including ascites, pleural and pericardial effusions, and diffuse skin thickening. Maternal physical exam was significant for 4+ pitting edema and mild range hypertension (155/95). Maternal laboratory evaluation revealed Rh+ blood type with negative antibody screen, mild anemia, a mild elevation of liver transaminases (AST/ALT 66/55), and elevated uric acid. Creatinine and platelets were within normal limits. These findings were suggestive of fetal hydrops with maternal mirror syndrome.

The recommendation was made to proceed with delivery, and JR was subsequently admitted to the hospital for induction of labor. The delivery management was discussed in depth with JR who was highly motivated for a vaginal delivery if this could be accomplished safely but was willing to accept cesarean if there was evidence of significant fetal compromise. The risk of shoulder dystocia in the setting of profound fetal hydrops was reviewed extensively.

Continuous external fetal monitoring was initially concerning for fetal distress but responded appropriately to intrauterine resuscitation efforts. When full dilation was reached, the patient was transferred to the operating room to optimize maternal positioning and space for neonatal resuscitation. The neonatal care team was updated throughout as to the progress of labor and was present for the delivery. The maternal positioning was optimized on the operating room table with Allen stirrups, the table extensions removed below the level of the maternal buttock, and additional staff on hand to assist.

Following delivery of the head, a shoulder dystocia was encountered. Multiple operators were required to perform seven iterations of standard shoulder dystocia reduction maneuvers with eventual resolution of the dystocia at just over 3 minutes following delivery of the head. The infant was passed to the awaiting care team who initiated resuscitative efforts. No episiotomy was placed due to the observation that adequate space was available for performance of shoulder dystocia maneuvers; however, there was noted to be spontaneous occurrence of a third-degree laceration which was repaired in usual fashion. The infant was initially evaluated by the NICU as per the patient and family plan but however was unable to be ventilated and was wrapped and handed back to the family as per the delivery plan. The infant passed away peacefully in the arms of the mother surrounded by family and friends.

Mild-range hypertension and edema persisted throughout JR's postpartum hospital course; however, lab abnormalities slowly began to resolve. She was discharged home on postpartum day #3, and evaluation in the office on postpartum day #10 revealed resolution of her hypertension and only trace edema. JR was referred to a local counseling group which specializes in infant bereavement. At the time of her visit on postpartum day #10, her mood was appropriate, and she declined any additional need for services or support. In addition to obstetric follow-up at 6 weeks of postdelivery, she was also called several times by the bereavement staff in the NICU to check on her after the loss of her infant.

Family Bonding at Birth

Although acute bereavement care is initiated at the time of delivery, planning for this, including delineation of family wishes during these limited times, should be done ahead of time as much as possible, especially for infants expected to pass away at birth or shortly thereafter. The goal is to support and promote bonding of the family and infant in the perinatal period [22]. This is guided by family preferences and goals but may be facilitated by assisting with bathing, accentuating the non-anomalous features of the infant, encouraging holding and dressing of the infant, and setting no limits to time with the infant both before and after death [7]. The utilization of refrigerated crib systems can allow extended time for the infant to remain with the family following the infant's death, if desired.

In contrast, the support of families electing aggressive care following delivery imparts different challenges. Given the anticipated separation of mother from infant, family bonding can be supported by taking care to show the baby to mom before transfer to the NICU, allowing the partner to accompany the baby to the NICU if appropriate, and providing the family updates over time with changes to the baby's condition if the mother and family are not yet able to visit.

Multidisciplinary support continues to be important at this juncture including the support of the obstetric providers, neonatal providers, palliative care team, social work, and chaplaincy if desired [7]. Families should be given the space they need, and labor and delivery staff may need to delay or defer some routine postpartum care (if safe) to allow this time. Additionally, staff should clarify ahead how the family will be handling visitation, as it is often helpful for immediate family to have limited visitors for a period of time for pictures, bonding, etc. If possible, dedicated spaces for patients with perinatal loss or life-limiting anomalies away from the families with healthy newborns can provide families with the privacy they need for their unique circumstances [9]. If a large family is expected, and the family needs privacy, then a secondary room outside the general waiting room may be helpful to provide separation and space for bereavement. Facilitating this period of bonding, family time, and memory-making can be additionally challenging when the mother has experienced medical complications requiring escalated maternal care interventions. When there will be maternal care requirements that interfere with postdelivery interactions between mother and infant, some families will offer preferences regarding the first person to view or hold the infant (mother versus family) or when to initiate memory-making activities such as dressing. If possible, antepartum discussion of these preferences can help to support individualized maternal goals. Most of the time, the need for interventions will be unknown, and the team should consider addressing this possibility in the birth plan to prevent misunderstandings and extended family decisions when the mother is unable to advocate for herself and the partner's attention is divided.

Physical Memories

Physical memory items can be collected for the patient regardless of route of delivery. Following a vaginal birth or cesarean section, a variety of items can be gathered to provide physical memories of the infant for the families to keep. These include outfits the infant wore, hats and blankets received at birth, hand and foot prints, locks of hair, blessing remembrances, and photographs. These items are traditionally placed into decorated boxes for the families to take home on discharge from the hospital [7]. If a patient has undergone a surgical evacuation of pregnancy, some of these physical memories can still be obtained. It may be appropriate to consider hospital policies to make and hold memory boxes for all perinatal loss patients. Occasionally, some patients will initially decline physical remembrances but subsequently ask for them later in their bereavement process.

Confirmation of Diagnosis: Genetic Testing and Autopsy

Genetic Testing

Ideally, a family with a baby with a life-limiting condition has met with a genetic counselor prior to delivery, and either undergone some testing, or made a plan for what testing is desired during the birth process (see Chap. 6). However, in many complex anomaly cases or unexpected findings at birth, the diagnosis may not be possible to make prior to delivery, and postnatal evaluation may be needed to guide testing. A multidisciplinary team is required to confirm the suspected diagnosis for many infants following their delivery. Experienced pediatricians can perform physical assessment to confirm findings and guide care planning, as applicable [2]. If the diagnosis remains uncertain, evaluation by a dysmorphologist may help guide genetic/metabolic testing [2]. If they are unavailable, good quality, well-lit, close range photographs of the face (front and profile) as well as ears, hands, feet, and any externally visualized anomalies may be helpful for later evaluation. Genetic testing should be offered if definitive diagnostic testing (e.g., via chorionic villus sampling or amniocentesis) had not been completed in pregnancy. Cytogenetics can be performed from blood sampling from the umbilical cord, from blood collected from the infant while living, or from samples collected from the placenta or fetal skin samples after a neonate passes away [2]. Genetic testing performed can range from simple karyotype to complex exome sequencing depending on the clinical questions that remain [23, 24]. For fetuses that arrive with an intrauterine demise, amniocentesis prior to induction has been shown to improve genetic yield and reduce the risk of "no call" or inconclusive results [25]. Genetic panels for some phenotype clusters also exist, such as hydrops and skeletal dysplasia. Further information on these testing options can be found in the genetic counseling chapter (see Chap. 6). If an anomalous infant is encountered unexpectedly, extra cord blood should be drawn in green and purple tops and saved until the appropriate evaluation and discussion can be completed.

Autopsy

If a fetal or neonatal demise occurs, autopsy can also provide important information for many infants. If the fetus is at high risk for this, then the team should have a discussion ahead of time if possible to review the benefits of this evaluation. This is best when performed by a pathologist with specialized experience in neonatal pathology and of particular importance when the diagnosis was uncertain or genetic testing was non-confirmatory of diagnosis [2]. When autopsy is performed following a diagnosis made by imaging alone, the findings on autopsy may change the estimated risk of recurrence in subsequent pregnancies in over one quarter of cases [26]. Of note, if comprehensive autopsy evaluation will be critical to confirming the diagnosis, this may be factored in to patient decision-making regarding mode of delivery. Although a gross evaluation can be performed following surgical extractions, the fetus will not be intact for evaluation as it will be following an induction of labor. However, the family planning literature suggests that with an experienced pathologist the difference in data obtained is minimal, so families should not feel that data cannot be obtained by D&E if this is their preferred method of delivery [27]. Autopsy is generally not a billed service at most academic medical centers, although exact billing and cost will vary by institution. Genetic testing, histologic evaluations, and special staining or slides that are done may have associated costs, however. For some anomaly groups, such as skeletal dysplasia, there exist national registries where samples and radiographs can be sent both to help obtain a diagnosis for the family, as well as to further research into these rare conditions. These are generally at no cost to families.

For families who decline comprehensive autopsy, there are less invasive alternatives that can provide at least partial analysis including external physical exam only and plain film X-ray. Advanced diagnostic techniques such as MRI, percutaneous organ sampling, endoscopic organ sampling, and/or high-field imaging may develop a future role for pathologic confirmation of anomalies; however, these are not yet considered within the standard of care for postmortem diagnosis [2]. If a family declines autopsy, the discussion should be had that this information cannot be obtained at a later date and that findings may guide genetic testing for other rare disorders that may not be possible to detect without direct knowledge of which genes are potentially affected. Even if the immediately affected family is not planning future pregnancies, they may wish to have this information for their other children or for extended family for future pregnancy planning.

Postpartum Care of Women and Their Families Following Fetal/Neonatal Demise in LLFC

Key Points

1. Ongoing support for emotional healing needs to be addressed.
2. Attention must be paid to physical recovery following delivery including breast care and postpartum healing.
3. Family planning following delivery is pivotal to consider as it is often overlooked during periods of stress. Appropriate inter-pregnancy interval is essential for maternal mental and physical health.

The loss of an infant, either through in utero demise or neonatal death, is a traumatic event. Families who have experienced a fetal or neonatal death often leave the hospital in a state of shock. It is essential for these women and their families to establish a support network and planned follow-up with their physician can be helpful. Women are encouraged to schedule a two-week follow-up appointment after their infant's death (rather than the typical six-week postpartum visit). This allows an early point of contact to answer any questions the family may have as well as to screen for depression which is more likely in families who have experienced a substantial loss. Predictors of complicated grief and post-loss depression include lack of social support, preexisting relationship difficulties, absence of surviving children, and needing to terminate a pregnancy due to fetal anomalies [28].

Grief and Emotional Healing

The loss of an infant or child is recognized as a traumatic life event. Grief is a deeply personal process and experienced uniquely among individuals. In a population-based study, individuals who had lost a child showed the highest prevalence of complicated grief [28]. More information on grief and normal grief process can be found in Chap. 12. All providers completing follow-up for women and their partners that have lost a child should be prepared to address these concerns. High levels of perceived emotional support from society are consistently associated with lower scores of perinatal grief [29]. Providers and support staff can significantly influence the impact of grief on these women and their families. Some suggestions for postpartum care and contact are reviewed in Table 5.2.

Assessment of Physical Healing and Medical Evaluation

Assessment of physical healing should take place at scheduled, regular intervals after delivery. This should be considered separate from postpartum follow-up visits for results of fetal or postnatal testing. Care should be taken to address normal postpartum concerns including normal lochia, perineal or cesarean scar healing, and activity level. Women should be counseled on when they can safely return to exercise and driving a vehicle depending on the circumstances surrounding their particular delivery and what medication(s) they may be taking. Maternal breast health should be included in these visits including methods for decreasing breast milk production (cold cabbage leaves, tight sports bra, lukewarm bathing). For women that have had medical complications of pregnancy, such as preeclampsia, cesarean or hemorrhage may need more and closer follow-up. The exact timing of the follow-up for these concerns will vary between pregnancy depending on the timing of when they deliver and medical conditions that occurred.

Post-loss Consult

All patients and their partners should be offered the opportunity to follow-up to review the pregnancy, any findings, and any testing results when they are ready. This consultation should include disease management of underlying medical conditions, should be undertaken with a maternal-fetal medicine physician, and, for complex genetic results, should include a genetic counselor. For some families, this may be relatively soon after delivery, but for others, this may be months later. This consult should include review of fetal or neonatal findings, review of their infant's diagnoses, and a full discussion of genetic and pathologic results when they are ready prior to attempting future pregnancies.

For women with underlying medical conditions or those who experienced complications during the pregnancy or labor and delivery, review of these events should be part of the discussion. For those with infants with genetic conditions, decision-making regarding testing or donor gamete options to avoid similar anomalies and risk of recurrence in the future may be something that families wish to pursue. For those with infants with neural tube disorders, planned pregnancy allowing for preconception folic acid therapy may help prevent recurrence. For those with fetal loss or poor outcomes related to maternal disease (such as severe preeclampsia and early growth restriction), evaluation and discussion of ways to avoid or reduce recurrent maternal risks should be discussed.

Family Planning After Delivery: Contraception and Pregnancy Spacing

Discussion and provision of contraception after delivery is key to facilitate physical and mental health following postpartum recovery from delivery of an infant with a life-limiting prognosis. This also allows time for results of diagnostic and autopsy testing to be completed and compiled and for postnatal consultations to be performed. Empowering women to plan a subsequent pregnancy may substantially decrease future pregnancy risks.

Not all women with complex fetal diagnosis will be ready to make a decision about contraception immediately following events of delivery. Therefore, this discussion should happen prior to delivery, ideally by the mid-trimester. It is important to remember that without the lactational amenorrhea that typically follows pregnancy (as lactation is not typically initiated after loss), there is a rapid return to fertility, and therefore, discussion of interval contraceptive methods is strongly recommended.

Even if an infant with a life-limiting prognosis is able to be home with the family, this is a significantly stressful time for the family, and time for self-care (daily pills, return to physician for visits to place contraceptive devices, etc.) may be limited. If these discussions can be initiated or reviewed in the months prior to delivery, this removes one potential stressor (unplanned pregnancy) from a family's life. Further, even if future children are desired, having time, space for healing, and full knowledge of final diagnosis may aid with planning.

Conclusion

Each year in the United States, approximately 15,000 infants are born with conditions incompatible with prolonged life, necessitating the need for a palliative care protocol for neonates and infants. Palliative care encompasses the entire milieu of care to prevent and treat suffering and improve conditions around death of an infant, both for the infant themselves and their families. Incorporating a palliative model into the antepartum, intrapartum, and postpartum care for pregnancies in which the infant has a life-limiting condition is essential in providing consistent, quality end-of-life care. Obstetric care providers along with pediatric care providers and palliative care specialists are pivotal in providing parents the highest-quality medical care they deserve. These providers, in addition to the network of resources, serve to ultimately create a birth plan which models their goals of care for both themselves and their infant.

References

1. Catlin AJ, Carter BS. Creation of a neonatal end of life palliative care protocol. J Perinatol. 2002;22(3):184–95.
2. Breeze ACG, Lees CC. Antenatal diagnosis and management of life-limiting conditions. Semin Fetal Neonatal Med. 2013;18:68–75.
3. Dialani V, Mehta T, Levine D. MR imaging of the fetal abdomen and pelvis. In: Levine D, editor. Atlas of fetal MRI. Boca Raton, FL: Taylor & Francis/CRC Press; 2005. p. 113–38.
4. Baile W, Buckman R, Lenzi R, Glober G, Beale E, Kudelka A. SPIKES – a six-step protocol for delivering bad news: application to the patient with cancer. Oncologist. 2000;5(4):302–11.
5. Denney-Koelsch E, Cote-Arsenault D. “My baby is a person”: parents’ experiences with life-threatening fetal diagnosis (313-A). J Pain Symptom Manag. 2012;43(2):340–1.
6. Hulac P. Creation and use of You are Not Alone, a video for parents facing difficult decisions. J Clin Ethics. 2001;12(3):251–3.
7. Calhoun BC, Napolitano P, Terry M, Bussey C, Hoeldtke NJ. Comprehensive care for the family of the fetus with a lethal condition. J Reprod Med. 2003;48(5):344–9.
8. Marty CM, Carter BS. Ethics and palliative care in the perinatal world. Semin Fetal Neonatal Med. 2018;23:35–8.
9. DiMiceli-Zsigmond M, Williams AK, Richardson MG. Expecting the unexpected: perspectives on stillbirth and late termination of pregnancy for fetal anomalies. Anesth Analg. 2015;121:457–64.
10. Tosello B, Haddad G, Gire C, Einaudi M. Lethal fetal abnormalities: how to approach perinatal palliative care? J Matern Fetal Neonatal Med. 2017;30(6):755–8.
11. Kavanaugh K, Roscigno CI, Swanson KM, Savage TA, Kimura RE, Kilpatrick SJ. Perinatal palliative care: parent perceptions of caring in interactions surrounding counseling for risk of delivering an extremely premature infant. Palliat Support Care. 2015;13(2):145–55.
12. Society of Family Planning. Cervical preparation for surgical abortion from 20 to 24 weeks’ gestation. Contraception. 2008;77:308–14.
13. Society of Family Planning. Cervical preparation for second-trimester surgical abortion prior to 20 weeks’ gestation. Contraception. 2014;89(2):75–84.
14. Society of Family Planning. Induction of fetal demise before abortion. Contraception. 2010;81:462–73.
15. Society of Family Planning. Labor induction abortion in the second trimester. Contraception. 2011;84:4–18.
16. Society of Family Planning. Interruption of nonviable pregnancies of 24–28 weeks’ gestation using medical methods. Contraception. 2013;88:341–9.
17. Society of Family Planning Clinical Guidelines webpage at https://www.societyfp.org/Resources/Clinical-guidelines.aspx.
18. Puia DM, Lewis L, Beck CT. Experiences of obstetric nurses who are present for a perinatal loss. J Obstet Gynecol Neonatal Nurs. 2013;42(3):321–31.
19. The Medical Task Force on Anencephaly. The infant with anencephaly. The medical task force on anencephaly. N Engl J Med. 1990;322(10):669–74.
20. Visvalingam G, Purandare N, Cooley S, Roopnarinesingh R, Geary M. Perinatal outcome after ultrasound diagnosis of anhydramnios at term. J Obstet Gynaecol. 2012;32(1):50–3.
21. Braun T, Brauer M, Fuchs I, Czernik C, Dudenhausen JW, Henrich W, Sarioglu N. Mirror syndrome: a systematic review of fetal associated conditions, maternal presentation and perinatal outcome. Fetal Diagn Ther. 2010;27:191–203.

22. Filges I, Fridman JM. Exome sequencing for gene discovery in lethal fetal disorders- harnessing the value of extreme phenotypes. Prenat Diagn. 2015;35:1005–9.
23. Cote-Arsenault D, Krowchuk H, Jenkins Hall W, Denney-Koelsch E. We want what's best for our baby: prenatal parenting of babies with lethal conditions. J Prenat Perinat Psychol Health. 2015;29(3):157–76.
24. Shamseldin HE, Kurdi W, Almusafri F, Alnemer M, Alkaff A, Baby Z, et al. Molecular autopsy in maternal-fetal medicine. Genet Med. 2018;20(4):420–7.
25. Reddy UM, Page GP, Saade GR. The role of DNA microarrays in the evaluation of fetal death. Prenat Diagn. 2012;32:371–5.
26. Boyd PA, Tondi F, Hicks NR, Chamberlain PF. Autopsy after termination of pregnancy for fetal anomaly: retrospective cohort study. BMJ. 2004;328(7432):137. Epub 2003 Dec 8
27. Ernst LM, Gawron L, Fritsch MK. Pathologic examination of fetal and placental tissue obtained by dilation and evacuation. Arch Pathol Lab Med. 2013;137(3):326–37.
28. Kersting A, Brahler E, Glaesmer H, Wagner B. Prevalence of complicated grief in a representative population-based sample. J Affect Disord. 2011;131:339–43.
29. Toedter LJ, Lasker JN, Janssen HJ. International comparison of studies using the perinatal grief scale: a decade of research on pregnancy loss. Death Stud. 2001;25(3):205–28.

Genetics and Genetic Counseling in Perinatal Palliative Care

6

Rebecca Carter and Blair Stevens

Key Points

1. Genetic counseling is a process that involves evaluating and communicating a family's risk for a genetic condition, providing education about testing and management options, and promoting informed decision-making [1].
2. Advancements in genetics knowledge and technology have improved prenatal diagnostic capabilities, but interpretation and application of genetic test results remain challenging, particularly in the prenatal setting.
3. Professional organizations increasingly recognize the perinatal palliative care model and the value of a multidisciplinary team, with genetic counselors (GCs) serving in the capacity of facilitating referrals, providing pre- and posttest counseling for genetic testing, and providing psychosocial support throughout the process.

Genetic Counseling

Background

Genetic counselors (GCs) are typically masters-prepared healthcare professionals with training in the field of genetics and psychosocial counseling. This profession has grown and evolved dramatically from Sheldon Reed's first introduction of the term "genetic counseling" in 1947, described then as a kind of "genetic social work" [2]. It was around this time that genetic counseling centers or "hereditary

R. Carter (✉) · B. Stevens
McGovern Medical School at the University of Texas Health Science Center at Houston, Department of Obstetrics, Gynecology, and Reproductive Services, Houston, TX, USA
e-mail: rebecca.d.sample@uth.tmc.edu; blair.k.stevens@uth.tmc.edu

E. M. Denney-Koelsch, D. Côté-Arsenault (eds.), *Perinatal Palliative Care*,
https://doi.org/10.1007/978-3-030-34751-2_6

counseling clinics" staffed by clinical geneticists were established, focusing primarily on providing recurrence risks to families with histories of genetic diseases or birth defects based on empirical observations [3]. In the early 1970s, a committee of the American Society of Human Genetics (ASHG) formally defined genetic counseling as "a communication process which deals with the human problems associated with the occurrence, or risk of occurrence, of a genetic disorder in the family" [4]. Thirty years later, a task force appointed by the National Society of Genetic Counselors (NSGC) revisited the definition adopted by ASHG and streamlined it to reflect changes in clientele and healthcare delivery. In 2006, NSGC published the following definition widely used today:

> Genetic counseling is the process of helping people understand and adapt to the medical, psychological and familial implications of genetic contributions to disease. This process integrates the following:
>
> - Interpretation of family and medical histories to assess the chance of disease occurrence or recurrence
> - Education about inheritance, testing, management, prevention, resources and research
> - Counseling to promote informed choices and adaptation to the risk or conditions [1] (p. 77).

Guidelines for the training and maintenance of competency of GCs are provided by the Accreditation Council for Genetic Counseling (ACGC) and fall into four domains: (1) genetics expertise and analysis; (2) interpersonal, psychosocial, and counseling skills; (3) education; and (4) professional development and practice [5]. These guidelines are applied across practice settings as the profession has expanded to meet the demands of rapidly changing technology and thus an increasingly diverse patient base, with multiple genetic counseling specialty areas including prenatal, pediatrics, and infertility, among others. The last few decades have seen significant growth of this field; as of May 2018, the American Board of Genetic Counseling (ABGC) (the organization that certifies genetic counseling professionals) has over 4600 certified GCs. The majority of GCs are affiliated with a medical center or facility, with 41% of those involved with direct patient care practicing in the prenatal specialty [6].

The ongoing expansion and diversification of the GC role is concurrent with perinatal palliative care's (PPC) significant strides as a healthcare model. GCs have the potential to make meaningful contributions to the multidisciplinary PPC approach designed to help families understand, cope, and make decisions related to a life-limiting fetal diagnosis.

Philosophy of Genetic Counseling

The framework for the practice, values, and conduct of the GC is based on the reciprocal-engagement model (REM) (see Fig. 6.1) and the ethical principles of autonomy, beneficence, non-maleficence, and justice; the professional principles

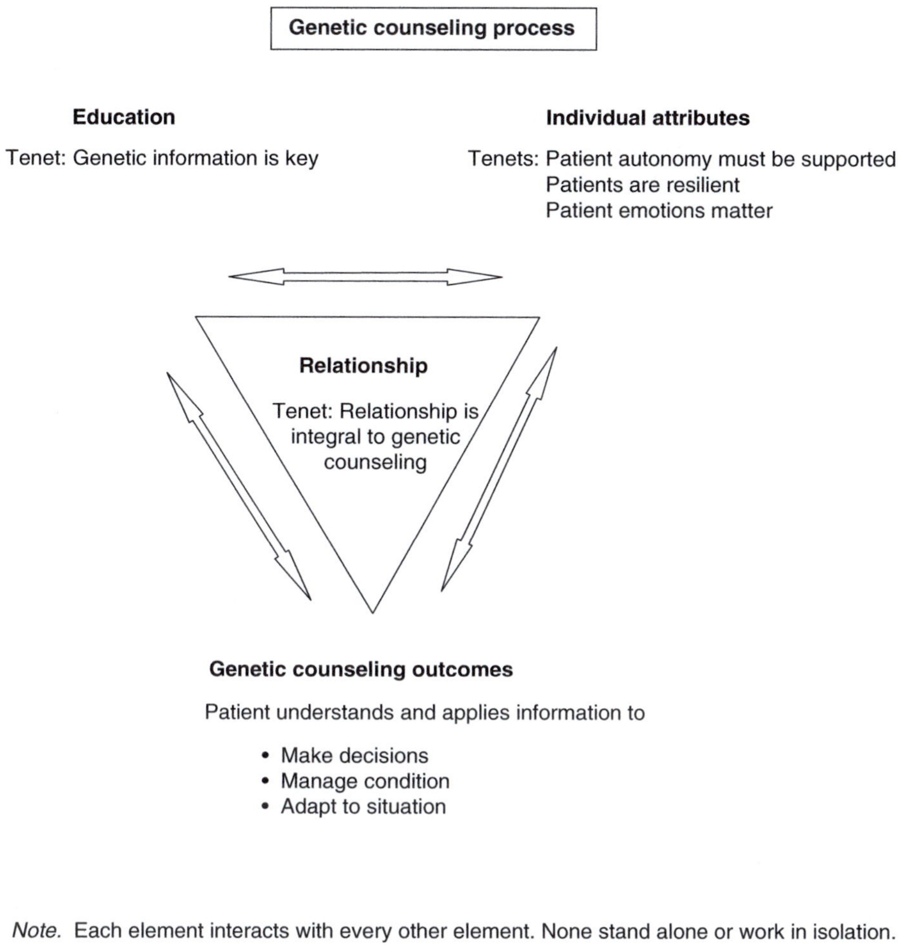

Fig. 6.1 The reciprocal-engagement model (REM) of genetic counseling practice [7]. (Reprinted by permission from Springer Nature, Veach et al. [7], © 2007)

of fidelity, veracity, integrity, dignity, and accountability as outlined in the NSGC Code of Ethics [7–10]. It is expected that there is significant overlap among healthcare professionals in conducting themselves according to the aforementioned ethical principles; therefore, this chapter will not explore them in-depth. The REM was developed by and for GCs as a unifying, validated model of practice specific to genetic counseling. The five tenets of genetic counseling include the following:

1. *Genetic information is key*: information focuses on what is known or thought to contribute to genetic disease. The provision and discussion of this type of information is considered one of the more unique aspects of genetic counseling and is based on the notion that knowledge is power [7].

2. *Patient autonomy must be supported*: the "patient knows best" and should be self-directed in making decisions. The GC values and respects the patient's sociocultural and family context in making an autonomous decision [7] (p. 721).
3. *Patients are resilient*: recognition of the strength and capabilities of patients to learn from and adapt to painful situations. GCs provide information and support to assist the patient in drawing upon their coping strategies and resources to make difficult decisions [7, 11].
4. *Patient emotions make a difference*: many emotions are experienced by the patient over the course of and following a counseling session, some of which may be intense. These emotions "interact with all facets of the genetic counseling processes and outcomes" [7] (p. 722).
5. *Relationship is integral to genetic counseling*: patient's genetic concerns are addressed most effectively when a strong alliance is formed. "Genetic counseling is a relationally based helping activity whose outcomes are only as good as the connection established between the counselor and the patient," with such a relationship being just as important to the outcomes as the genetic information provided [7].

This model demonstrates how the patient/GC relationship is central to the counseling process, with the above elements interacting to achieve the outcome of patient comprehension and autonomous application of the information to making decisions, managing the condition, and adapting to the situation. Empathic communication is a hallmark of this model, defined as "the vicarious experiencing of another person's feelings and situation and an ability to communicate one's understanding of another's feelings and experience" [12] (p. 77). Importantly, the GC takes a nonprescriptive approach, which "is perhaps the most defining feature of genetic counseling" [9] (p. 10) and refers to the firm belief that information conveyed in the genetic counseling session is presented fairly without encouraging a particular course of action. In taking this approach, GCs must still equip patients with effective tools to make decisions, thus striking a balance between promoting self-directedness of the patient and providing guidance in the situation where genetic and medical issues are complicated, data are limited, and choices raise moral or psychosocial issues [9, 13, 14].

There has been significant and ongoing effort put forth by the genetic counseling profession to ensure that those providing "genetic counseling" services have specific training and, in some states, licensure. Clinical or medical geneticists and genetic nurses with training from a medical genetics educational program accredited by the ABGC or the American Board of Medical Genetics and Genomics are also known to provide genetic counseling. Clinical geneticists have completed a fellowship or other advanced training in medical genetics and, as physicians, may perform physical evaluations and will often make the genetic diagnosis in a pediatric or adult clinic setting. The title and practice of genetic counseling requires protection, with documented instances of patient harm when education and guidance are given under the guise of genetic counseling by those with little or no training in medical genetics or psychosocial counseling [15, 16].

Components of the Genetic Counseling Session

Patients present for prenatal and preconception genetic counseling with a variety of indications. Obstetricians often refer pregnant women for genetic counseling to discuss screening and diagnostic testing options for genetic conditions or to review concerns based on age, teratogen exposures, or a family history of a birth defect or genetic disease. Some patients present for genetic counseling for the first time after receiving an abnormal genetic test result or ultrasound from the obstetrician's office.

Because a life-limiting diagnosis may be ascertained in numerous ways, the role and level of involvement of the GC will vary, and each session must be tailored to meet the needs of that particular patient. The interactions between the genetic counselor and the patient are unique to the presenting circumstances, varying in length and complexity, and may be limited to a one-time conversation or involve numerous encounters in person and by telephone over the course of the pregnancy and after birth [13]. The diagnosis of a life-limiting condition may be disclosed initially by the GC when obtained through genetic testing of a seemingly healthy pregnancy or may be discussed with the patient by the obstetrician or maternal-fetal medicine (MFM) physician who identifies anomalies on ultrasound and then refers to a GC. The use of a multidisciplinary team is ideal for the care of patients and may involve collaboration of the GC with the obstetrician, MFM, and ultrasound technician at the most basic level. Depending on the fetal diagnosis, the team can expand to involve others including a neonatologist, radiologist, nurse, social worker, surgeon, chaplain, pediatric geneticist, palliative care provider, and other specialists.

The typical components of the genetic counseling process are listed in Table 6.1 and involve contracting; collecting pertinent medical, pregnancy, and family history; presenting information; discussing genetic testing options; facilitating decision-making; and establishing a plan for follow-up [9, 12]. Psychosocial counseling and support are provided as needed. The order of these components and time spent doing each are adapted based on the clinical circumstances and may be influenced by the patient's comprehension level and emotional responses.

Table 6.1 Components of genetic counseling session

Component	Definition
Contracting	Establish mutually agreed-upon goals of the session
Collecting pertinent medical, pregnancy, and family history	Review medical records for medical history, obtain three-generation pedigree, and evaluate for possible teratogenic exposures
Presenting information	Provide risk assessment based on history and perform risk counseling
Discussing genetic testing options	Discuss personalized testing options, including screening and diagnostic testing, based on risk assessment
Facilitating decision-making	Decision-making regarding genetic testing as well as prenatal and neonatal management may be facilitated by counselor
Establishing a plan for follow-up	Confirm and facilitate genetic testing plan, make a plan for results disclosure, and provide referrals related to pregnancy management

- *Contracting* allows the patient and the GC to mutually agree upon the goals of the session. By exploring the patient's perspective through the use of open-ended questions, the GC can begin to assess patient comprehension, what vocabulary is being used or avoided, and the expectations of what will be gained through the interaction [12, 13, 17]. The establishment of mutual trust through effective contracting is crucial in the asking and answering of personal questions and assessing and expression of emotions. Such trust is essential to the patient's belief in the information and guidance provided by the GC [13].
- *Collecting pertinent history* includes information about potential teratogenic exposures or obstetric complications in a pregnancy as well as family history. Gathering family history information through the use of a three-generation pedigree allows for visualization of family members and degree of relatedness and serves as a psychosocial tool to help understand that impact of the condition on the family and provide insight into family dynamics [12].
- *Presenting information* often involves assessing and explaining risks and the implications of the likely or confirmed diagnosis. A *risk assessment* incorporates what is known and unknown about the clinical picture (i.e., results of genetic testing, ultrasound findings) to determine the likelihood that a genetic condition is present and, if so, which conditions are included in the differential. Roles central to genetic counseling are analyzing clinical information, calculating risks, and effectively communicating this risk [18]. Such *risk counseling* or *risk communication* utilizes different methods of explaining the risk for a genetic condition or a known diagnosis in terms best understood by the patient. Sometimes, this involves presenting the risk in numerical terms with a percentage or fractions or through the use of visual aids.
- A review of basic genetic concepts is provided to the patient, typically including a description of chromosomes, genes, DNA, and modes of inheritance. A common approach to this explanation is using the encyclopedia analogy. The 46 individual chromosomes of 23 pairs of chromosomes found in the cells of the body contain the genetic information inherited from one's parents and can be thought of as set of encyclopedias. Half of the chromosomes come from one parent and the other half from the other parent. The genes contained in those chromosomes are made up of DNA that instructs the body how to grow and develop. Like chromosomes, genes come in pairs and are inherited from the parents. In this analogy, the genes are the pages, and the letters of the words on each page represent the DNA bases. An entire extra or missing copy of a book is a numerical chromosome change (aneuploidy), such as an extra chromosome 21 that causes trisomy 21. A paragraph can be repeated (duplication) or missing (deletion) or a word itself can be misspelled (single-gene mutation). Many GCs develop their own explanations or analogies in order to enhance patient comprehension. The presentation and explanation of such medical-genetic information is complicated; this lies at the heart of genetic counseling as it represents a convergence of the medical and psychosocial domains at a level that is commensurate with the oftentimes low health literacy of the patient [12, 13]. This flows into *information giving*, which follows the diagnosis or risk assessment in order to assist the patient with understanding

the implications for the family. Information giving when the risk for a condition is high or has been confirmed may be described as "breaking bad news," an approach which emphasizes the importance of providing some forewarning that bad news is coming to allow for cognitive and emotional preparation (commonly referred to as a "warning shot"). It also involves avoiding the use of medical jargon, checking reception frequently through the use of open-ended questions, and assessing communication level [12, 17, 19, 20]. The GC has the unique opportunity to introduce troubling information in a direct and empathic manner that will be viewed over time as caring and supportive [20]. It is essential that the GC recognizes, appreciates, and responds appropriately to the emotional reactions and coping styles that unexpected and devastating news may bring forth in the patient [11]. It is also important that healthcare providers demonstrate respect and truth in the information delivered and provide the level of certainty surrounding the diagnosis with empathy and transparency [21, 22].

- *Discussing genetic testing options* is a complicated component of the genetic counseling process and must be highly personalized. A more thorough description of genetic testing can be found in Section II.
- *Decision-making* is frequently complex, time constrained, and emotionally demanding [14]. Decisions such as those surrounding pregnancy management or whether or not to pursue genetic testing are being made during times of stress with potentially lifelong consequences. The GC should be prepared to explore all options with the patient in a nonjudgmental manner in the context of a life-limiting diagnosis, including termination of pregnancy and continuation of pregnancy with options of intervention or palliative care. Knowledge of logistics surrounding termination of pregnancy includes its accessibility, state law(s), safe and reliable abortion providers, and support groups. When the decision is made to continue the pregnancy, the GC often serves initially as a liaison in orienting the patient to the palliative care team. Facilitating decision-making requires knowledge of how decisions are made and relies on the concept of informed shared decision-making, which supports the patient's crucial role in making the final decision while utilizing the GC's experience and insight [14]. Language and word choice surrounding options are important as this appears to influence decision-making, especially in situations that involve uncertainty [14]. The GC's role is to motivate patients to think through possible scenarios, provide a safe place to discuss fears, encourage patients to react, and reassure them that they are capable of making the best decisions for themselves [12, 14].
- Concluding the interaction involves a summary of what was discussed to allow for confirmation of the patient's comprehension and an agreement on the next step by making a *plan for follow-up*. Such follow-up may include facilitating genetic testing, making a plan for results disclosure, or providing referrals related to pregnancy management. Here is an opportunity to determine the patient's available support structure, emotional and spiritual needs, and who is available to the patient after the session. Regardless of next steps, closing the session with a plan for follow-up should reassure the patient that, as appropriate, the GC will remain involved and accessible, as needed [13].

Psychosocial counseling and *support* are fundamental to the genetic counseling process, as the GC serves as sometimes the only intermediary between the patient and vast, complicated, and often unanticipated genetic information. The GC is faced with the task of balancing attention to the science and attention to the needs of the patient to understand, cope with, and integrate the information [13]. The extent to which psychosocial counseling and support are provided varies significantly; however, three critical elements derived from Carl Rogers' person-centered counseling form the basis of any psychosocial interaction: unconditional positive regard, empathy, and genuineness [13]. The interested reader is directed to the resources on this topic listed in the references.

Making the Diagnosis

Congenital malformations and chromosomal abnormalities account for 21% of infant deaths, making ultrasound screening and genetic testing fundamental to perinatal palliative care [23]. Ultrasound detection of such fetal anomalies ranges widely (15–85%) and depends on multiple factors including gestational age, the fetal structure being evaluated, the sonographer, and maternal body mass index [24, 25]. Some anomalies require additional assessment through serial ultrasounds, fetal echocardiogram, or fetal magnetic resonance imaging (MRI). The yield of genetic testing increases when ultrasound abnormalities are identified because genetic conditions are more common in the setting of structural fetal abnormalities [26]. When counseling patients about the use of genetic testing, many genetics terms are utilized and often need to be defined in a session. Please see Table 6.2 for a list of commonly used genetic terms.

When parents are informed of a fetal abnormality on ultrasound, they face the decision of whether or not to pursue genetic testing and, if so, which test is the best choice for them. Risk assessment and determining a differential diagnosis is the first step in determining the most appropriate type of genetic test to offer. Genetics expertise is essential in determining the most appropriate test as the number of genetic testing options is rapidly expanding. Nearly 70,000 genetic testing products are available in the United States, with an average of 10 new testing products entering the market every day [29]. Selection of the most appropriate genetic test(s) depends upon the differential diagnosis which is determined by several factors, including maternal age, family history, screening test results, or ultrasound findings. Test selection may also be influenced by turnaround time, insurance coverage, amount of sample available, impact on management, and the patient's desires. Risk assessment and determination of the best testing strategy are components of the pretest genetic counseling session, which should also include a discussion of the benefits and limitations of prenatal and postnatal testing.

Both *screening* and *diagnostic* tests are available in the prenatal period. *Screening* tests are performed on maternal blood and assess the risks for a number of

Table 6.2 Glossary of common genetics terms [27, 28]

Term	Definition
Amniocentesis	An invasive, transabdominal procedure performed during pregnancy to collect a sample of amniotic fluid
Aneuploidy	The presence of an additional chromosome or missing chromosome producing an unbalanced chromosome set
Cell-free DNA (cfDNA) screening	Prenatal screening method for certain fetal conditions via small fragments of DNA derived from the placenta, present in the maternal bloodstream
Chorionic villus sampling (CVS)	An invasive, transabdominal or transcervical procedure performed during pregnancy to collect tissue (chorionic villi) from the placenta
Chromosomal microarray (CMA)	A method for detecting increased or decreased copies of a chromosome region with resolution down to ~5 Kb
Chromosome	An intracellular structure consisting of a long molecule of double-stranded DNA, nucleoproteins, and RNA that is able to reproduce its molecular structure through successive cell divisions
Deletion/duplication	Loss or gain of genetic material that may encompass part of a gene, an entire gene, or a set of genes
Fluorescence in situ hybridization (FISH)	A method for detecting presence or absence of specific chromosomal region (e.g., aneuploidy FISH detects copies of chromosomes 21, 18, 13, X, and Y)
Gene	Unit of inheritance, consisting of a DNA sequence coding for a specific protein or component of a protein, arranged in a linear manner on chromosomes
Karyotype	The chromosome constitution as displayed by a microscopic preparation of dividing chromosomes photographed and arranged in homologous pairs
Microdeletion/ microduplication	Submicroscopic loss or gain of genetic material detectable by CMA or FISH
Maternal serum screening (MSS)	A prenatal screen that estimates the chances for certain chromosome conditions and/or birth defects such as spina bifida using analytes in maternal blood
Sequencing test	A method for detecting single-gene disorders using sequencing technology (such as Sanger or next-generation sequencing)
Single-gene disorder	A genetic condition caused by a molecular change within a single gene
Syndrome	A combination of clinical features forming a recognizable entity

conditions. Cell-free DNA (cfDNA)-based screening is increasingly utilized over diagnostic testing in routine pregnancies; however, it is limited to only increasing or decreasing the chances for a limited number of genetic conditions and requires follow-up diagnostic testing to confirm or rule out the presence of a suspected condition. While such screening is becoming available for an increasing number of conditions, limited data exists on the accuracy of these blood tests for conditions other than trisomy 21, 18, and 13. Screening tests are not discussed in detail in this chapter as they are not diagnostic, and medical management decisions, such as pregnancy continuation or termination or place of delivery, should not be made based on screening test results alone.

Table 6.3 Screening vs diagnostic testing characteristics, advantages, and disadvantages

Test characteristics	Screening test	Diagnostic test
Definition	Provides a risk assessment	Determines definitively whether specific genetic conditions are present or not
Examples	First trimester screening Quad screen Maternal serum alpha-fetoprotein screen Cell-free DNA screening	Chorionic villus sampling Amniocentesis Cordocentesis
Methodology	Performed on maternal blood May be combined with ultrasound measurements	Requires invasive procedure to obtain placental tissue, amniotic fluid, or umbilical cord blood
Advantages	No risk for procedure-related pregnancy complications Provides a personalized risk assessment for specific conditions (detection rate varies based on screen)	Most definitive prenatal tests (accuracy varies based on test) Can test for chromosome conditions, open neural tube defects (amniocentesis), and additional genetic syndromes
Disadvantages	Subject to false positives and false negatives Limited to select conditions	Carries procedure-related risks including miscarriage

While *screening* provides a risk assessment, *diagnostic* testing determines whether a condition is present or not. Diagnostic testing holds the added benefit of accuracy and the ability to evaluate for a greater number of conditions. Diagnostic testing is performed on samples obtained via ultrasound-guided invasive procedures, such as chorionic villus sampling (CVS) and amniocentesis. CVS involves sampling of placental tissue often performed in the first trimester, and amniocentesis is the sampling of amniotic fluid typically after 16 weeks' gestation. Both procedures carry risks for pregnancy complications such as miscarriage, which occur with a frequency of less than 1% [30] (Table 6.3).

Depending upon the testing indication, several diagnostic testing options can be performed on the samples obtained from the CVS or amniocentesis procedure. Various genetic etiologies exist, such as chromosome aneuploidy, deletions/duplications, and single-gene disorders. Not all genetic conditions can be detected by all genetic tests; therefore, the genetic test must be carefully selected based upon the differential diagnosis. For example, Down syndrome is caused by an extra chromosome 21 (i.e., an extra encyclopedia in the set) and can be detected by creating a picture of the chromosomes via a genetic test called the karyotype. On the other hand, autosomal recessive polycystic kidney disease (ARPKD) is typically due to both copies of a gene having a single-letter change (misspelling of a single word of one page in the encyclopedia) and requires a genetic test that entails sequencing, or spell checking, the gene (see Case 6.1 for example). See Table 6.4 for a list of common diagnostic tests and examples of the conditions they can detect. Despite advancing technology, there is no genetic test that can rule out every genetic condition.

Case 6.1

A routine ultrasound performed at 20 weeks identifies bilaterally enlarged and polycystic kidneys, small bladder, enlarged abdomen, and severe oligohydramnios. The patient and her husband are informed by the MFM that these findings are concerning for poor outcome due to pulmonary hypoplasia and that there is suspicion for a genetic cause. The couple meets with the GC, where they express their disbelief in light of having already received normal aneuploidy screening results in the first trimester and feeling reassured of a normal outcome.

Patient: *We felt like everything was going to be fine since we got the negative results.*

Counselor: *I imagine that makes getting today's difficult news that much more shocking. I'm sorry something this unexpected has come up.*

The GC reviews the findings in detail and the possibility of autosomal recessive polycystic kidney disease (ARPKD). Due to the low fluid, placental biopsy is offered and accepted. Sequencing of the *PKHD1* gene identifies two pathogenic variants in the baby, consistent with a diagnosis of ARPKD. Termination is declined. The couple asks about renal replacement therapies and neonatal respiratory support based on their research on ARPKD.

Patient: *We've been doing some reading, and it sounds like babies with this condition can actually get kidney transplants and do okay.*

Counselor: *While you're absolutely right that some babies with ARPKD are able to get treatment to improve their outcome, unfortunately, this isn't necessarily an option for all babies. One reason it may not be an option is because there is so little fluid that the babies are too sick when they are born for the treatment to help. This is a concern we have right now for your baby. It sounds like you've been really trying to educate yourself on ARPKD; tell me what else you have found.*

The counselor discusses the option of meeting with the PPC team to allow the couple to ask this question of the neonatologist, nephrologist, and pulmonologist in order to best address it. A referral to PPC is facilitated by the GC and MFM, who make the team aware of the prenatal diagnosis and the questions surrounding intervention. The family meets with the PPC team and establishes a plan of supportive care at the time of delivery, with an understanding that if the baby does better than anticipated the plan of care can be reassessed. Follow-up ultrasounds are concerning for worsening oligohydramnios and the baby is stillborn at 38 weeks. The parents were understandably devastated.

Follow-up testing of the parents confirms they are carriers of the identified mutations and have a 25% risk of recurrence for this condition in each pregnancy. Genetic counseling is provided at the couple's request regarding the recurrence risk and options of in vitro fertilization (IVF) so that embryos can be tested for the heritable condition through preimplantation genetic testing (PGT) as well as prenatal diagnostic testing for the known familial mutations.

This case highlights the following:

- Limitations of aneuploidy screening: pre- and often posttest counseling for routine aneuploidy screening involves a discussion of the scope of the screening, emphasizing that it is not diagnostic and does not assess for all genetic conditions.
- The utility of genetic testing: mutation-specific testing provided a genetic diagnosis, which allowed for accurate recurrence risk information to be provided to the couple as well as the option of IVF with preimplantation genetic testing (PGT) or prenatal testing in future pregnancies.
- Variable outcomes of genetic conditions: ARPKD is associated with risk for neonatal mortality but is not universally lethal. Prognosis is highly dependent upon the clinical picture.

Table 6.4 Genetic etiologies and testing options

Genetic etiology	Diagnostic testing options	Examples
Aneuploidy	Aneuploidy FISH, karyotype, chromosomal microarray	Down syndrome, Turner syndrome, trisomy 18
Chromosome deletions or duplications	Karyotype, chromosomal microarray	Wolf-Hirschhorn syndrome, 1p36 deletion syndrome
Microdeletions/ microduplications (copy number variants)	Chromosomal microarray	22q11 deletion syndrome (DiGeorge)
Single-gene disorders	Sequencing test	Thanatophoric dysplasia, Smith-Lemli-Opitz syndrome, Noonan syndrome

FISH fluorescence in situ hybridization

Limitations of Genetic Testing

Pretest counseling is essential in educating patients on the benefits as well as the risks and limitations of genetic testing. While the benefit of obtaining information about the health of a pregnancy may be obvious, patients must be made aware of the possibilities of uncertain or incidental results, the need for additional testing on the fetus or family members, and the possibility of not obtaining results and requiring a repeat procedure. Results may be uncertain because they have not been described previously or have not been fully described, or they have been reported with variable expressivity (e.g., variations in the way a genetic change manifests in a patient, such as a child with abnormalities and an asymptomatic parent with the same genetic change). Incidental findings from testing may include nonpaternity, consanguinity, diagnosis of an adult onset condition, diagnosis of asymptomatic carriers, or diagnosis of conditions not relevant to the testing indication. For example, a deletion that may predispose a person to mental illness or intellectual disabilities may be detected in a pregnancy affected with multiple anomalies. Although this finding may be important to the family, it does not explain the fetal anomalies and could create additional anxiety. Furthermore, if this deletion goes on to be identified in a parent, it may have implications for that parent's health and well-being.

An additional limitation of prenatal testing is insurance coverage and cost. Routine tests such as karyotype and chromosome microarray should be covered based on recommendations by professional societies such as the American College of Obstetricians and Gynecologists (ACOG) [31]; however, a patient's coinsurance or deductible may result in a significant financial obligation. More specialized tests, such as sequencing panels or whole exome sequencing, may not be covered by all insurance plans and may result in an out-of-pocket cost for the patient. Many laboratories offer preauthorization or benefits investigation services to providers and patients, the exploration of which often falls under the GC's responsibility as part of the patient's care.

Declining Prenatal Testing

While many patients may feel information obtained from genetic testing is helpful, prenatal genetic testing has also been reported in some patients to cause anxiety and stress [32] and has been described as "toxic knowledge" or knowledge the patient wished they did not have [33]. Prenatal testing is most frequently declined due to the risk of physical complications related to the diagnostic procedures [34]. For all of these reasons, parents should be given the *option* of pursuing genetic testing, and the decision to decline it should be supported.

In counseling about the utility of genetic testing, it should be discussed that prenatal genetic testing may provide the patient and her medical team important information that could impact prenatal management, delivery plans, and immediate neonatal management. When prenatal testing is declined, patients should be informed that immediate management options may be limited by the lack of genetic test results. Depending on the type of genetic test ordered after delivery, results may take anywhere from 24 hours to several weeks to return; therefore, postnatal management may not be tailored to the results of the genetic testing for up to weeks after delivery. Finally, patients who decline prenatal testing and prefer to obtain genetic information through postnatal testing should be informed of the possibility that genetic testing may not be successfully ordered or performed after birth, particularly in the case of a stillbirth or neonatal demise (see Case 6.2 for example). Some questions to consider when counseling about prenatal genetic testing include the following:

- What are the chances of identifying a genetic condition?
- Will a genetic diagnosis impact the prognosis?
- Will a genetic diagnosis impact prenatal or postnatal management?
- Can postnatal testing be performed?
- What are the drawbacks of waiting until after birth to undergo testing?

Case 6.2

An early anatomy scan at 18 weeks is performed for the indication of advanced maternal age. This ultrasound detects severe micromelia; abnormal head shape; a small, bell-shaped chest; and polyhydramnios. The patient is informed that the ultrasound raises significant concern for a skeletal dysplasia with a likely lethal prognosis due to the small chest size. The GC meets with the patient to discuss the suspected diagnosis of thanatophoric dysplasia type I. Prenatal testing of the *FGFR3* gene (responsible for thanatophoric dysplasia) is possible through amniocentesis but is declined by the patient based on the risk for pregnancy complications. She further expresses that, while she really wants to know more information, testing seems pointless as it cannot improve her baby's outcome and will just cause increased stress. The GC discusses that while this information may not change the likely lethal prognosis in the current pregnancy, testing has the potential to find an answer as to why it is occurring and provide clarification on risks in future pregnancies if pursued.

Patient: *Of course, I want to know why this is happening. But the idea of putting the pregnancy at any more risk terrifies me. Plus, it sounds like whether I find out at this point or not won't change the fact that she's going to die.*

Counselor: *What I'm hearing is that, while you want more information, the fact that we are concerned that the baby has a life-limiting condition based on the ultrasound findings makes it feel like a test, particularly one that carries a risk, is not something you're comfortable with right now. Would you be open to discussing the option of testing after delivery? Some parents consider this when they want more information but don't want testing during the pregnancy.*

She reviews the option of testing after delivery, which the patient states she will consider. The GC obtains a brief pregnancy history, during which time the patient becomes emotional and discloses that she had been drinking socially prior to learning of her pregnancy and fears that this could have caused the abnormalities.

Counselor: *From the form you filled out, it looks like you haven't had any infections, medications, or other exposures of concern during the pregnancy.*

Patient: *Yes… well, I had a few drinks the weekend before I found out I was pregnant. (Tearfully) Is there any way that could have caused this?*

Counselor: *Having a few drinks before you knew you were pregnant would not have caused what we are seeing in the baby right now on ultrasound, and it certainly would not have caused the baby to have a genetic condition. But it is normal to have these fears when you get news like this.*

Patient: *I had no idea. I should have taken a pregnancy test.*
Counselor: *It sounds like you are very worried that you could have caused this.*

A referral to PPC is facilitated by the GC and MFM, who make the team aware of the suspected diagnosis. The patient and her family meet with the PPC team and establish a plan of supportive care at the time of delivery. At that time, the patient also makes the decision to pursue genetic testing after birth. The baby is delivered, receives comfort care, and dies peacefully at 6 hours of life. A plan for obtaining cord blood at delivery had been confirmed with the patient and care team in advance, and testing was sent out. This confirms an *FGFR3* mutation, which occurs spontaneously in the majority of cases. Despite the grief the patient is experiencing surrounding the death of her child, she is relieved that she did not cause the abnormalities to occur. The patient is counseled that the risk of recurrence in future pregnancies is very low; however, IVF with PGT and/or prenatal diagnostic testing is available for this mutation if desired.

This case highlights the following:

- The utility of genetic testing: mutation-specific testing provided a genetic diagnosis, which allowed for accurate recurrence risk information to be provided to the couple as well as the option of IVF with PGT or prenatal testing in future pregnancies. Confirming the diagnosis also provided reassurance that the alcohol consumed early in the pregnancy did not cause the abnormalities.

Pursuing Genetic Testing

When patients elect to pursue genetic testing, informed consent should be obtained and include a discussion of the possible outcomes, including normal, uncertain, or abnormal results.

Normal Results

Normal results may either rule out the particular condition(s) evaluated by the test or only reduce the risk in some cases. For example, if an omphalocele is detected on ultrasound, a normal karyotype will rule out chromosome aneuploidy, such as trisomy 18. However, a normal chromosomal microarray analysis (CMA) will only reduce the chance that the diagnosis is Beckwith-Wiedemann syndrome, an additional genetic condition associated with omphalocele, since not all forms of Beckwith-Wiedemann syndrome can be detected by chromosome microarray. While most patients celebrate normal results, a normal result may actually be frustrating when a fetus is known to have structural anomalies, and genetic testing does not determine the underlying etiology. A patient's expectations and hopes regarding their genetic test results and acknowledgment of residual risks should be explored during pretest counseling to ensure results disclosure can be sensitive to these needs and goals.

It should be noted that there is no test that can rule out *all* genetic conditions. Therefore, while a normal result reduces the chance of a genetic etiology, it cannot eliminate the possibility completely. Depending on what testing has been performed and the differential diagnoses, additional testing may be offered to the patient who is motivated to receive this information. Knowledge of the amount of DNA available for testing from the prenatal sample is important, as a postnatal sample may not be readily obtained in the event of stillbirth or neonatal demise. It is ideal to obtain a postnatal sample when possible in case more DNA is needed for testing. Collecting a sample of DNA and storing or "banking" it may also be recommended if a diagnosis is not made. This type of long-term storage is available at an affordable rate and allows for future testing to be performed, if death occurs before an etiology has been determined or if additional testing is indicated in the future. If fetal demise, stillbirth, or neonatal death occurs, the option of full or limited autopsy should be sensitively addressed and offered to the patient seeking additional information. Autopsy can provide clarification on the cause of death and confirmation or identification of birth defects, which can potentially lead to a diagnosis and more accurate assessment of recurrence risks for future pregnancies [27]. See also Chap. 5, section "Autopsy", for additional information.

Uncertain Results

Uncertain results may include genetic changes that are detected in a gene or chromosome but that have an uncertain effect on the function of the gene. These uncertain genetic changes may not result in a damaging effect and may be considered normal variation (benign) or may cause abnormalities (pathogenic). An uncertain result may require follow-up evaluations, such as additional genetic testing, MRI, or autopsy, but results can remain uncertain even after all testing options are exhausted. Patients should be counseled that while results may be uncertain at the time of their disclosure, they may be reclassified as benign or pathogenic at a later time. For this reason, most laboratories offer reanalysis of results after a certain amount of time has passed. Patients should be informed of this possibility so they can contact their healthcare provider in the future to obtain any updates to the interpretation of their results.

Abnormal Results

Patients respond in a variety of ways to news of abnormal genetic test results. An abnormal result may be distressing in its confirmation of an underlying problem, which may worsen the prognosis due to comorbidities often associated with genetic disorders (see Case 6.3 for example) [35]. Some families may find relief in abnormal genetic test results as it provides a definitive answer for the prenatal findings and can often confirm that no action or inaction on their part could have caused the abnormality. The variability in patient responses highlights the need for anticipatory guidance and an exploration of patient needs and desires during pretest counseling.

Case 6.3

A routine ultrasound at 20 weeks identifies a ventricular septal defect (VSD), two-vessel cord, and growth lag. The MFM discusses the fact that the heart defect is repairable and generally carries a very good prognosis; however, there is additional concern that seeing the heart defect in conjunction with the other findings carries an increased risk for a chromosome condition. The GC meets with the patient and her husband, whose questions are mostly related to postnatal management of the VSD. They request consultation with the pediatric cardiologist as soon as possible. The GC states that she is happy to facilitate this referral, gently reminding the couple that if there is an underlying chromosome condition the plan for management and treatment will be different compared to the plan for an otherwise healthy infant. The couple decides to pursue amniocentesis, the results of which indicate trisomy 18. The couple is shocked by this diagnosis and the life-limiting nature of the condition, as they had been preparing questions for the cardiologist and focusing on surgery after delivery. The couple expresses the desire to continue the pregnancy and asks if it is still an option to speak to the cardiologist. Through this discussion, the GC confirms that the couple understands that surgery will not change the chromosome abnormality and that the option may or may not be available to them through the facility.

Patient: *We'd like to meet with the cardiologist.*

Counselor: *I think we can make that happen. Can you tell me more about what you hope to discuss?*

Patient: *Well, the baby has a heart defect. So it would be helpful to talk to a heart specialist.*

Counselor: *You did a lot of research on how to manage the heart defect that we see. I know it is very unexpected that the baby has trisomy 18, which we believe to be the reason for the heart problem.*

Patient: *Yes. But that doesn't mean we are just going to give up. If her heart can be fixed, we should fix it.*

Counselor: *I think any parent would want to do anything they can to help their baby. For many parents who learn their baby has trisomy 18, it's helpful to come up with a birth plan and explore all their options. We know that heart surgery cannot change the diagnosis of trisomy 18 and all of the life-limiting health problems that come along with it, but that doesn't mean it can't be explored as an option. But perhaps discussing this with the heart specialist can allow you to feel like you have as much information as possible to make the best choice for your family. Please know that no matter what you decide, you won't be giving up on her.*

The GC facilitates a referral to the PPC team, informing the team of the diagnosis and the couple's request to speak to a cardiologist. A meeting between the parents and the cardiologist occurs that involves a discussion of the pros and cons of cardiac surgery in babies with trisomy 18. A birth plan is created and involves comfort care only, per the parents' request. The baby is born at 36 weeks' gestation and lives for 48 hours.

This case highlights the following:

- The utility of genetic testing: a genetic diagnosis can greatly impact prognosis, as the expected outcome is altered from management of a heart defect and growth lag to a life-limiting condition

Even when a genetic abnormality is detected, uncertainty remains in predicting the exact outcome. Parents should be informed of the most accurate and up-to-date information surrounding the condition's natural history, chances of survival, length of survival, and the possibility of related comorbidities, when known. Healthcare providers should also ensure the information from studies and research provided to the patient is representative of their patient's clinical circumstances. For example, when discussing chances for survival of a pregnancy diagnosed with trisomy 18 at 12 weeks' gestation via CVS, outcome data should be based on prenatal diagnosis in the first trimester. In this instance, informing the patient of the commonly quoted 10% chance of survival to 1 year of life can be misleading. Alternatively, patients should be informed of the 30% chance of even having a live-born child when diagnosed in the first trimester. If the baby is live-born, only then is there an approximately 10% chance of surviving the first year [36]. In other words, patients need evidence-based information relevant to their clinical circumstances.

While data are available on natural history and survival for some conditions, such as trisomy 18 and trisomy 13, this information may not be readily available for many other genetic conditions. Data may not exist or may be insufficient for many reasons. First, some genetic conditions are so rare that the literature may only contain case reports or a small number of cases that make it difficult to generalize to all cases. Secondly, some conditions are primarily diagnosed after delivery, and this ascertainment bias may not allow for accurate counseling about the prenatal natural history and survival statistics when the condition is detected prenatally. Finally, some conditions have a wide range of variability so even if abundant data exist it may be very difficult to predict the outcome for a specific case. For example, up to 20% of babies with Beckwith-Wiedemann can die in the neonatal period due to complications of prematurity, hypoglycemia, cardiomyopathy, macroglossia, or tumors, but 80% of babies survive. These complications can be very difficult to predict in the prenatal setting, making the ability to counsel families challenging. When accurate information is not available for a particular condition or when outcomes are highly variable, patients should be informed of what is known about the condition as well as the relevant limitations of this information. Patients should also be provided with written information and support network resources, when available. After results are disclosed, GCs or other healthcare providers should check in with the family periodically to assess for informational and emotional needs [33].

Recurrence Risks and Future Testing

Fetal anomalies may be nongenetic, genetic, or multifactorial (due to a combination of genetic and environmental factors) in etiology. If a genetic etiology is determined, the patient can be counseled about the natural history, prognosis, and management recommendations associated with that condition. Recurrence risks in subsequent pregnancies can also be addressed. Parental testing may be indicated to clarify whether the genetic abnormality occurred sporadically or was inherited. Due to the complexity of inheritance and recurrence risk counseling, a consultation with a healthcare provider with genetics expertise, such as a GC, is recommended to discuss future reproductive options.

When a parent or parents are found to be asymptomatic carriers of a genetic condition, the risk for recurrence may be up to 50%. Prenatal testing through CVS or amniocentesis in future pregnancies is available, if desired. Patients may also consider undergoing in vitro fertilization (IVF) so that embryos can be tested for the heritable condition through preimplantation genetic testing (PGT). IVF with donor egg or sperm, as well as adoption, may also be considered once a genetic condition has been identified in a family.

If an underlying genetic etiology is not determined for a fetal condition, accurate recurrence risks and genetic testing for that condition are not available in future pregnancies. In such scenarios, ultrasound screening and occasionally further evaluations (such as fetal echocardiogram) may be recommended. Some fetal conditions are known to be multifactorial, such as isolated congenital heart defects or spina bifida. While genetic testing cannot evaluate for recurrence in these cases either, empiric recurrence risk data can be provided. For example, in the case of heart defects and spina bifida, the recurrence risk is increased over the general population risk at approximately 3%.

The Genetic Counselor and Perinatal Palliative Care

There remains limited literature on the GC's role in PPC, despite the fact that both fields have a "client centered framework upon an ethical foundation" [37] (p. 542). There appears to be an overwhelmingly positive perception of PPC and broad endorsement of the PPC concepts by GCs [37]. Parents experiencing a pregnancy in which a life-limiting diagnosis has been made report a desire for "supportive counseling to help them understand medical conditions, make informed decisions, and communicate with multiple providers" [38] (p. 1307) along with transparency regarding prognostic uncertainty and nonjudgmental advice [38]. The GC is often one of the first healthcare providers to disclose the news of a suspected or known life-limiting diagnosis. As such, the GC can serve to bridge the patient and the PPC team by making one aware of the other, facilitating the referral, and providing continuous support to the patient in the form of emotional support or knowledge gained from testing as the pregnancy progresses and following delivery. The required psychosocial skills and knowledge of the complex issues surrounding genetic testing, coupled with their presence in the prenatal diagnosis setting, make GCs an ideal included discipline to complement and serve on PPC multidisciplinary teams.

Conclusion

Genetic counselors are experts in risk assessment, facilitating discussions regarding the benefits and limitations of genetic testing, and interpretation and communication of test results. These skills are critical in helping families understand the prognosis related to a potentially life-limiting diagnosis. Additionally, the GC serves as an advocate and a source of support for patients and their families. The degree of support and advocacy is tailored to the parents' informational and psychosocial needs, and counselors can continue to serve in this capacity if and when the parents transition to receiving support from the PPC team. The combined services of the GC and members of the PPC team guide and empower families as they learn of the diagnosis and transition from pregnancy to delivery of a child with a life-limiting diagnosis.

References

1. National Society of Genetic Counselors' Definition Task F, Resta R, Biesecker BB, Bennett RL, Blum S, Hahn SE, et al. A new definition of Genetic Counseling: National Society of Genetic Counselors' Task Force report. J Genet Couns. 2006;15(2):77–83.
2. Reed SC. A short history of genetic counseling. Soc Biol. 1974;21(4):332–9.
3. Resta RG. Eugenics and nondirectiveness in genetic counseling. J Genet Couns. 1997;6(2):255–8.
4. Genetic counseling. Am J Hum Genet. 1975;27(2):240–2.
5. Practice-based competencies for genetic counselors: accreditation council for genetic counseling; 2015. Available from: http://www.gceducation.org/Documents/ACGC%20Core%20Competencies%20Brochure_15_Web.pdf.
6. Professional Status Survey: National Society of Genetic Counselors; 2018. Available from: https://www.nsgc.org/d/do/8436.
7. Veach PM, Bartels DM, Leroy BS. Coming full circle: a reciprocal-engagement model of genetic counseling practice. J Genet Couns. 2007;16(6):713–28.
8. NSGC Code of Ethics: National Society of Genetic Counselors; 2018. Available from: https://www.nsgc.org/p/cm/ld/fid=12.
9. Walker AP. A guide to genetic counseling. In: Uhlmann WR, Schuette JL, Yashar BM, editors. 2nd ed. Hoboken: Wiley-Blackwell; 2009. 1 online resource (648 p.).
10. Schmerler S. A guide to genetic counseling. In: Uhlmann WR, Schuette JL, Yashar BM, editors. 2nd ed. Hoboken: Wiley-Blackwell; 2009.
11. Veach PM, LeRoy B, Bartels DM. Genetic counseling practice: advanced concepts and skills. Hoboken: Wiley-Blackwell; 2010. x, 415 pages.
12. McCarthy Veach P, LeRoy B, Callanan N. Facilitating the genetic counseling process: practice based skills. 2nd ed. Cham, Switzerland: Springer International Publishing; 2018.
13. Weil J. Psychosocial genetic counseling. New York: Oxford University Press; 2000. Available from: http://search.ebscohost.com/login.aspx?direct=true&scope=site&db=nlebk&db=nlabk&AN=315032.
14. Zanko A, Fox M. Genetic counseling practice: advanced concepts and skills. In: Veach PM, LeRoy B, Bartels DM, editors. Hoboken: Wiley-Blackwell; 2010. x, 415 pages.
15. Brierley KL, Blouch E, Cogswell W, Homer JP, Pencarinha D, Stanislaw CL, et al. Adverse events in cancer genetic testing: medical, ethical, legal, and financial implications. Cancer J. 2012;18(4):303–9.

16. Brierley KL, Campfield D, Ducaine W, Dohany L, Donenberg T, Shannon K, et al. Errors in delivery of cancer genetics services: implications for practice. Conn Med. 2010;74(7):413–23.
17. Buckman R, Kason Y. How to break bad news: a guide for health care professionals. Baltimore: Johns Hopkins University Press; 1992. x, 223 pages
18. Baty BJ. A guide to genetic counseling. In: Uhlmann WR, Schuette JL, Yashar BM, editors. 2nd ed. Hoboken: Wiley-Blackwell; 2009.
19. Luz R, George A, Spitz E, Vieux R. Breaking bad news in prenatal medicine: a literature review. J Reprod Infant Psychol. 2017;35(1):14–31.
20. Djurdjinovic L. A guide to genetic counseling. In: Uhlmann WR, Schuette JL, Yashar BM, editors. 2nd ed. Hoboken, NJ: Wiley-Blackwell; 2009.
21. Gunderman RB. Patient communication: what to teach radiology residents. AJR Am J Roentgenol. 2001;177(1):41–3.
22. Alkazaleh F, Thomas M, Grebenyuk J, Glaude L, Savage D, Johannesen J, et al. What women want: women's preferences of caregiver behavior when prenatal sonography findings are abnormal. Ultrasound Obstet Gynecol. 2004;23(1):56–62.
23. Matthews TJ, MacDorman MF. Infant mortality statistics from the 2010 period linked birth/infant death data set. Natl Vital Stat Rep. 2013;62(8):1–26.
24. Edwards L, Hui L. First and second trimester screening for fetal structural anomalies. Semin Fetal Neonatal Med. 2018;23(2):102–11.
25. Rao R, Platt LD. Ultrasound screening: status of markers and efficacy of screening for structural abnormalities. Semin Perinatol. 2016;40(1):67–78.
26. Donnelly JC, Platt LD, Rebarber A, Zachary J, Grobman WA, Wapner RJ. Association of copy number variants with specific ultrasonographically detected fetal anomalies. Obstet Gynecol. 2014;124(1):83–90.
27. Mathiesen A, Roy K. Foundations of perinatal genetic counseling. New York: Oxford University Press; 2018.
28. Harper PS. Practical genetic counselling. 7th ed. London: Hodder Arnold; 2010. 407 p.
29. The current landscape of genetic testing: concert genetics; 2017. Available from: https://www.concertgenetics.com/wp-content/uploads/2017/05/10_ConcertGenetics_CurrentLandscapeofGeneticTesting_2017Update.pdf.
30. Akolekar R, Beta J, Picciarelli G, Ogilvie C, D'Antonio F. Procedure-related risk of miscarriage following amniocentesis and chorionic villus sampling: a systematic review and meta-analysis. Ultrasound Obstet Gynecol. 2015;45(1):16–26.
31. American College of O, Gynecologists' Committee on Practice B-O, Committee on G, Society for Maternal-Fetal M. Practice bulletin no. 162: prenatal diagnostic testing for genetic disorders. Obstet Gynecol. 2016;127(5):e108–22.
32. Allison SJ, Stafford J, Anumba DO. The effect of stress and anxiety associated with maternal prenatal diagnosis on feto-maternal attachment. BMC Womens Health. 2011;11:33.
33. Bernhardt BA, Soucier D, Hanson K, Savage MS, Jackson L, Wapner RJ. Women's experiences receiving abnormal prenatal chromosomal microarray testing results. Genet Med. 2013;15(2):139–45.
34. Liamputtong P, Halliday JL, Warren R, Watson F, Bell RJ. Why do women decline prenatal screening and diagnosis? Australian women's perspective. Women Health. 2003;37(2):89–108.
35. De Groote K, Vanhie E, Roets E, Ramaekers P, De Wilde H, Panzer J, et al. Outcome after prenatal and postnatal diagnosis of complex congenital heart defects and the influence of genetic anomalies. Prenat Diagn. 2017;37(10):983–91.
36. Cavadino A, Morris JK. Revised estimates of the risk of fetal loss following a prenatal diagnosis of trisomy 13 or trisomy 18. Am J Med Genet A. 2017;173(4):953–8.
37. Wool C, Dudek M. Exploring the perceptions and the role of genetic counselors in the emerging field of perinatal palliative care. J Genet Couns. 2013;22(4):533–43.
38. Cote-Arsenault D, Denney-Koelsch E. "My baby is a person": parents' experiences with life-threatening fetal diagnosis. J Palliat Med. 2011;14(12):1302–8.

The Neonatologist's Role in Prenatal Counseling

7

Stephanie K. Kukora and Steven R. Leuthner

Abbreviations

CDH	Congenital diaphragmatic hernia
ECMO	Extracorporeal membrane oxygenation
MFM	Maternal fetal medicine
NICU	Neonatal intensive care unit

When End of Life Is at the Beginning

Technological advances in neonatal intensive care have led to significant improvement in neonatal survival since the inception of neonatal-perinatal medicine as a subspecialty in 1960; however, the neonatal period continues to have the highest rate of morbidity and mortality of pediatric patients. Of the nearly 4 million births that happen in the United States each year, over 20,000 infants do not survive the neonatal period. This is an infant mortality rate of nearly 6 per 1000

S. K. Kukora (✉)

University of Michigan, Division of Neonatal-Perinatal Medicine, Department of Pediatrics, Ann Arbor, MI, USA

Center for Bioethics and Social Sciences in Medicine, University of Michigan, Ann Arbor, MI, USA
e-mail: skukora@med.umich.edu

S. R. Leuthner
Medical College of Wisconsin, Department of Pediatrics and Bioethics, Wauwatosa, WI, USA

Children's Hospital of Wisconsin, Medical College of Wisconsin, Department of Pediatrics, Wauwatosa, WI, USA

E. M. Denney-Koelsch, D. Côté-Arsenault (eds.), *Perinatal Palliative Care*,
https://doi.org/10.1007/978-3-030-34751-2_7

infants [1]. The majority of these deaths, approximately 4800 per year, are attributed to congenital anomalies, followed closely by deaths from prematurity, which is responsible for approximately 4000 infant deaths annually [2]. Other causes, including perinatal asphyxia, meconium aspiration/pulmonary hypertension, and neonatal sepsis, also make a significant contribution to morbidity and mortality. For perspective, though pediatric cancers garner considerable media attention, only approximately 1200 deaths in children under age 18 occur annually in the United States from malignancies, about 20 times fewer than from neonatal causes [3].

Complicating the morbidity and mortality of the neonatal population are the challenges stemming from diagnostic and prognostic uncertainty. Though antenatal imaging and genetic testing have greatly improved the ability to identify infants anticipated to be critically ill at delivery, at times definitive diagnosis is delayed until after the child is born and sometimes until autopsy. Even in situations in which the diagnosis is clear, and some population data exist for the particular neonatal conditions, prognostication for any single infant remains imperfect. In situations in which variation in specific characteristics of the infant is likely to impact survival, as in many congenital anomalies, population data may not exist at all, and decisions regarding what treatments should ethically be withheld, offered, encouraged, or obligated fall to the clinician.

In decisions as high stakes as these, neonatologists must use the information they have (either from existing data or gestalt based on their clinical experience) and interpret how the likelihood of a potential outcome intersects with parents' perceptions of those outcomes. Both benefits and harms exist with treatment and nontreatment and when the neonatologist fails to prognosticate under the guise of uncertainty, parents are left without adequate information for informed decision-making. Instead, neonatologists must be open and honest about what is known and unknown, and what is or is not expected in that situation, to help parents make a decision that best aligns with their values. For example, if expectant parents express that they perceive a severely handicapped survival as being worse than death, the discussion must consider that providing intensive care increases the likelihood of this outcome.

To address these complicated clinical scenarios, neonatologists must be proficient in ethical reasoning, to determine where the limits of parental authority fall, as well as in communication, including the disclosure of bad news, values elicitation, and shared decision-making. Though there is variation between clinicians regarding comfort and experience level with these conversations, the necessary skills to engage parents with honesty, authenticity, and empathy can be learned and developed. Capacity building in this area is not straightforward as traditional techniques used in medical education like readings and didactic lectures have limited utility in imparting this knowledge. Initiation of experiential learning through observation, simulation, and supervised practice in fellowship may lay the foundation for competency in these realms. Subsequent career-long commitment to thoughtful reflection, perspective taking, and learning from past experiences to ensure quality care provision is also essential.

Though neonatologists encounter end-of-life care frequently, they may have differing levels of proficiency, and deaths in the delivery room and neonatal ICU are heterogeneous, with some occurring after planned redirection of care and others after CPR for cardiac arrest. At the same time, pediatric palliative care providers are well versed in the communication skills of end-of-life care. For this reason, partnerships between these providers and neonatologists both in clinical care of expectant parents and in education can improve providers' comfort and parents' experiences with these encounters.

In this chapter, we will explore the role of the neonatologist in the care of the critically ill infant in the antenatal and perinatal period. Though debate exists regarding the appropriate goals and approach to antenatal consultation, empirical studies continue to emerge endorsing strategies in neonatology practice such as supporting parents and parental hope, providing information and encouraging parents' understanding, eliciting parents' personal and spiritual values, and engaging in shared medical decisions [4, 5].

The Timeline of Antenatal Decisions

Though the vast majority of pregnancies result in an uneventful delivery at term, identification that an expected infant will likely be imperiled may occur at any time during the pregnancy (Fig. 7.1). Neonatologists often meet with parents antenatally one or multiple times to provide information and engage in shared decision-making for the many complex decisions that arise.

While some of these visits may be planned with ample time and preparation for the parents and clinicians, others may arise urgently, when delivery is imminent, and neonatologists must be skilled and flexible to communicate under the additional pressure of rushed or emotional situations. The neonatal provider can contribute to the comprehensive care of these patients by gaining comfort and trust, supporting the parents in these decisions, helping families explore their goals for their expectant child, and giving advice on whether those goals are feasible and which option best achieves it. Only then can they provide antenatal, perinatal, and neonatal care that is consistent with those decisions or tasks (Table 7.1).

When a severe fetal anomaly, chromosomal/genetic disorder, or extreme multiple gestation is discovered on routine testing (typically between 10 and 20 weeks' gestation), pregnancy termination or fetal reduction may be offered. Such choices are sometimes emotionally charged or even religiously prohibited by expectant parents. Perceptions of parents regarding obligation to the fetus vary widely, and parents rely heavily on personal values, long-term family planning, and their perception of prognosis in their decisions [6, 7]. Discussion with parents must focus on these issues, so that recommendations may be offered to guide parents to the decision that most aligns with their values and preferences. For parents for whom termination is morally prohibitive, early diagnosis still confers benefits including providing time for parents to plan and adjust, identifying candidates for fetal therapies, and planning location of delivery [8, 9].

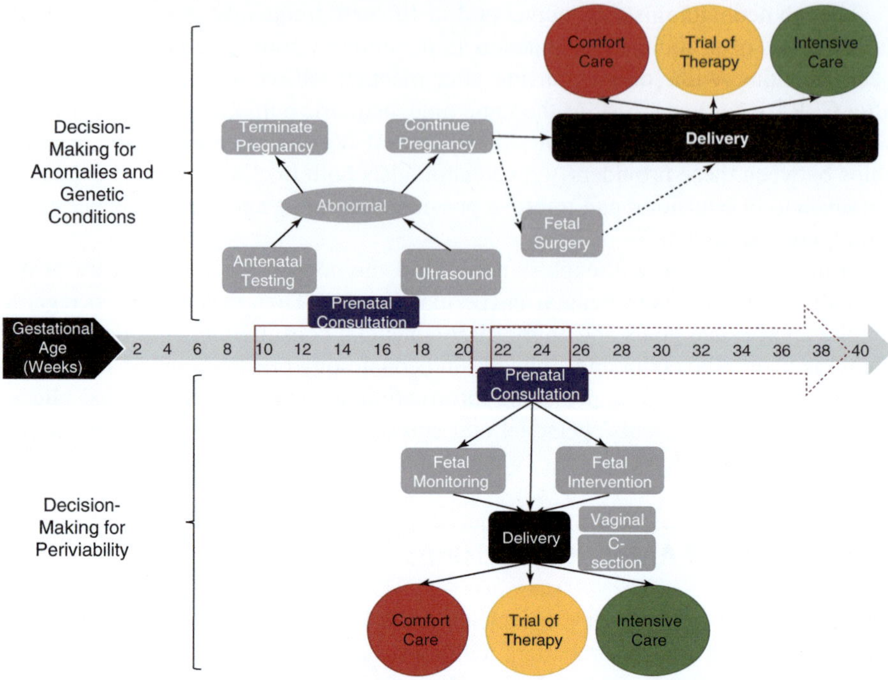

Fig. 7.1 Timeline and decisions in prenatal counseling. If an anomaly is noted on ultrasound or genetic testing, counseling may include decisions about termination or continuing pregnancy, fetal interventions or surgery, and plans for resuscitative therapy at delivery, depending on anticipated prognosis and gestational age. Prenatal counseling in these instances may occur any time after the diagnosis is made throughout the pregnancy, and often multiple encounters are warranted. If a pregnancy is threatened with extreme prematurity, often the prenatal consultation occurs at the time of the complication, between 22 and 25 weeks' gestation, and decisions faced include whether or not to undergo fetal monitoring or intervention, mode of delivery, and resuscitation provision

In certain congenital anomalies, for example, neural tube defects, in which there is anticipated benefit from in utero surgery, the mother and fetus may be eligible for an antenatal procedure which could lessen the extent of future morbidity [10, 11]. These are also complex decisions, as these procedures involve risk to the health of the mother and threaten the pregnancy with the risk of fetal demise or induction of premature delivery [10, 12, 13].

In addition to decisions about pregnancy termination and fetal therapy, expectant women who continue pregnancies with antenatally diagnosed congenital anomalies, genetic conditions, and severe feto-maternal disorders may also face the decision of what degree of postnatal resuscitation to provide and at what gestational age, as the age of viability of these infants may differ from that of an unaffected fetus [14, 15]. This is similar to when an obstetric complication threatens preterm delivery 22 and 25 weeks' gestation in a pregnancy in which antenatal screening had been normal, and decisions about what interventions to provide at the time of delivery must be made. In the case of threatened premature birth, the

Table 7.1 Steps in a neonatologist's prenatal consultation

Step	Rationale
Introduce self to parents	Parents in these situations often meet with multiple obstetric and other subspecialty providers to address a myriad of maternal and fetal/infant concerns. Clarifying your role as a physician who cares for sick infants in the ICU can help reduce confusion and prepare parents that you may not be able to answer all of their questions.
Ask baby's sex and name	Parents report that having their fetus treated as a person with a name in these visits is extremely meaningful particularly when the prognosis is poor.
Ask parents' understanding of condition	Have parents articulate, in their own words, what they understand of their infant's condition. By listening to their version, rather than providing a summary as the clinician, a neonatologist can gain clues about what aspects parents are most focused on and whether they have misconceptions or misunderstandings of medical information.
Establish goals and expectations for the visit	Sometimes the expectant parents' goals for the prenatal encounter are different than those anticipated by the neonatologist. Parents may prioritize different questions and decisions or think about them differently than their physician. Clear discussion about the family's expectations for the visit can help guide the neonatologist in addressing the aspects important to the expectant parents and avoid leaving them with unanswered questions.
Clarify any questions about diagnosis and prognosis	If any areas of misinformation were identified in the parents' summary of the infant's condition, make efforts to correct or clarify these issues, and ask whether there is more medical information they want to know or wish to better understand.
Ask what family is hoping for/ is worried about	Asking about hopes and worries is a good way to begin exploring parents' values around decision-making for their infant if a difficult decision is anticipated.
Discuss decisions that may need to be made; offer ethically permissible options	If the parents are faced with a complicated decision regarding goals of care and resuscitation options at delivery, clear delineation of what options exist, as well as the risks and benefits of pursuing each option, is warranted. If parents ask about an option that would not be medically or ethically permissible, sensitively and honestly explain why this option is not a choice.
Engage in discussion with family around their values around potential outcomes of these options	While population-level statistical outcome data have historically been recommended to guide these conversations, there is increasing evidence that the utility of this information to help parents in decision-making is limited. Instead, discussing what possible outcomes look like and discussing parents' perspectives on quality of life, potential regrets, faith tradition, and beliefs about suffering may be more helpful.
Offer recommendation, if appropriate, based on medical factors and parents' values	Some parents will want recommendations from their clinicians, while others will want to make the decision on their own. Clinicians are often poor at gauging parental desires to share the burden of decision-making, so it is appropriate to simply ask whether they would want a recommendation and then offering one based on the medical information and their values.

(continued)

Table 7.1 (continued)

Step	Rationale
Discuss anticipated course for the chosen option; confirm that parents agree that this is consistent with their values	Physician recommendations can influence patient decisions, even when the recommendation is counter to their values. Take the time to double-check whether expectant parents are comfortable with the recommended plan.
Describe additional information about the NICU; offer a tour	For many expectant parents, the NICU may be a frightening and unknown place. Offering information about who will be at the delivery, who they will encounter on their care team, typical policies and procedures such as visiting hours, rounding times, breastfeeding support, and the physical space and equipment common to the NICU may be helpful in relieving parental anxiety.
Ask if there are other questions or ways in which the neonatologist can be helpful	Offering referral to other subspecialists, including palliative care, spiritual care, or social work providers, may also help address additional concerns the expectant parents may have.
Offer additional meeting if time permits; provide contact information in case additional questions arise	Often the prenatal consultation is emotionally overwhelming for parents, and they may have additional questions or wish to further discuss the diagnosis/prognosis, care goals, options and decisions, or the anticipated NICU stay.

parents and care team may also be faced with a decision of when to monitor and intervene on behalf of the fetus, which requires deliberation not only about the long-term anticipated outcome of the infant, but also risks to the mother and her future fertility from a classical cesarean section. Likewise, therapies to prolong the pregnancy may also pose risks to the mother and fetus which must be weighed against the benefit of gained gestational time. For example, prolonging pregnancy with tocolytic therapy in the context of ruptured membranes poses the threat of chorioamnionitis. Also, ablation of vessels in twin-twin transfusion (a complication arising from sharing of placental blood flow between the twins) and fetal transfusion increases risk of fetal demise and exposes the mother to an invasive procedure.

Of all decisions faced by parents and clinicians in the antenatal period, arguably the most difficult and well-studied is that of care provision at the time of delivery. In situations of extreme prematurity, congenital anomalies, and genetic conditions, prognostic uncertainty in survival and neurologic morbidity outcomes may permit a spectrum of ethically appropriate care options for the infant. The most aggressive of these options is the provision of full resuscitative interventions to preserve life at all costs. While this option may provide the infant the greatest chance at long-term survival, it may be at the expense of burdensome suffering and the opportunity for parents to hold their child alive. On the other end of the spectrum is the provision of comfort care, in which the focus is on quality of life rather than prolongation of life. For some parents, this approach allows for a peaceful death for their infant and an opportunity for holding and memory-making. For other parents, squandering an opportunity for survival of their infant, no matter how small, is unacceptable (see Chap. 4, Fig. 4.2, Spectrum of Care Options).

Between these two extremes is the option of a "trial of therapy," in which initial resuscitative efforts are provided with continued reassessment of the infant's status and redirection to comfort care if a poor outcome is anticipated based on the clinical presentation. Likewise, a "middle ground approach" may also be considered, in which some, limited resuscitative interventions are provided, but clear boundaries are set prenatally regarding which interventions are appropriate and which are not based on the individual infant's prognosis. For example, it may be most appropriate to provide positive pressure ventilation at delivery to allow parents to potentially meet their infant alive, but not pursue intubation and mechanical ventilation. Determining the medically appropriate thresholds that correspond to parents' values-based preferences is one of the responsibilities of the neonatologist in counseling. Setting expectations during the antenatal consultation for limits to intensive care trials when an infant is anticipated to have poor prognosis can assist in postnatal decision-making. In situations when prognosis is extremely uncertain, an infant's clinical response to intensive care may provide more information to inform predictions of survival [16]. When it becomes clear that continued provision of supportive interventions will not achieve a desired outcome, having established this foundation may help parents accept the decision to redirect to comfort goals. It is important to note that while withdrawing and withholding intensive therapies are ethically equivalent, many providers and parents find removing a treatment modality that has been initiated to feel morally worse than not providing it in the first place [17]. For this reason, it is essential to preemptively discuss parents' personal views on withdrawing therapies and setting expectations regarding what constitutes a reasonable trial of a therapy.

Antenatal Consultation for Extreme Prematurity

Case 7.1

Mrs. W is a 30-year-old woman with a history of fetal loss who is referred at an estimated gestational age of 22 1/7 weeks on the date of your consultation. Her prenatal labs are all normal screens.

Prenatal ultrasound has confirmed a monochorionic-diamniotic twin gestation and growth discordance. Twin B is noted to be severely growth restricted, with a current estimated weight of 339 g at 22 1/7 weeks. Twin A was noted to be 489 g at 22 1/7 weeks. There is no evidence of twin-twin transfusion syndrome. It is felt that the growth discordance is due to Twin B having a small share of the placenta. Umbilical artery Doppler studies revealed there is absent end diastolic flow, with intermittent reversal of flow in Twin B, indicating that this twin is potentially getting an insufficient blood supply. She was counseled by the maternal fetal medicine (MFM) physicians that if there was persistent reversal in flow, the concern would be that Twin B would die, and Twin A would then have a 20% chance of neurological injury or death.

Options the MFM has offered include (1) termination by umbilical cord radiofrequency ablation (RFA) of Twin B to preserve Twin A or (2) expectant management with inherent risks for being the death of Twin B, death or neurologic injury to twin A death or neurologic injury, and prematurity if they reach a viable gestational age and size.

Mrs. W was referred for antenatal consultation with a neonatologist to discuss complications of prematurity, limits of viability, and growth restriction in order to help make obstetrical decisions regarding options of RFA versus *expectant management and monitoring and timing of delivery. At the antenatal consultation visit, Mrs. W is confused and scared. She has been doing everything in her power to try to have two healthy babies, Parker (Twin A) and Sammy (Twin B). She is fearful of the possibility of having both babies die or survive with many medical or developmental concerns. She expresses that though she wants to try and salvage at least one baby with the best neurodevelopmental outcome possible, RFA feels like she is choosing to kill one of her babies. After discussion, she indicates that she is leaning toward wanting to make every effort to save both babies and would like further information about what decision that entails.*

In cases of threatened extreme prematurity, parents and physicians may have hours to days to make resuscitation decisions about the infant. The American Academy of Pediatrics (AAP) and other national organizations worldwide provide guidelines for antenatal counseling [18–20]. These recommend that key features of counseling include provision of information to expectant parents regarding outcomes and ethically permissible options. While historically the guidelines encouraged disclosure of statistical estimates for morbidity and mortality to guide these discussions, this has been de-emphasized in recent iterations [21]. This is largely because of the challenges that arise in using outcome data in predicting the prognosis of a specific neonate. Much of the population data that exists reports survival and neurodevelopmental impairment with respect to gestational age alone. Not only are there limitations in the ability to accurately estimate gestational age by last menstrual period and ultrasonography but wide variability exists between institutions in outcomes in these infants [22, 23]. Additionally, other characteristics, such as infant sex, birthweight, single vs. multiple gestation, and provision of maternal antenatal steroids, have been demonstrated to impact survival of these patients. It is likely that additional factors including the reason for delivery (e.g., chorioamnionitis) play a significant role in shaping a premature infant's clinical outcome, though this has not been empirically confirmed [24].

Challenges also arise in communicating statistical survival data to parents. Mortality and long-term disability have been found to be overestimated by clinicians at gestational ages lower than 28 weeks, and when correct data are conveyed, the manner of presentation influences parental decisions [25, 26]. Positively or negatively framing information, such as reporting the proportion of intact survivors rather than neurologically impaired and nonsurvivors or vice versa, influences parents' resuscitation decisions [27]. Likewise, parental decisions can be influenced by presenting default courses of action (opt out) as opposed to presenting available options from which the parents may choose (opt in) [28]. Even when the correct data are known and presented in an unbiased fashion by clinicians, parental comprehension of statistical outcomes may be suboptimal. According to the National Assessment of Adult Literacy, approximately 36% of adults in the United States are estimated to have limited health literacy, 22% have basic health literacy, and 14% have a below basic health literacy. Only 12% of the population has a proficient health literacy level [29]. Likewise, only 13% of adults perform at a proficient numeracy level, and those who do not struggle especially with quantifying risks and probabilities, precisely the information conveyed in antenatal consultation [30]. The stress and time pressure experienced by parents faced with threatened premature delivery also inhibit their ability to recount information discussed in counseling, and recollection decreases as anxiety increases [31].

In addition to providing parents with statistical outcome data, the existing guidelines for antenatal counseling for extremely preterm delivery also bestow the responsibility on clinicians to discuss with parents the ethically permissible resuscitation care options for delivery [18]. These guidelines advise that at gestational ages in which survival is extremely poor, such as below 22 weeks' gestation, intensive supportive therapies should not be offered, as the burdens of treatment clearly outweigh benefits and are not in the best interests of the infant. Likewise, at gestational ages that boast survival rates of about 50% with about half of survivors intact neurologically, such as 25 weeks' gestation or higher, treatment benefits outweigh burdens and resuscitation is obligated due to the best interests of the infant. In between, in the range of 22–25 weeks' gestation, these guidelines recommend that decisional autonomy be ceded to parents because outcomes are uncertain (see also Chap. 3, Fig. 3.2). Interestingly, most published guidelines suggest gestational age thresholds, despite the aforementioned limitations to gestational dating and variation in morbidity and mortality attributable to other infant characteristics.

Case 7.1: Resolution

The neonatologist, in meeting with Mrs. W, explains the different levels of risk for each of the twins. If they perform an RFA, the risk to B is certain death, and the risk to A is a 20% rate of stillbirth from the procedure. At the same time, if they provide expectant management, the risk to Twin A is 20% chance of significant neurologic injury or death if twin B does die in utero *(not certain but "high" chance). Mrs. W notes that she still feels very uncomfortable at the idea of "killing" Twin B, especially since the risks to Twin A are equivalent for RFA and expectant management with demise of Twin B. The question then becomes when to deliver the infants, weighing the prematurity risk on Twin A at various gestational ages. The neonatologist proposes that due to the overall survival rate without neurological impairment at 28 weeks (approaching 80%*

reasonably intact survival), waiting at least until then to deliver Twin A would not dramatically increase the risk of morbidity and mortality for that twin, though it is still uncertain whether Twin B could survive until then. The neonatologist also notes that Twin B will likely have a poorer chance of survival after delivery at 28 weeks' gestation than his twin, due to the growth restriction. Mrs. W and the neonatologist discuss the family's ultimate goals and the trade-offs of trying to achieve the best outcomes for one versus *both babies. Together, they determine that trying to continue the pregnancy with delivery at 28 weeks best aligns with her values, allowing Twin B a chance while not placing additional risk on Twin A. The twins are born and cared for in the NICU; Twin A survives without impairment, and Twin B dies following withdrawal of intensive therapies after 3 days of life.*

Antenatal Consultation for Congenital Anomalies

Case 7.2

Mr. and Mrs. Q are scheduled to meet a neonatologist prenatally for consultation about their fetus with genetically determined trisomy 18, a left-sided congenital diaphragmatic hernia (CDH), and a large perimembranous ventricular septal defect (VSD). On ultrasound determination, the lung to head ratio for the CDH is 1.76, which has a reasonably good predictive outcome for a fetus with CDH. Also, the VSD will not need immediate intervention, but has a high likelihood of resulting in congestive heart failure within a few months. These conditions were diagnosed at a different facility, and the parents are seeking care after having discussed their baby's condition with a mother of a 4-year-old surviving child with trisomy 18 who has a tracheostomy, ventilator, and G-tube. The mother with whom Mr. and Mrs. Q have spoken has been known to be a staunch advocate for aggressive care in the trisomy 18 community. However, she has been forcibly removed from the NICU in the past for being verbally abusive, accusing providers of not offering a baby all treatment evaluations and options and demanding medically unnecessary and inappropriate therapies.

The expectant parents enter the consult with a fairly aggressive and defensive tone. They verbalize understanding that there are birth defects that would require surgery, but are concerned that the medical team will not be honest about what options there are for any other child with these defects and will discriminate based on the diagnosis of trisomy 18. They note that they have heard stories about patients with their baby's condition being denied common therapies, as well as mistreatment of parent supporters. When the neonatologist engages in discussion of the possible needs for extracorporeal membrane oxygenation (ECMO) and heart surgery, the parents share that they are strict Jehovah's witnesses. They wish to pursue these interventions, but without any blood transfusions given to their baby.

Just as for extremely premature infants, resuscitation decisions for infants with uncertain outcomes due to severe genetic conditions or congenital anomalies are often based on informed choices made by the patient's parents. For this reason, accurate information and clear communication from the medical team at the time of counseling is critical. Counseling for infants with these conditions presents considerably more challenges than for extreme prematurity. Fortunately, parents and physicians often have a longer timeline of weeks to months to engage in decision-making. Despite significant improvements in identification of lesions on antenatal imaging via ultrasound and MRI over the past two decades, accurate prognostication with these entities remains difficult [32, 33]. Likewise, the severity and distribution of anomalies varies between infants, making it difficult to provide an accurate and precise prognosis based on population-level data. Furthermore, what outcome data exist may be biased by non-resuscitation practices of these infants in the past, causing the "lethality" of the anomaly to become a self-fulfilling prophecy [34].

Guidelines for counseling expectant parents for severe anomalies exist similarly to the guidelines for extreme prematurity and call for disclosure of information and assistance with decision-making on the part of the clinicians [14, 33, 35–37]. Unlike the guidelines for prematurity, however, these do not provide specific prognostic thresholds at which various resuscitation options are ethically permissible. Instead it is often the role of the neonatologist as the antenatal counselor to determine thresholds for offering and obliging intensive care. The considerable diagnostic and prognostic uncertainty for these infants obscures the boundary between lethality and survivability, and treatments offered for these patients may vary widely between providers and centers [38, 39]. Added complexity to prognostication arises when infants with congenital anomalies and genetic disorders have a higher propensity to deliver preterm than other infants; outcome data for premature neonates with these conditions are extremely limited, but suggest poorer prognoses than their term counterparts [40–47].

For certain conditions, outcome data are available to inform parents in decision-making. Unfortunately, for some of these conditions, such as trisomy 13 and 18, the broad range of outcomes spanning from neonatal death to survival greater than 10 years does not resolve the prognostic uncertainty [48]. Recent studies investigating individual characteristics, however, may assist in differentiating those infants with a relatively better chance at survival [49]. Likewise, there are conditions for which antenatally measurable severity scores exist, such as lung area to head circumference ratio (LHR) in infants with congenital diaphragmatic hernia, but these too are imprecise predictors of survival [50]. In the absence of condition-specific population outcome data and clinical practice guidelines, neonatologists must infer an individual infant's prognosis based on the severity of anomalies on imaging and their intuition from personal experience. Limited evidence suggests that, though imperfect, neonatologists' predictions of poor or nonsurvivable prognosis correlate with neonatal death and that provision of resuscitative therapies do not avert, prevent, or prolong death [51–54].

Multidisciplinary teams are often involved in the counseling of these cases, as they often require the expertise of pediatric and surgical subspecialists in addition to neonatologists for decision-making [55–58]. Joint counseling with pediatric palliative care specialists can be helpful for both parents and neonatologists. Input from palliative care specialists is especially important when there will be anticipated needs for home hospice coordination. Additionally, their expertise is pivotal when the neonatologist is uncomfortable or unfamiliar with guiding families through values elicitation and decision-making around end-of-life. In these situations, the palliative care provider can support parents in navigating complex situations when goals of care include aggressive interventions, care limitations, or a focus on comfort. The palliative care provider can serve to reduce the tension by trading off with the neonatal provider, who discusses available interventions, by discussing when to consider the limits to those interventions. Though involvement of subspecialists in the antenatal period can have positive effects on parental anxiety, the increased number of providers creates opportunities for presenting parents with mixed or inconsistent information. Presentation of divergent prognostic predictions by multiple specialists throughout the pregnancy may result in heightened decisional conflict for expectant parents considering complex goals of care choices [59]. An important role of the neonatologist is to assist in assembling the pieces and tailoring a unified plan for the family, especially when multiple specialists are involved (genetic, cardiac, and general surgery, for example). In that sense, the neonatologist serves as the general "fetiatrician" or primary provider coordinating subspecialists and managing the care of the whole infant for the family in the NICU.

Case 7.2: Resolution

The neonatologist explores how to align this family's wishes for their child not to be discriminated against (which they view offering only comfort care as being) and identify some level of appropriate care that is medically feasible within restrictive parental wishes. Over many meetings of different subspecialists, the neonatologist serves as the primary care provider to help the family navigate possibilities. The decision-making team included genetics, cardiology and cardiovascular surgery, general surgery, and palliative care, as well as the parents and their spiritual support system. Everyone agreed that ECMO was not to be initiated if needed. The surgical team agreed they would support doing a CDH repair without blood products, and the family understood the risks. While the family understood the baby might not need a transfusion for the initial CDH repair surgery, this would not be the case for open cardiac repair, and there was precedent to not operate on the cardiac condition without their consent for transfusion. Following a late preterm birth and an uneventful CDH repair on day 2 of life, the family held firm to their refusal of blood products. The medical team opted not to pursue a court order, since blood products would be only a temporizing measure in an ultimately dismal prognosis, and a goal of the intensive care provided was to honor the parents' values. The infant died at a week of life, before heart surgery could be performed, with the parental spiritual wish for no transfusion supported.

Postnatal Goals of Care Discussion for Severe Complications from Birth

Case 7.3

Baby S is a 2-day-old baby girl who was delivered urgently for fetal bradycardia when her mother presented for her 39-week obstetric visit. She required aggressive resuscitation, including intubation and chest compressions at birth. Her Apgar scores were 1/1/1/5/7. She was noted to have moderate to severe encephalopathy on neurologic exam and was severely acidotic on blood gas. She has undergone therapeutic hypothermia with EEG monitoring, with very abnormal baseline brain activity; the neurologists predict likely long-term neurologic impairment, though they cannot be certain of the degree. She has had no urine output since birth and has been developing worsening respiratory failure due to pulmonary hypertension. She is now severely hypoxic on high-frequency ventilation, and her parents are called to the bedside to discuss the possibility of extracorporeal membrane oxygenation (ECMO) therapy.

After being told the risks and benefits of ECMO for severe pulmonary hypertension, baby S's parents verbalize concern about her long-term prognosis. They note that while they desperately want their daughter to survive, they feel it would be selfish to have her to endure suffering for a life with severe neurological impairment and renal failure requiring dialysis or transplant. They ask if there is a way to tell with more certainty whether their daughter will be doomed to significant morbidity. The mother becomes tearful and says her worst fear is that her daughter will die never having been held.

In addition to sharing difficult decisions with parents antenatally, neonatologists are called at times to engage with parents about care goals after an infant has been delivered and resuscitated. The timeline for these decisions are variable, with some occurring very shortly after birth in the delivery room while others may occur after several days or weeks. Unlike antenatal conversations which essentially always include the expectant mother, in some cases in which the delivery necessitated general anesthesia, the mother is unable to partake in decision-making and the father or other family members may take a heightened role instead. Postnatal decision-making also differs from that in antenatal counseling in terms of parental expectations. Though they may not have all of the pertinent information before meeting the neonatologist in the antenatal encounter, expectant parents of an infant with known anomaly or threatened premature delivery suspect or have been explicitly warned that their infant is imperiled and difficult decisions are anticipated. Parents of term infants who are critically ill from complications of delivery often receive the bad news from the neonatologist after aggressive resuscitation has already occurred. Due to the time pressure of the situation and substantial possibility of a good outcome following revival of a depressed infant, these measures are assumed in the best interest of the infant and provided without explicit parental input.

The burden of postnatal goals of care decision on parents differs considerably than an antenatal one. While the provision of intensive care at delivery precludes the possibility that parents will feel guilt from denying their infant a chance at survival, their decision now entails whether to withdraw a therapy that has already been initiated, which many individuals perceive as more troubling than never providing it in the first place [60]. Additionally, in the antenatal encounter parents have only seen ultrasound images of their infant, not a living baby. Infants injured by delivery complications rarely have visible manifestations of their illness, unlike many infants with congenital anomalies, genetic conditions, or extreme prematurity. As parents require concrete evidence of their infant's bleak prognosis to prevent subsequent doubt or regret, this lack of observable abnormalities may introduce additional challenges to the decision-making process [61].

Prognostic certainty in these infants is limited. Severe multiorgan failure in the first hours of life, evidenced by anuria, coagulopathy, and cardiac dysfunction, portends a more ominous outcome than in cases with mild or absent organ injury. Degree of organ dysfunction does not predict neurologic injury, however, and substantial tissue recovery is not unusual within the first several days of life. Brain MRI and EEG are the best predictors of long-term neurologic impairment, though a poor outcome is certain only in cases in which severe persistent encephalopathy is noted [62]. Neonatologists engaged in these decisions may feel time-pressured to come to a decision for fear of missing a "window of opportunity" to redirect care before breathing reflexes return [63]. Given the gravity and potential lifelong effects on parents of making such a decision, though, parents should be given sufficient time to make a thoughtful decision based on their values. Spontaneous respiration after a terminal extubation is not unusual. Parents should be informed of this possibility and that survivors with extreme neurologic impairment often do not live long without medical support, and provision of artificial nutrition is not ethically obligated [64]. If parents are adequately informed of this possibility, comfort care may still be provided, and this may allow an unexpected opportunity for a desirable outcome for parents such as additional time with their child or the ability to bring their child home with hospice care.

Case 7.3: Resolution

Despite the time pressure to make a decision to pursue ECMO or not, the neonatologist feels the gravity of this decision warrants further reflection by the parents to ensure that it is guided by their values. The family notes that their faith is deeply important to their consideration of this decision. The neonatologist asks whether a spiritual leader from their faith community is able to come and join in the decision-making. The family's pastor arrives a short time later and engages in discussion with the parents about their personal beliefs and shared faith tradition regarding suffering and the afterlife.

Following this discussion, the parents feel more confident in articulating their values that heavy dependence on medical technology for survival is not conducive with the quality of life they find acceptable for their daughter and that missing a chance to hold her alive would be more regrettable than forgoing a very small chance of intact survival. Baby S is held by her mother, father, aunts, uncles, and siblings, as their pastor offers prayers and readings from scripture. Her father whispers that he looks forward to meeting her again in heaven, as she is compassionately extubated in her mother's arms.

Shared Decision-Making

As discussed above, neonatologists must participate in complex decision-making in many contexts and for diverse diagnoses. In decisions that are complex, high stakes, uncertain, with values-laden outcomes, like decisions about goals of care for critically ill neonates, shared decision-making between physicians and parents is appropriate. Shared decision-making has been defined as "a collaborative process that allows patients, or their surrogates, and clinicians to make health care decisions together, taking into account the best scientific evidence available, as well as the patient's values, goals, and preferences" [65]. It falls on a spectrum of decisions between paternalistic decision-making, in which physicians provide medical information and recommendations that are assumed to be in the patient's best interest, with little input from the patients themselves, and informed decision-making, in which the physician provides all relevant medical information, and the patient is responsible for choosing between options (Fig. 7.2) [66]. For a decision to be shared, it requires at least two parties, the patient and physician, both of whom participate in the process [67].

Before engaging in the shared decision process, the neonatologist must determine whether the decision at hand is suitable to be shared between physicians and parents. Many decisions encountered by clinicians on a daily basis are low stakes and do not have particularly uncertain or values-laden outcomes; parents report that in these circumstances it is appropriate for physicians to make the decision [68]. In high-stakes decisions, such as whether to provide intensive care at delivery, parental authority is bounded by relative prognostic certainty (Fig. 7.3).

When provision of intensive therapy is anticipated to result in a reasonable chance of unimpaired survival, providers are obligated to attempt resuscitation in the best interests of the child even over parental objection. In the antenatal encounter, this should not be presented to parents as a choice at all, as explaining the option of comfort care and then not allowing parents to choose this option can be damaging to trust and the therapeutic relationship. Likewise, when fetal conditions are severe enough that intensive interventions are felt to be medically futile with certainty, intensive intervention should not be offered to parents as a choice. In this situation, framing an end-of-life conversation for a child as a decision when there really is no

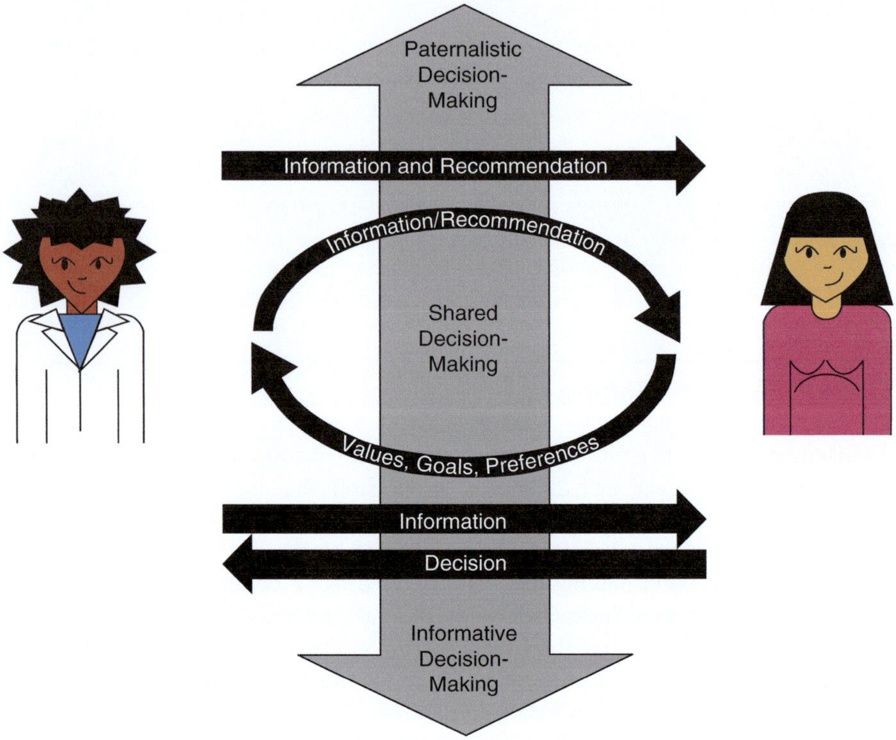

Fig. 7.2 The decision-making spectrum. In paternalistic decision-making, the physician provides information and a recommendation to the patient. In informative decision-making, the physician provides information, and the patient makes a decision. Between these two models is the spectrum of shared decision-making, in which the physician provides information; the patient describes their values, goals, and preferences; and the physician may make recommendations or share in decision deliberations with the patient so that the decision made is based on both the medical information and the patient's values, goals, and preferences

decision to be made places an unnecessary burden of responsibility on parents and puts them at risk of long-term grief and guilt. It is important, however, not to conflate certainty of physiologic or quantitative futility (survival is unlikely despite all available medical treatments) with qualitative futility (survival with a good quality of life is unlikely despite available medical treatments). The determination of qualitative futility is dependent on perceptions of what an acceptable quality of life entails and is often values-based; denying expectant parents an opportunity for a trial of therapy based on a clinician's values is inappropriately paternalistic [69] (see Chap. 3).

Once a resuscitation or continued goals of care decision has been identified as appropriate to be shared, the neonatologist must then determine the parents' preferences for decisional authority (Fig. 7.3). In shared decision-making, the decisional burden and responsibility to ultimately decide on the treatment can be shared equally or unequally between the parent and physicians. Current guidelines in

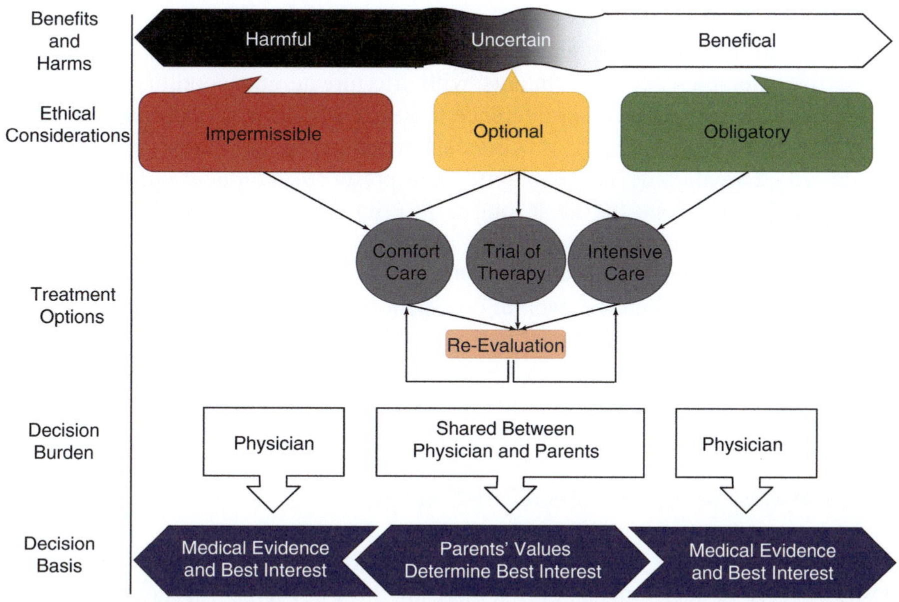

Fig. 7.3 Ethical framework for considering prenatal decisions. The harms and benefits of resuscitation and intensive care should be considered based on the anticipated prognosis of the individual infant. If the harms clearly outweigh benefits, then only comfort care should be offered; the decision burden falls on the clinician and is based on medical evidence and the best interests of the infant. Conversely, if the benefits clearly outweigh harms, active treatment is obligatory, and only intensive care should be offered. Again, the decision burden falls on the physician, and the decision is based on medical evidence and the best interest of the infant. In between, when benefits and harms are uncertain, therapies are optional, and intensive care, comfort care, or the "middle ground" approach of a trial of therapy (with reevaluation after delivery) should be offered. The decision burden in these situations is shared between physicians and parents, and the decision should be based on the parents' values determining the infants' best interest

shared decision-making acknowledge significant variability in parental preferences for decisional authority and recommend that physicians tailor the process to meet the needs of individual parents [65]. However, physicians and parents report a wide range of perceptions regarding how much parental input does and should affect these decisions, and clinicians are poor at judging parental desire for decisional autonomy in the clinical context [31, 70–74]. The majority of surrogate decision makers for critically ill ICU patients prefer an approach that shares decision responsibilities somewhere in the middle, between themselves and physicians. But a nontrivial minority prefer either significantly greater control or to cede control to clinicians [65]. When parents demonstrate clear understanding of the pertinent medical information and their relevant values to the decision, physicians should allow independence in choosing between the medically acceptable options. Conversely, if a parent is struggling to assume decisional responsibility emotionally or psychologically, additional physician guidance and responsibility in the decision is warranted.

Exploring parents' desired level of decisional authority poses several challenges, however. Parents often report a desire for responsibility in high-stakes decisions for supportive therapies for their infants with life-threatening conditions, but it is unclear whether this is truly a preference to bear this decisional burden or a desire for transparency and honesty from clinicians when engaging in these decisions [68, 71, 75, 76]. Parents have more anxiety when presented treatment options without guidance [77] and have the most long-term grief if they perceive that they have made a decision to withdraw supportive therapies alone [78]. Additionally, preferences for decisional authority are not static and may change over the antenatal and perinatal period based on the evolving medical information, clinical scenario, and parental values. Over the antenatal period, additional counseling sessions between the parents and medical team may foster or damage trust, causing parents to cede more or less control to physicians across the decision-making period.

Three Stages of Shared Decision-Making

After establishing that the decision should be shared and determining the parents' desired degree of decisional authority, there are three key temporal stages to sharing decisions, including information exchange, deliberation, and making a treatment decision [65]. In the first phase, it is the responsibility of the physician to provide information about the ethically permissible treatment options and the risks and benefits of each option. The patient or surrogate is then responsible for disclosing information about personal values and preferences that inform their perceptions of the potential outcomes. The physician and the patient or surrogate share in discussion about which option optimally aligns with the goals for the patient, based on those values (Fig. 7.2). This discussion may include deliberating between differing opinions, asking questions, correcting misperceptions, and perspective taking on both parts. Ultimately, this process concludes as the physician and patient/surrogate agree on a treatment plan for implementation.

The first phase of the shared decision-making process seems straightforward; it is the portion with which neonatologists are most comfortable, and they may erroneously equate it with full counseling. However, determination of ethically permissible options for resuscitation and explanation of risks, benefits, and prognosis to expectant parents in antenatal counseling is complex. As detailed in previous sections for specific conditions, limitations in available population outcome data obfuscate accurate prognostication for imperiled infants. Additionally, antenatal consultation is fraught with opportunities for miscommunication of these data and their implications, including provision of misinformation by physicians and misunderstanding by parents. Fortunately, there is current research being conducted on potential improvements to these issues, including decision-aids which standardize and visually depict outcome information [79].

Approaches to improving the second phase of shared decision-making in the antenatal context are less well developed. Models of shared decision-making call for the physicians to help patients by "elucidating and interpreting relevant patient values" or even "articulating and persuading the patient of the most admirable values" before informing the patient and implementing the patient's self-selected intervention [66]. What precisely values are and how to elicit them, however, is not yet clearly understood. Values in general have been defined as the "enduring belief that a specific mode of conduct or end-state of existence is personally or socially preferable to an opposite or converse mode of conduct or end state of existence" [80]. They are beliefs which are prescriptive or proscriptive and acted upon by preference. Paradoxically, values are both enduring and changing and transcend specific situations [81].

In medical decisions and neonatal resuscitation decisions specifically, values may be considered the aspects of one's personality and belief system that influence how negatively or positively they perceive a potential outcome [82]. Though there is general agreement at a societal level that survival is generally preferred to death, and intact health and development is favored over impairment, outcomes for neonates with serious conditions are more nuanced [83]. Survivors of extreme prematurity, congenital anomalies, or genetic conditions face a broad range of potential impairments, ranging from developmental delays and autism spectrum disorders to severe visual or auditory impairment, to significant motor disabilities or profound cognitive impairment. While some families may prefer survival of their infant at all costs, other families may find a wheelchair-bound, noncommunicative existence intolerable for their child. There is, however, no consensus on what degree of impairment is worse than death, and even if there were, it would be difficult to predict the likelihood of this outcome in the antenatal or early neonatal period, to determine if interventions would be more helpful or harmful. In the short term, trade-offs may be between alternatives like having a chance to hold their child alive, allowing dignified death, avoiding suffering, forgoing a slim chance at their infant's survival, or feeling that they have "tried everything" or remained faithful or hopeful. Parents in these situations must be guided by clinicians to consider their values and what it means to be a "good parent" and to inform a decision that will minimize long-term regret [59, 84].

Unfortunately, discussing parents' values for these difficult decisions is fraught with challenges. For many expectant parents this may be the first time that they have faced a decision of this gravity and may be unaware of or unable to articulate these values and how they relate to the decision at hand. They may also express values that are confusing or contradictory, such as wanting to "try all possible interventions" but also to "not cause suffering." Furthermore, though factors such as family considerations and opinions, faith and religion/spirituality, the condition of infant, financial issues, and influences from the community and media likely impact parents' values in these contexts, neonatologists report reluctance to discuss these issues in counseling [85].

Failure to discuss parents' values in shared decision-making is particularly problematic, as physicians and parents' values often differ. Physicians are a self-selected population, who often place high value on logic, rationality, evidence, and trust in technology. Their personal choices to pursue higher education and professional career often translate to views on quality of life that emphasize the importance of cognitive functioning and independent living [82, 86]. Furthermore, their experience with severely disabled children is often based on their observations providing medical care to these patients in the inpatient or ICU setting; not seeing these children in their homes, with their families, or in other enjoyable contexts may negatively bias their perceptions of quality of life [86].

Parents, on the other hand, are more willing than physicians to save an infant at all costs, regardless of anticipated morbidity and mortality outcome [87, 88]. Hope, spirituality, and compassion are more likely to influence expectant parents' decisions than empirical outcome data [89], and other family members' input and religious beliefs are highly influential factors when making life and death decisions for infants [74, 89–92]. Parents faced with urgent decisions tend to opt for treatments aimed to prolong life and perceive quality of life of NICU survivors as better than providers do [93–95]. Additionally, though many physicians would characterize death of an infant after intensive care as burdensome or futile, parents report that knowing that all interventions were attempted is rarely regretted [96].

Lack of insight into these disparate perspectives grounded in values may lead to physicians misattributing values' differences to poor numerical comprehension of statistical outcome data on the part of the expectant parents. This not only endangers shared decision-making and the therapeutic alliance, it can lead to preference misdiagnosis, or misunderstanding the parents' wishes, and selecting an option other than what the patient or surrogate would choose if he or she were a fully informed decision-maker [97]. Additionally, physicians' personal values can bias counseling and pose a threat to autonomy. In hypothetical case scenarios, physicians are more willing to forgo resuscitation of these patients compared to older patients with equivalent expected outcomes, and personal preferences regarding life-sustaining treatments have been noted to influence provider decisions in other pediatric critical care scenarios [98, 99]. There are also conditions, such as hypoplastic left heart syndrome, in which clinicians have reported being disinclined to offer comfort options based on institutional practices or personal beliefs rather than outcome data [100]. Counseling biased toward overtreatment in these scenarios also hampers parental authority in high-stakes life and death decisions that should be shared between clinicians and parents [101].

Though evidence on how to effectively engage parents in antenatal shared decision-making, identify and provide the desired level of parental authority in these decisions, and elicit parents' values and discriminate personal values from medically based recommendations is limited, research to address these gaps is in progress. In the interim, physicians engaging in antenatal decision-making can focus on active listening, honesty, and authenticity in these conversations, particularly in regard to prognostic certainty and uncertainty. Neonatologists should be curious about the lives and perspectives of expectant parents and ask: what they are hoping for, what they worry about, what they would regret, who they turn to for advice, what their faith tells them, or what their family is like. Empathic communication and attempts to foster trust are crucial to these encounters.

Conclusion

Neonatologists, as with any medical subspecialty, are trained to manage a variety of illnesses and develop several skill sets, with the goal of healing and improving the life of a baby. They are necessary partners in antenatal counseling, as potential treatment options, and the anticipated neonatal course and outcome are vital pieces of information for prospective parents to understand. With this counseling comes issues of uncertainty and infant morbidity and mortality. Unfortunately, neonatologists' comfort and aptitude in counseling and supporting parents through these most critical situations is variable, as these skills have historically not been emphasized in training. For these reasons palliative care specialists have been increasingly involved in perinatal and neonatal services. Neonatologists, however, should continue to work toward advancing training in counseling and shared decision-making and remain a critical team member to any perinatal palliative care program.

References

1. Murphy S, Xu J, Kochanek K, Curtin S, Arias E. Deaths: final data for 2015. In: National vital statistics reports. Vol 66 no 6. Hyattsville: National Center for Health Statistics; 2017.
2. Kochanek KD, Murphy SL, Xu JQ, Arias E. Mortality in the United States, 2016. NCHS Data Brief, no 293. Hyattsville: National Center for Health Statistics; 2017.
3. Siegel RL, Miller KD, Jemal A. Cancer statistics, 2015: cancer statistics, 2015. CA Cancer J Clin. 2015;65(1):5–29. https://doi.org/10.3322/caac.21254.
4. Lantos JD. What is the purpose of antenatal counseling? J Pediatr. 2018;196:8–10. https://doi.org/10.1016/j.jpeds.2017.12.060.
5. Kharrat A, Moore GP, Beckett S, Nicholls SG, Sampson M, Daboval T. Antenatal consultations at extreme prematurity: a systematic review of parent communication needs. J Pediatr. 2018;196:109–115.e7. https://doi.org/10.1016/j.jpeds.2017.10.067.
6. Bijma HH, Wildschut HIJ, van der Heide A, Passchier J, Wladimiroff JW, van der Maas PJ. Parental decision-making after ultrasound diagnosis of a serious foetal abnormality. Fetal Diagn Ther. 2005;20(5):321–7. https://doi.org/10.1159/000086806.
7. Kuppermann M, Feeny D, Gates E, Posner SF, Blumberg B, Washington AE. Preferences of women facing a prenatal diagnostic choice: long-term outcomes matter most. Prenat Diagn. 1999;19(8):711–6.
8. American College of Obstetricians and Gynecologists, Committee on Ethics, American Academy of Pediatrics, Committee on Bioethics. Maternal-Fetal intervention and fetal care centers. Pediatrics. 2011;128(2):e473–8. https://doi.org/10.1542/peds.2011-1570.
9. Berndl A, Pearce K, Mondal T. Fetal echocardiography assists in determining optimal delivery site. J Obstet Gynaecol Can. 2014;36(3):210–5.
10. Fadel HE. Ethical aspects of prenatal diagnosis of fetal malformations. J IMA. 2011;43(3):182–8. https://doi.org/10.5915/43-9560.
11. Danzer E, Johnson MP. Fetal surgery for neural tube defects. Semin Fetal Neonatal Med. 2014;19(1):2–8. https://doi.org/10.1016/j.siny.2013.09.004.
12. Dickens BM, Cook RJ. Legal and ethical issues in fetal surgery. Int J Gynaecol Obstet. 2011;115(1):80–3. https://doi.org/10.1016/j.ijgo.2011.07.007.
13. Chervenak FA, McCullough LB, Levene MI. An ethically justified, clinically comprehensive approach to peri-viability: gynaecological, obstetric, perinatal and neonatal dimensions. J Obstet Gynaecol. 2007;27(1):3–7. https://doi.org/10.1080/01443610601133605.

14. Chervenak FA, McCullough LB. An ethically justified, clinically comprehensive management strategy for third-trimester pregnancies complicated by fetal anomalies. Obstet Gynecol. 1990;75(3 Pt 1):311–6.
15. ACOG Committee on Practice Bulletins. ACOG Practice Bulletin No. 77: screening for fetal chromosomal abnormalities. Obstet Gynecol. 2007;109(1):217–27.
16. Meadow W, Meadow X, Tanz RR, Lagatta J, Lantos J. The value of a trial of therapy - football as a "proof-of-concept". Acta Paediatr. 2011;100(2):167–9. https://doi.org/10.1111/j.1651-2227.2010.02113.x.
17. Weise KL, Okun AL, Carter BS, et al. Guidance on forgoing life-sustaining medical treatment. Pediatrics. 2017;140(3):e20171905. https://doi.org/10.1542/peds.2017-1905.
18. Cummings J, Committee on Fetus and Newborn. Antenatal counseling regarding resuscitation and intensive care before 25 weeks of gestation. Pediatrics. 2015;136(3):588–95. https://doi.org/10.1542/peds.2015-2336.
19. Nuffield Council on Bioethics. Critical care decisions in fetal and neonatal medicine: ethical issues. London: Nuffield Council on Bioethics; 2006.
20. Management of the woman with threatened birth of an infant of extremely low gestational age. Fetus and Newborn Committee, Canadian Paediatric Society, Maternal-Fetal Medicine Committee. Society of Obstetricians and Gynaecologists of Canada. CMAJ. 1994;151(5):547–53.
21. Batton DG, Committee on Fetus and Newborn. Antenatal counseling regarding resuscitation at an extremely low gestational age. Pediatrics. 2009;124(1):422–7. https://doi.org/10.1542/peds.2009-1060.
22. Committee opinion no 611: method for estimating due date. Obstet Gynecol. 2014;124(4):863–6. https://doi.org/10.1097/01.AOG.0000454932.15177.be.
23. Rysavy MA, Li L, Bell EF, et al. Between-hospital variation in treatment and outcomes in extremely preterm infants. N Engl J Med. 2015;372(19):1801–11. https://doi.org/10.1056/NEJMoa1410689.
24. Tyson JE, Parikh NA, Langer J, Green C, Higgins RD, National Institute of Child Health and Human Development Neonatal Research Network. Intensive care for extreme prematurity--moving beyond gestational age. N Engl J Med. 2008;358(16):1672–81. https://doi.org/10.1056/NEJMoa073059.
25. Blanco F, Suresh G, Howard D, Soll RF. Ensuring accurate knowledge of prematurity outcomes for prenatal counseling. Pediatrics. 2005;115(4):e478–87. https://doi.org/10.1542/peds.2004-1417.
26. Morse SB, Haywood JL, Goldenberg RL, Bronstein J, Nelson KG, Carlo WA. Estimation of neonatal outcome and perinatal therapy use. Pediatrics. 2000;105(5):1046–50.
27. Haward MF, Murphy RO, Lorenz JM. Message framing and perinatal decisions. Pediatrics. 2008;122(1):109–18. https://doi.org/10.1542/peds.2007-0620.
28. Haward MF, Murphy RO, Lorenz JM. Default options and neonatal resuscitation decisions. J Med Ethics. 2012;38(12):713–8. https://doi.org/10.1136/medethics-2011-100182.
29. Kutner M, Greenberg E, Jin Y, Paulsen C. The Health Literacy of America's Adults: results From the 2003 National Assessment of Adult Literacy (NCES 2006–483).U.S. Department of Education. Washington, DC: National Center for Education Statistics; 2006.
30. Nelson W, Reyna VF, Fagerlin A, Lipkus I, Peters E. Clinical implications of numeracy: theory and practice. Ann Behav Med. 2008;35(3):261–74. https://doi.org/10.1007/s12160-008-9037-8.
31. Zupancic JAF, Kirpalani H, Barrett J, et al. Characterising doctor-parent communication in counselling for impending preterm delivery. Arch Dis Child Fetal Neonatal Ed. 2002;87(2):F113–7.
32. American College of Obstetricians and Gynecologists. ACOG Practice Bulletin No. 101: ultrasonography in pregnancy. Obstet Gynecol. 2009;113(2 Pt 1):451–61. https://doi.org/10.1097/AOG.0b013e31819930b0.

33. Santos XM, Papanna R, Johnson A, et al. The use of combined ultrasound and magnetic resonance imaging in the detection of fetal anomalies. Prenat Diagn. 2010;30(5):402–7. https://doi.org/10.1002/pd.2481.
34. Wilkinson D. The self-fulfilling prophecy in intensive care. Theor Med Bioeth. 2009;30(6):401–10. https://doi.org/10.1007/s11017-009-9120-6.
35. Lakhoo K. Fetal counselling for surgical conditions. Early Hum Dev. 2012;88(1):9–13. https://doi.org/10.1016/j.earlhumdev.2011.11.004.
36. Hansen AR, Madsen JR. Antenatal neurosurgical counseling: approach to the unborn patient. Pediatr Clin N Am. 2004;51(2):491–505. https://doi.org/10.1016/S0031-3955(03)00209-8.
37. Lepigeon K, Van Mieghem T, Vasseur Maurer S, Giannoni E, Baud D. Gastroschisis - what should be told to parents? Prenat Diagn. 2013;34:316. https://doi.org/10.1002/pd.4305.
38. Wilkinson DJC, Thiele P, Watkins A, De Crespigny L. Fatally flawed? A review and ethical analysis of lethal congenital malformations. BJOG. 2012;119(11):1302–8. https://doi.org/10.1111/j.1471-0528.2012.03450.x.
39. Brown SD, Donelan K, Martins Y, et al. Differing attitudes toward fetal care by pediatric and maternal-fetal medicine specialists. Pediatrics. 2012;130(6):e1534–40. https://doi.org/10.1542/peds.2012-1352.
40. Honein MA, Kirby RS, Meyer RE, et al. The association between major birth defects and preterm birth. Matern Child Health J. 2009;13(2):164–75. https://doi.org/10.1007/s10995-008-0348-y.
41. Purisch SE, DeFranco EA, Muglia LJ, Odibo AO, Stamilio DM. Preterm birth in pregnancies complicated by major congenital malformations: a population-based study. Am J Obstet Gynecol. 2008;199(3):287.e1–8. https://doi.org/10.1016/j.ajog.2008.06.089.
42. Tsao K, Allison ND, Harting MT, Lally PA, Lally KP. Congenital diaphragmatic hernia in the preterm infant. Surgery. 2010;148(2):404–10. https://doi.org/10.1016/j.surg.2010.03.018.
43. Nembhard WN, Salemi JL, Ethen MK, Fixler DE, Canfield MA. Mortality among infants with birth defects: joint effects of size at birth, gestational age, and maternal race/ethnicity. Birth Defects Res Part A Clin Mol Teratol. 2010;88(9):728–36. https://doi.org/10.1002/bdra.20696.
44. Archer JM, Yeager SB, Kenny MJ, Soll RF, Horbar JD. Distribution of and mortality from serious congenital heart disease in very low birth weight infants. Pediatrics. 2011;127(2):293–9. https://doi.org/10.1542/peds.2010-0418.
45. Pappas A, Shankaran S, Hansen NI, et al. Outcome of extremely preterm infants (<1,000 g) with congenital heart defects from the National Institute of Child Health and Human Development Neonatal Research Network. Pediatr Cardiol. 2012;33(8):1415–26. https://doi.org/10.1007/s00246-012-0375-8.
46. Dees E, Lin H, Cotton RB, Graham TP, Dodd DA. Outcome of preterm infants with congenital heart disease. J Pediatr. 2000;137(5):653–9. https://doi.org/10.1067/mpd.2000.108568.
47. Tanner K, Sabrine N, Wren C. Cardiovascular malformations among preterm infants. Pediatrics. 2005;116(6):e833–8. https://doi.org/10.1542/peds.2005-0397.
48. Nelson KE, Rosella LC, Mahant S, Guttmann A. Survival and surgical interventions for children with trisomy 13 and 18. JAMA. 2016;316(4):420–8. https://doi.org/10.1001/jama.2016.9819.
49. Acharya K, Leuthner S, Clark R, Nghiem-Rao TH, Spitzer A, Lagatta J. Major anomalies and birth-weight influence NICU interventions and mortality in infants with trisomy 13 or 18. J Perinatol. 2017;37(4):420–6. https://doi.org/10.1038/jp.2016.245.
50. Snoek KG, Peters NCJ, van Rosmalen J, et al. The validity of the observed-to-expected lung-to-head ratio in congenital diaphragmatic hernia in an era of standardized neonatal treatment; a multicenter study. Prenat Diagn. 2017;37(7):658–65. https://doi.org/10.1002/pd.5062.
51. Kukora S, Gollehon N, Weiner G, Laventhal N. Prognostic accuracy of antenatal neonatology consultation. J Perinatol. 2016;37:27. https://doi.org/10.1038/jp.2016.171.

52. Courtwright AM, Laughon MM, Doron MW. Length of life and treatment intensity in infants diagnosed prenatally or postnatally with congenital anomalies considered to be lethal. J Perinatol. 2011;31(6):387–91. https://doi.org/10.1038/jp.2010.124.
53. Parravicini E, Lorenz JM. Neonatal outcomes of fetuses diagnosed with life-limiting conditions when individualized comfort measures are proposed. J Perinatol. 2014;34(6):483–7. https://doi.org/10.1038/jp.2014.40.
54. Kukora S, Gollehon N, Laventhal N. Antenatal palliative care consultation: implications for decision-making and perinatal outcomes in a single-centre experience. Arch Dis Child Fetal Neonatal Ed. 2016;102:F12. https://doi.org/10.1136/archdischild-2016-311027.
55. Bijma HH, Van der Heide A, Wildschut HIJ, Van der Maas PJ, Wladimiroff JW. Impact of decision-making in a multidisciplinary perinatal team. Prenat Diagn. 2007;27(2):97–103. https://doi.org/10.1002/pd.1598.
56. Raboei EH. The role of the pediatric surgeon in the perinatal multidisciplinary team. Eur J Pediatr Surg. 2008;18(5):313–7. https://doi.org/10.1055/s-2008-1038641.
57. Aite L, Trucchi A, Nahom A, Spina V, Bilancioni E, Bagolan P. Multidisciplinary management of fetal surgical anomalies: the impact on maternal anxiety. Eur J Pediatr Surg. 2002;12(2):90–4. https://doi.org/10.1055/s-2002-30164.
58. Kemp J, Davenport M, Pernet A. Antenatally diagnosed surgical anomalies: the psychological effect of parental antenatal counseling. J Pediatr Surg. 1998;33(9):1376–9.
59. Hickman RL Jr, Daly BJ, Lee E. Decisional conflict and regret: consequences of surrogate decision making for the chronically critically ill. Appl Nurs Res. 2012;25(4):271–5. https://doi.org/10.1016/j.apnr.2011.03.003.
60. Singh J, Lantos J, Meadow W. End-of-life after birth: death and dying in a neonatal intensive care unit. Pediatrics. 2004;114(6):1620–6. https://doi.org/10.1542/peds.2004-0447.
61. McHaffie HE, Lyon AJ, Hume R. Deciding on treatment limitation for neonates: the parents' perspective. Eur J Pediatr. 2001;160(6):339–44.
62. Bonifacio SL, deVries LS, Groenendaal F. Impact of hypothermia on predictors of poor outcome: how do we decide to redirect care? Semin Fetal Neonatal Med. 2015;20(2):122–7. https://doi.org/10.1016/j.siny.2014.12.011.
63. Kon AA. The "window of opportunity:" helping parents make the most difficult decision they will ever face using an informed non-dissent model. Am J Bioeth. 2009;9(4):55–6. https://doi.org/10.1080/15265160802716811.
64. Diekema DS, Botkin JR, Committee on Bioethics. Forgoing medically provided nutrition and hydration in children. Pediatrics. 2009;124(2):813–22. https://doi.org/10.1542/peds.2009-1299.
65. Kon AA, Davidson JE, Morrison W, Danis M, White DB. Shared decision making in ICUs: an American College of Critical Care Medicine and American Thoracic Society Policy Statement. Crit Care Med. 2016;44(1):188–201. https://doi.org/10.1097/CCM.0000000000001396.
66. Emanuel EJ, Emanuel LL. Four models of the physician-patient relationship. JAMA. 1992;267(16):2221–6.
67. Charles C, Gafni A, Whelan T. Shared decision-making in the medical encounter: what does it mean? (or it takes at least two to tango). Soc Sci Med. 1997;44(5):681–92.
68. Weiss EM, Barg FK, Cook N, Black E, Joffe S. Parental decision-making preferences in neonatal intensive care. J Pediatr. 2016;179:36–41.e3. https://doi.org/10.1016/j.jpeds.2016.08.030.
69. Morata L. An evolutionary concept analysis of futility in health care. J Adv Nurs. 2018;74(6):1289–300. https://doi.org/10.1111/jan.13526.
70. Doron MW, Veness-Meehan KA, Margolis LH, Holoman EM, Stiles AD. Delivery room resuscitation decisions for extremely premature infants. Pediatrics. 1998;102(3):574–82. https://doi.org/10.1542/peds.102.3.574.
71. McHaffie HE, Laing IA, Parker M, McMillan J. Deciding for imperilled newborns: medical authority or parental autonomy? J Med Ethics. 2001;27(2):104–9.
72. Singh J, Fanaroff J, Andrews B, et al. Resuscitation in the "gray zone" of viability: determining physician preferences and predicting infant outcomes. Pediatrics. 2007;120(3):519–26. https://doi.org/10.1542/peds.2006-2966.

73. Brinchmann BS, Førde R, Nortvedt P. What matters to the parents? A qualitative study of parents' experiences with life-and-death decisions concerning their premature infants. Nurs Ethics. 2002;9(4):388–404.
74. Kavanaugh K, Moro TT, Savage TA, Reyes M, Wydra M. Supporting parents' decision making surrounding the anticipated birth of an extremely premature infant. J Perinat Neonatal Nurs. 2009;23(2):159–70. https://doi.org/10.1097/JPN.0b013e3181a2cacc.
75. Madrigal VN, Carroll KW, Hexem KR, Faerber JA, Morrison WE, Feudtner C. Parental decision-making preferences in the pediatric intensive care unit. Crit Care Med. 2012;40(10):2876–82. https://doi.org/10.1097/CCM.0b013e31825b9151.
76. Johnson SK, Bautista CA, Hong SY, Weissfeld L, White DB. An empirical study of surrogates' preferred level of control over value-laden life support decisions in intensive care units. Am J Respir Crit Care Med. 2011;183(7):915–21. https://doi.org/10.1164/rccm.201008-1214OC.
77. Orfali K, Gordon EJ. Autonomy gone awry: a cross-cultural study of parents' experiences in neonatal intensive care units. Theor Med Bioeth. 2004;25(4):329–65.
78. Caeymaex L, Jousselme C, Vasilescu C, et al. Perceived role in end-of-life decision making in the NICU affects long-term parental grief response. Arch Dis Child Fetal Neonatal Ed. 2013;98(1):F26–31. https://doi.org/10.1136/archdischild-2011-301548.
79. Guillén Ú, Suh S, Munson D, et al. Development and pretesting of a decision-aid to use when counseling parents facing imminent extreme premature delivery. J Pediatr. 2012;160(3):382–7. https://doi.org/10.1016/j.jpeds.2011.08.070.
80. Rokeach M. The nature of human values. New York: The Free Press; 1973.
81. Schwartz SH. An overview of the Schwartz theory of basic values. Online Readings Psychol Culture. 2012;2(1) https://doi.org/10.9707/2307-0919.1116.
82. Kukora SK, Boss RD. Values-based shared decision-making in the antenatal period. Semin Fetal Neonatal Med. 2017;23:17. https://doi.org/10.1016/j.siny.2017.09.003.
83. Kipnis K. Harm and uncertainty in newborn intensive care. Theor Med Bioeth. 2007;28(5):393–412. https://doi.org/10.1007/s11017-007-9051-z.
84. Feudtner C, Walter JK, Faerber JA, et al. Good-parent beliefs of parents of seriously ill children. JAMA Pediatr. 2015;169(1):39–47. https://doi.org/10.1001/jamapediatrics.2014.2341.
85. Bastek TK, Richardson DK, Zupancic JAF, Burns JP. Prenatal consultation practices at the border of viability: a regional survey. Pediatrics. 2005;116(2):407–13. https://doi.org/10.1542/peds.2004-1427.
86. Wilfond BS. Tracheostomies and assisted ventilation in children with profound disabilities: navigating family and professional values. Pediatrics. 2014;133(Suppl 1):S44–9. https://doi.org/10.1542/peds.2013-3608H.
87. Streiner DL, Saigal S, Burrows E, Stoskopf B, Rosenbaum P. Attitudes of parents and health care professionals toward active treatment of extremely premature infants. Pediatrics. 2001;108(1):152–7.
88. Lam HS, Wong SPS, Liu FYB, Wong HL, Fok TF, Ng PC. Attitudes toward neonatal intensive care treatment of preterm infants with a high risk of developing long-term disabilities. Pediatrics. 2009;123(6):1501–8. https://doi.org/10.1542/peds.2008-2061.
89. Boss RD, Hutton N, Sulpar LJ, West AM, Donohue PK. Values parents apply to decision-making regarding delivery room resuscitation for high-risk newborns. Pediatrics. 2008;122(3):583–9. https://doi.org/10.1542/peds.2007-1972.
90. Feudtner C. The breadth of hopes. N Engl J Med. 2009;361(24):2306–7. https://doi.org/10.1056/NEJMp0906516.
91. Xafis V, Wilkinson D, Sullivan J. What information do parents need when facing end-of-life decisions for their child? A meta-synthesis of parental feedback. BMC Palliat Care. 2015;14(1):19. https://doi.org/10.1186/s12904-015-0024-0.
92. Roscigno CI, Savage TA, Kavanaugh K, et al. Divergent views of hope influencing communications between parents and hospital providers. Qual Health Res. 2012;22(9):1232–46. https://doi.org/10.1177/1049732312449210.
93. Kirschbaum MS. Life support decisions for children: what do parents value? ANS Adv Nurs Sci. 1996;19(1):51–71.

94. Saigal S, Stoskopf BL, Feeny D, et al. Differences in preferences for neonatal outcomes among health care professionals, parents, and adolescents. JAMA. 1999;281(21):1991–7.
95. Saigal S, Stoskopf B, Pinelli J, et al. Self-perceived health-related quality of life of former extremely low birth weight infants at young adulthood. Pediatrics. 2006;118(3):1140–8. https://doi.org/10.1542/peds.2006-0119.
96. Arnolds M, Xu L, Hughes P, McCoy J, Meadow W. Worth a try? Describing the experiences of families during the course of care in the neonatal intensive care unit when the prognosis is poor. J Pediatr. 2018;196:116–122.e3. https://doi.org/10.1016/j.jpeds.2017.12.050.
97. Mulley AG, Trimble C, Elwyn G. Stop the silent misdiagnosis: patients' preferences matter. BMJ. 2012;345:e6572.
98. Laventhal N, Spelke MB, Andrews B, Larkin LK, Meadow W, Janvier A. Ethics of resuscitation at different stages of life: a survey of perinatal physicians. Pediatrics. 2011;127(5):e1221–9. https://doi.org/10.1542/peds.2010-1031.
99. Needle JS, Mularski RA, Nguyen T, Fromme EK. Influence of personal preferences for life-sustaining treatment on medical decision making among pediatric intensivists*. Crit Care Med. 2012;40(8):2464–9. https://doi.org/10.1097/CCM.0b013e318255d85b.
100. Kon AA, Ackerson L, Lo B. How pediatricians counsel parents when no "best-choice" management exists: lessons to be learned from hypoplastic left heart syndrome. Arch Pediatr Adolesc Med. 2004;158(5):436. https://doi.org/10.1001/archpedi.158.5.436.
101. Kon AA. Healthcare providers must offer palliative treatment to parents of neonates with hypoplastic left heart syndrome. Arch Pediatr Adolesc Med. 2008;162(9):844. https://doi.org/10.1001/archpediatrics.2008.3.

Neonatal Pain Management

8

Jeffrey M. Meyers, Andrew S. Decker, and Chris Tryon

Introduction

As the field of neonatology has continued to progress over the last several decades, so too has our understanding of the neonatal pain experience. As recently as the 1970s major surgery was reported in neonates without the use of analgesia [1] as a result of the belief that neonates were unable to experience pain owing to immaturity of the central nervous system [2]. However, it is now well recognized that neonates experience and respond to pain, including those born at the limits of viability. In addition, evidence demonstrates that pain has untoward effects on the neonatal brain during a critical time of development, which underscores the importance that clinicians recognize and treat pain appropriately. Despite this knowledge, significant challenges remain when caring for infants who experience pain. Pain assessment is difficult in a nonverbal population, therapies for neonatal pain are not as well studied compared to those used in older children and adults, and concerns exist regarding potential adverse effects from exposure to these therapies (such as opioids) on the developing brain. In this chapter, we will provide guidance on assessing pain, include a summary of

J. M. Meyers (✉)
Department of Pediatrics, University of Rochester Medical Center, Rochester, NY, USA

Division of Neonatology, Golisano Children's Hospital, University of Rochester Medical Center, Department of Pediatrics, Rochester, NY, USA
e-mail: jeff_meyers@urmc.rochester.edu

A. S. Decker
Department of Pharmacy, University of Rochester Medical Center, Golisano Children's Hospital, Rochester, NY, USA

C. Tryon
Department of Child Life, Golisano Children's Hospital, University of Rochester Medical Center, Rochester, NY, USA

E. M. Denney-Koelsch, D. Côté-Arsenault (eds.), *Perinatal Palliative Care*,
https://doi.org/10.1007/978-3-030-34751-2_8

pharmacologic and non-pharmacologic pain management, and attempt to assist clinicians with balancing the risks of undertreating pain and unwanted effects from pharmacologic therapies.

Case 8.1

You are part of the team caring for Lacey, a female infant born at 24 weeks' gestation, who is now 1 day old. Since birth, Lacey has been requiring mechanical ventilation through an endotracheal tube and has received 2 doses of surfactant. Attempts to place an umbilical venous catheter were unsuccessful, and thus a percutaneous central catheter was inserted. As part of her care, Lacey has required heel sticks every 2–4 hours for blood gas and blood glucose monitoring and frequent suctioning of secretions from her endotracheal tube. During rounds, Lacey's mother inquires about her daughter's comfort, especially because "she can't tell you if something hurts." Specifically, her questions include:

- *What do we know about how Lacey experiences pain, given that she is so premature?*
- *How can you determine if she is in pain?*

Neonatal Pain Experience

To experience pain, an individual must have the ability to sense a noxious stimulus through chemical, mechanical, and/or thermal nociceptors. This stimulus must then be propagated to the central nervous system and processed by a complex network of neurochemical pathways in the cortical and subcortical tissues. It is recognized that the processing of noxious stimuli (i.e., nociception) and the transmission of noxious stimuli into a painful experience can occur independently from one another [3]. For the purposes of this review, however, nociception and the experience of pain will be considered as one entity.

Neonates, even those born extremely preterm, have the ability to experience pain. Cutaneous sensory receptors are present in some areas as early as 7 weeks' gestation and by 20 weeks are widespread in the growing fetus [4]. Likewise, synaptic connections between sensory fibers in the spinal cord develop as early as the sixth week of gestation and are fully developed by 30 weeks' gestation [2, 5]. Cortical development of connections important in the processing pathway of noxious stimuli has occurred by 20–24 weeks of gestation [2, 6]. In a study of 18 infants ranging from 25 to 45 weeks' postmenstrual age (PMA), cortical activity following noxious stimuli was demonstrated using near-infrared spectroscopy in all study subjects [7]. Altered physiologic responses to noxious stimuli have also been described in neonates, particularly those born prematurely [8]. Altogether, these data confirm that even those infants born at the limits of viability are capable of sensing and experiencing pain.

It is important to consider aspects of the pain experience unique to neonates. First, while neonates are able to sense noxious stimuli, their ability to modulate pain through inhibitory feedback mechanisms is immature. Descending pathways that act to inhibit pain experiences are not developed until sometime after 32 weeks' gestation, but even in term neonates are still functionally immature [9]. Thus, the balance between excitation and inhibition in response to noxious stimuli is altered in the neonate. Second, the pain experience itself influences processing and response to future stimuli. For example, after having experienced painful stimuli, preterm infants were noted to have increased indicators of stress, such as facial expression and heart rate reactivity, even after non-noxious stimuli such as routine care [10]. However, similar responses were not observed when the initial stimulus was not painful [10]. A greater number of painful procedures occurring early in life in extremely preterm infants were correlated with a blunted behavioral and cortisol response following a painful procedure elicited at 32 weeks' PMA [8]. Term-born infants undergoing repeated heel sticks shortly after birth demonstrated more intense responses to pain during a subsequent painful procedure [11]. Third, localization and discrimination of pain in neonates is also less mature than that of adults, demonstrated by both animal and human studies, which in turn may result in altered development of inhibitory and excitatory pain pathways and influence the response to future noxious stimuli [9]. Overall, these data suggest that premature infants who are exposed to painful stimuli may process pain differently for the rest of their lives.

Painful experiences are common shortly after birth, even in healthy newborns, as nearly all newborns receive injections (hepatitis B vaccine, vitamin K) and blood draws (newborn metabolic screen) before leaving the hospital. For those infants requiring admission to a neonatal intensive care unit (NICU), the number of painful experiences increases substantially, owing largely to various interventions necessary as part of the medical care provided in these ill newborns. As demonstrated in large observational studies, infants cared for in the NICU experience 10–14 painful procedures each day, and those born most prematurely experience these procedures most frequently [12, 13]. Common painful procedures occurring in the NICU are shown in Table 8.1. Despite the frequency with which painful procedures occur in these infants, only 50% of these procedures were preceded by some form of analgesia [12].

Table 8.1 Common painful procedures in the NICU

Nasal/tracheal suctioning
Heel stick
Gastric tube insertion
Venipuncture
IV insertion
Chest physiotherapy
Tracheal intubation
Adhesive removal
Central line placement
Surgical procedure

Clinicians and other caregivers may be faced with situations where determining the presence of pain is challenging. Examples of these situations might include infants with significant brain injury, such as that following hypoxic-ischemic injury or those with congenital malformations of the central nervous system. In these situations, the ability of the brain to process painful stimuli, and thus the infant to experience pain, may be blunted or altogether nonexistent. However, at present there is little data to support a conclusion that infants with these conditions cannot experience pain, and thus we believe it appropriate to anticipate painful experiences to be similar to that observed in otherwise healthy infants.

Effects of Pain on the Developing Neonatal Brain

External influences play an important role in the growth and development of the brain, and the experience of pain is no exception. This is particularly true when that experience occurs during a critical and unexpected window of brain development, such as in those infants born prematurely. Immediately following a noxious stimulus, acute physiologic responses occur in the neonate such as tachycardia, increased blood pressure, increased oxygen demand, and elevated levels of the stress hormones cortisol and epinephrine [2]. In critically ill premature neonates, these alterations in cardiorespiratory status following pain, especially if occurring in the first few days after birth, may contribute to risk of complications such as intraventricular hemorrhage and periventricular leukomalacia [14].

Evidence is now emerging that pain experienced during the neonatal period, particularly repeated experiences, has long-lasting impacts on brain growth, processing, and development. In infants born between 24 and 32 weeks' gestation, a greater number of skin breaks were associated with reduced white matter and subcortical gray matter maturation measured with MRI at term-equivalent age [15]. Painful procedures also influence brain growth into childhood, where in a similar population of preterm infants, a greater number of skin breaks during the neonatal period correlated with significantly thinner cortex at 7 years of age, most notably in the frontal and parietal regions (Fig. 8.1) [16]. Furthermore, differing responses to painful stimuli have been noted among adolescents born preterm, who were presumably exposed to pain while in the NICU, when compared with adolescents born at term. Using functional MRI, Hohmeister et al. noted greater numbers of brain regions activated, as well as higher brain activation, following painful heat stimulation in adolescents born preterm when compared with those born at term [17]. Unlike those born at term, adolescents born prematurely demonstrated no habituation (the body's ability to suppress the response to repeated pain) following repeated painful stimuli, suggesting that each subsequent stimulus was perceived as equally painful as the last [17]. Neurodevelopmental outcomes measured in childhood also appear linked to pain experiences during the neonatal period. In a study of 137 preterm infants, a greater number of skin-breaking procedures during hospitalization were associated with poorer cognitive and motor function at both 8 and 18 months' corrected age [18]. Poorer visual-perceptual abilities at school age

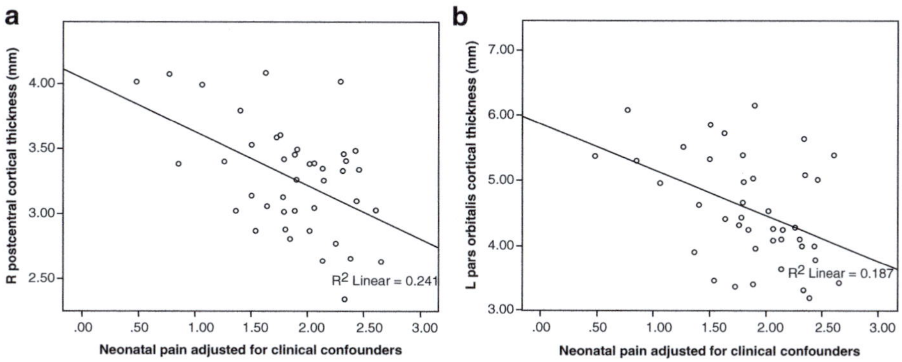

Fig. 8.1 Scatterplots demonstrating strong inverse correlation between neonatal pain and cortical thickness in the right postcentral (**a**) and left pars orbitalis (**b**) regions of the brain in former preterm infants measured at 7 years of age, after adjustment for clinical confounders. Pain is represented as the number of skin-breaking procedures log transformed [16]. (Reprinted from Ranger et al. [16])

were also noted in preterm infants experiencing greater numbers of painful procedures [19]. Internalizing behaviors, such as anxiety/depression, were expressed more commonly at 18 months' corrected age in those born preterm who experienced greater skin-breaking procedures as neonates; this relationship persisted to school age [20, 21]. Altogether, it is clear that pain experienced during the neonatal period can impact future brain processing, growth, and development and underscores the important role care providers play in mitigating painful experiences whenever possible.

Pain Assessment in Neonates

When painful stimuli occur as part of necessary medical care, clinicians must be able to assess pain properly and prescribe appropriate therapies to treat pain. Unlike older children and adults, however, neonates lack the ability to communicate their pain experience to their care provider, making the gold standard of pain assessment (self-report) unavailable to clinicians. As a surrogate for self-report, physiologic and behavioral responses that occur following pain have been incorporated into scales used to assess pain in neonates. While numerous neonatal scales have been developed, historically all have limitations in their application to various types of pain (acute vs chronic, intermittent vs persistent) and to the neonatal population itself (preterm vs term). For example, the Premature Infant Pain Profile (PIPP) has excellent internal consistency and both inter- and intra-rater reliability for use in acute pain [22, 23]. However, it cannot assess prolonged pain and, based on the population studied, is limited to use in infants 28 weeks and older. Examples of pain scales that have been well studied and tested in neonates, including their application in clinical settings, are shown in Table 8.2. Clinicians should weigh the strengths

Table 8.2 Common neonatal pain scales

Name of scale	Physiologic and behavioral parameters	Population studied	Clinical use	Limitations
Behavioral Indicators of Infant Pain (BIIP) [24]	Sleep/wake state 5 facial actions 2 hand actions	$N = 92$ 24–32 weeks at birth Majority (88 of 100) of assessments performed at 32 weeks' corrected age	Acute procedural pain	Not validated for use with prolonged pain Cannot be readily applied to infants less than 32 weeks' corrected age Does not incorporate readily measured physiologic parameters
Neonatal Facial Coding System (NFCS) [25]	10 discrete facial actions (brow bulge, eye squeeze, nasolabial furrow, open lips, horizontal mouth stretch, vertical mouth stretch, taut tongue, lip purse, chin quiver, tongue protrusion)	$N = 40$ 24–32 weeks at birth Assessed at 32 weeks corrected age	Acute procedural pain	Not validated for use with prolonged pain Does not incorporate readily measured physiologic parameters
Neonatal Pain, Agitation and Sedation Scale (NPASS) [26, 27]	Crying, behavior state, facial expression, extremities/tone, vital signs Also accounts for GA	$N = 42, 46$ 23–42 weeks at birth 0–100 days of age at assessment	Acute procedural pain Chronic/prolonged pain Degree of sedation	
Premature Infant Pain Profile (PIPP) [22, 23, 28]	Behavioral state, brow bulge, eye squeeze, nasolabial furrow, vital sign changes	$N = 43, 238, 24$ 28–40 weeks at birth	Acute procedural pain	Not validated for use with prolonged pain Cannot be readily applied to infants less than 28 weeks' corrected age

and limitations of each scale within their clinical setting and patient population to determine the most appropriate pain scale for use. Regardless of the scale chosen, consistency in its application is critical to monitor and detect pain in neonates.

Like Lacey in the case, neonates cannot provide a self-report of their pain; therefore, assessment of pain by care providers requires both physiologic monitoring and careful observation of the infant's behavioral state. In the NICU, this task is most often carried out by nurses owing to their nearly constant presence at the infant's bedside. Pain assessments are typically carried out as part of routine care, similar to vital sign monitoring. However, adequate assessment of pain requires more than the presence of a care provider at the bedside. To assess pain properly, each clinical team should consider the following:

- Appropriate education of staff on:
  - Recognition of procedures or care practices unique to neonates that can elicit pain (see Table 8.1 for examples)
  - When and how frequently to assess for pain
  - The pain scale(s) chosen for use in their setting, including how to use and interpret
- Consistent use of 1, or at most 2, pain scales that have been validated for use in neonates
- Assessing for inter-rater reliability with the pain scale within their own care setting

Case 8.2
Lacey is now approximately 4 weeks old, is tolerating gavage feedings through a nasogastric tube, and remains intubated and on mechanical ventilation. Heel sticks are performed daily to obtain a sample for blood gas monitoring. She is active and has previously dislodged her endotracheal tube once and nasogastric tube several times. Occasionally Lacey has received an opioid before a procedure, or to "calm her down." While Lacey's mother recognizes that some of the medications Lacey has been given achieved their desired effect, she wants to know if there are different ways to treat Lacey's pain, other than medications.

Consider the following questions:

- *What non-pharmacologic strategies exist to treat pain in neonates?*
- *How and when should these strategies be applied to treating pain in neonates?*
- *Are certain strategies more, or less, appropriate based on the infant's postmenstrual age?*

Non-pharmacologic Pain Management

Non-pharmacologic Interventions

Non-pharmacologic interventions are strategies known to help alleviate mild to moderate pain and discomfort associated with routine procedures and caregiving tasks while supporting the infant's regulatory and coping capabilities. These strategies play an important role when considering the spectrum of pain management in neonates (Fig. 8.2).

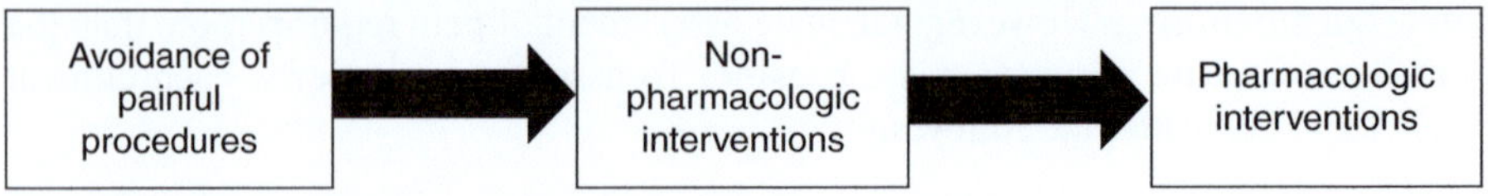

Fig. 8.2 Spectrum of pain management in neonates

Known non-pharmacologic interventions effective in neonates include: facilitated tucking, swaddling, nonnutritive sucking, oral sucrose or glucose, breast milk, breast or bottle feeding, sensorial saturation, and kangaroo care, also known as skin-to-skin care [29–31]. Those interventions best suited to alleviate pain from common procedures are listed in Table 8.3. Additional strategies that can and should be considered when striving to reduce the effects of painful events for neonates are reducing the number of procedures whenever possible, respecting sleep states and minimizing interruptions, clustering care and procedures based on behavioral cues, and reducing environmental sources of stress by lowering light and sound levels [32]. Many of these strategies will be discussed below (for more information about non-pharmacologic soothing techniques, please refer to Chap. 9).

Oral Sucrose or Glucose

Oral sucrose or glucose administered via a pacifier dipped in the solution, and used in combination with other non-pharmacologic strategies, has been well documented to produce an analgesic effect for mild to moderately painful procedures. Research has determined that as little as 0.05–2 ml of sucrose administered in conjunction with using a pacifier for infants as young as 25 weeks' gestational age 2 minutes prior to the procedure can produce optimal pain reduction response that lasts up to 4 minutes [29]. The two-minute interval seems to coincide with endogenous opioid release triggered by the sweet taste of sucrose. Multiple doses administered both before and after the painful procedure was found to be more effective than a single dose [31]. Less-concentrated doses are recommended for preterm infants as higher concentrations (24–33%) are thought to be associated with adverse outcomes such as increased risk of necrotizing enterocolitis [31].

Breastfeeding and Breast Milk

Breastfeeding and the administration of sucrose have been found to be equally effective in preterm infants that possess appropriate oral motor skills. However, sucrose proved to be a more effective analgesia than breast milk over multiple procedures [34]. Expressed breast milk on a pacifier or bottle fed to an infant was found to be less effective at reducing pain than breastfeeding [35]. Guidelines for using breast milk for pain relief mimic those of sucrose in that breastfeeding or administration of expressed milk should be initiated prior to the start of the procedure.

Kangaroo Care and Facilitated Tucking

Kangaroo care initiated 30 minutes prior to a procedure and continued 10 minutes afterward has proven to be an effective strategy for pain relief in preterm

Table 8.3 Non-pharmacologic interventions to relieve pain from common procedures and care tasks in neonates [32]

	Non-pharmacologic intervention[a]						
Procedure/care task	Facilitated tucking/hand containment ≥ 23 weeks	Nonnutritive sucking ≥ 25 weeks	Oral sucrose or breast milk ≥ 25 weeks	Kangaroo care ≥ 29 weeks	Swaddling ≥ 32 weeks	Sensorial saturation ≥ 36 weeks	Breastfeeding ≥ 40 weeks
Heel/finger stick	X	X	X	X	X	X	X
Subcutaneous/intramuscular injection	X	X	X	X	X	X	X
Venipuncture/arterial puncture/PIV placement	X	X	X		X	X	
Adhesive tape/PIV removal	X	X	X	X	X	X	X
Dressing change/wound treatment	X	X	X		X	X	
Central line placement	X	X	X		X	X	
PICC placement	X	X	X		X	X	
Nasal/oral or nasoduodenal gastric tube insertion	X	X			X	X	
Bladder catheter insertion		X	X		X	X	
Lumbar puncture	X	X	X			X	
Chest tube removal	X	X	X			X	
Circumcision		X	X		X	X	
ET tube or nasal/oral suction[b]	X				X		
Retinopathy of prematurity screen		X	X		X		

Adapted from Kenner and McGrath [33]

Physicians, nurses, child life specialists, parents, or virtually any healthcare team member that has patient care contact (e.g., occupational, physical, speech, and respiratory therapists) can be trained to provide the non-pharmacologic interventions discussed in this section. It is important, however, that members of the healthcare team and parents work together whenever possible to support infants during painful procedures, or caregiving tasks, to minimize the pain and maximize infants' coping skills

[a]Gestational age indicates infant's postmenstrual age at the time of the intervention

[b]ET = endotracheal tube

infants [36, 37]. Similarly, facilitated tucking, where the infant is gently held in a flexed and tucked position with one hand on the head and the other on the infant's bottom, has proven beneficial in reducing pain scores in preterm infants experiencing frequent painful procedures, such as endotracheal suctioning, including when facilitated tucking is performed by parents [38, 39] (see Chap. 9, Fig. 9.2, for picture of facilitated tucking).

Sensorial Saturation

Sensorial saturation is the use of taste (sucrose or breast milk offered on a pacifier), touch, talk and visual stimulation (such as a human face) to support the infant before, during, and after a procedure to reduce the effects of the painful event. In combination, these interventions work better than sucrose alone, but are recognized to be more labor intensive [40].

Vibration

The strategy of vibration to manage pain has been adopted for use in both adult and pediatric populations. It is theorized that mechanical vibration modulates peripheral and spinal afferent impulses and that when utilized during a painful procedure can dull or prevent afferent pain impulses from reaching the brain [41]. While there is emerging literature that indicates that the use of mechanical vibration in conjunction with oral sucrose can be an effective non-pharmacologic intervention [41], more research is needed to determine the optimal intervention strategy (age group, length of vibration) and long-term effects of this intervention.

Music Therapy

Music therapy is the use of structured interventions by a board-certified music therapist to provide music with the purpose of meeting a patient's specific medical or psychosocial goals to enhance and/or improve clinical outcomes [42, 43]. A growing body of research indicates that the provision of music therapy not only helps to reduce a neonate's overall irritability, but may also be an effective intervention to help reduce stress and the perception of pain often associated with caregiving tasks or procedures [32, 42, 43]. Studies also indicate that live music facilitated by a board-certified music therapist is often more effective in calming neonates than recorded music and that music therapy was more effective for some neonates when used in conjunction with another non-pharmacologic intervention [32, 42, 44]. However, due to inconsistent methodology and small sample sizes, more rigorous research is needed to determine the true efficacy of music therapy as a non-pharmacologic pain management intervention before it is adopted for routine use [32, 42–44].

Procedures Appropriate for Non-pharmacologic Interventions

Procedures appropriate for non-pharmacologic interventions include heel sticks, finger stick, adhesive removal, dressing change, wound treatment, venipuncture, arterial puncture, subcutaneous injection, intramuscular injection, peripheral IV insertion/removal, central line placement, gastric tube insertion, bladder catheterization, tracheal extubation, lumbar puncture, peripheral arterial line, PICC line placement, circumcision, and chest tube insertion/removal [31]. It is also important to minimize routine care procedures that can cause pain such as endotracheal tube suctioning, nasal and oral suctioning, and nasogastric, orogastric, or nasoduodenal tube placement and identify strategies to mitigate associated pain.

Administration of Non-pharmacologic Interventions

How procedures are performed, when they are performed, and whether or not they are necessary should all be considered part of non-pharmacologic pain management in the NICU. Research has revealed that preterm infants benefit from procedural or caregiving task support before, during, and after the pain-eliciting event until they return to their physiologic and behavioral baseline [32]. It is often the case that two non-pharmacologic interventions offered in tandem produce a greater calming effect than when only one is offered [36]. For most interventions, it is important to have at least two people available for one patient: one to provide the support and one to perform the procedure. The patient should be supported before, during, and after the procedure without interruption.

Providing the most effective, age-appropriate supportive intervention for a painful procedure, or care-giving task, is essential for the infant's overall wellbeing. Table 8.3 provides gestational age-based guidelines for applying non-pharmacologic interventions for preterm and term neonates.

Case 8.3

Lacey is now corrected to 40 weeks' postmenstrual age, is taking nearly all her feeds by mouth, and has weaned off respiratory support. Tomorrow she will be having surgery to repair bilateral inguinal hernias. During rounds you are discussing the options for pharmacologic pain management during surgery, as well as in the postoperative period while Lacey recovers in the NICU.

- *What medications can be used to treat pain in the neonate?*
- *What are the indications, contraindications, and side effects of these medications?*

Pharmacologic Pain Management

In situations that warrant levels of analgesia and/or sedation beyond what non-pharmacologic treatments can provide, pharmacologic treatment is the next step. Although analgesic and sedative medications are prevalent in NICUs across the country, it is important to remember that these treatments are not without their short-term and long-term risks. In order to limit these risks, there are a few principles of pharmacologic treatment that should be followed.

- Use the lowest dose for the shortest duration as possible to achieve the desired effect [45].
- Balance the benefit of the treatment to the potential adverse effects.
- Avoid polypharmacy if possible; optimize treatment with one medication before adding another.

Dosing recommendations and conversions are found in Tables 8.4 and 8.5.

Table 8.4 Dosing recommendations for analgesic medications used in neonates

Medication	Corrected gestational age	Starting dose	Frequency	Maximum dose
Acetaminophen, oral	28–32 weeks[a]	12–15 mg/kg	Every 6, 8, or 12 hours	40 mg/kg/day
	33–37 weeks[a]	12–15 mg/kg	Every 6–8 hours	60 mg/kg/day
	38 weeks and greater [a]	10–15 mg/kg	Every 4–6 hours	75 mg/kg/day
Acetaminophen, IV	28–32 weeks[b]	10 mg/kg 7.5 mg/kg	Every 12 hours Every 8 hours	22.5 mg/kg/day
	32–36 weeks[b]	7.5–10 mg/kg	Every 6–8 hours	40 mg/kg/day
	37 weeks and greater[b]	10 mg/kg	Every 6 hours	50 mg/kg/day
Acetaminophen, rectal	28–32 weeks	12–20 mg/kg	Every 12 hours	40 mg/kg/day
	33–38 weeks	12–20 mg/kg	Every 8 hours	50–60 mg/kg/day
	38 weeks and greater	12–20 mg/kg	Every 6 hours	50–75 mg/kg/day
Fentanyl, IV intermittent	All	0.5–3 mcg/kg	Every 2–4 hours	3 mcg/kg/dose[c]
Fentanyl, IV continuous	All	0.5–2 mcg/kg/hour	Continuous	3 mcg/kg/hour[c]
Gabapentin, PO[d]	23 weeks and greater	5–10 mg/kg	Every 8–24 hours	35 mg/kg/day
Ketamine, IV[d]	Not specified	0.5–2 mg/kg	As needed for procedural sedation	Use minimal amount needed
Morphine, IV intermittent	All	0.05–0.1 mg/kg	Every 4–6 hours	0.2 mg/kg/dose[c]
Morphine, PO intermittent	All	0.08 mg/kg	Every 4–6 hours	0.08 mg/kg/dose[c]
Morphine, IV continuous	All	0.01–0.02 mg/kg/hour	Continuous	0.03 mcg/kg/hour[c]

[a]May load with 20–25 mg/kg once
[b]May load with 20 mg/kg once
[c]May exceed due to tolerance with pharmacy and/or palliative care consultation
[d]Limited data available

Table 8.5 Conversion of continuous opioids to methadone [46]

Fentanyl (mcg/kg/hour)	Morphine (mg/kg/hour)	Enteral methadone (mg/kg/dose)	Intravenous methadone (mg/kg/dose)	Comments
1–2	0.1	0.1	0.05	
3–4	0.2	0.3	0.15	Consider adjuvants
5–6	0.3	0.5	0.25	Consider adjuvants and opioid rotation
7–8	0.4	0.6	0.3	Palliative care consult recommended
9–10	0.5	0.6	0.3	Palliative care consult recommended

Non-opioid Analgesia

Topical Anesthetics

Local anesthetics work by inhibiting ion channels in nerve cells, preventing the pain signal from being transmitted [47]. There are multiple agents and formulations available, with the most common being lidocaine. Topical anesthetics are most commonly used for blood draws, lumbar punctures, or circumcisions. The topical products should be applied for 20–60 minutes before the procedure and tend to last at least 30 minutes depending on the active ingredient/formulation [47]. While these agents have a low side effect profile, due to the nature of the neonatal skin, there is an increased risk of systemic absorption. Although rare, high blood levels of these agents can have serious effects such as arrhythmias, seizures, and other neuropathic symptoms [48]. To decrease the amount of systemic absorption, the smallest amount over the smallest area should be applied.

Acetaminophen

Acetaminophen is a non-opioid analgesic available over the counter and marketed for the treatment of mild to moderate pain and fever [49, 50]. Despite being first marketed in 1953, the exact mechanism of action remains unknown. Although it is thought to inhibit the cyclooxygenase (COX) family of enzymes, it has minimal anti-inflammatory effects. The antipyretic effects are thought to be due to the inhibition of the hypothalamic heat-regulating center [49, 51].

Acetaminophen is metabolized by the liver; however, the mechanism is different in neonates compared to older children and adults [52, 53]. Neonates primarily metabolize acetaminophen via sulfate conjugation, while infants and older children metabolize it by glucuronidation [49, 51, 52]. The difference in metabolism may play a role in protecting neonates against hepatotoxicity, one of the most serious adverse effects of acetaminophen. Hepatotoxicity is due to the buildup of toxic metabolites. The sulfation pathway decreases the likelihood of accumulating toxic metabolites, which in turn decreases the likelihood that toxicity will develop in the neonate [54].

Neonatal pharmacokinetic models have been developed using patients as young as 23 weeks' corrected gestational age. Acetaminophen is thought to have an extended half-life of 7 hours (4–10 hours) in neonates compared to 4 hours in infants [49, 50, 55]. Studies have also shown that the rate of acetaminophen clearance is directly correlated to the patient's weight and less so with gestational age [55]. Minimal gestational age cutoffs and initial dosing recommendations vary depending on the route (Table 8.4). There is debate in the literature whether a loading dose of 20–25 mg/kg is necessary [49, 55, 56]. Pharmacokinetic studies have shown that a loading dose of 20 mg/kg leads to acetaminophen levels of 11 mcg/mL which is within the therapeutic range [55, 57]. Data supporting the safety of a loading dose is, however, limited. Due to the incomplete absorption of the rectal suppositories, doses range from 20 to 30 mg/kg per dose with frequencies similar to the oral formulations [49, 55, 57].

Although acetaminophen is considered a cornerstone of pain management in the pediatric population, its role in neonatal analgesia is not universally agreed upon, with studies showing a wide range of efficacy. Oral acetaminophen was shown to be equally effective as topical lidocaine cream on physical response and facial expressions during heel sticks [58]. However, in two studies comparing acetaminophen to oral sucrose during heel sticks, acetaminophen was found to be inferior when comparing pain scores and showed no difference in crying time or facial actions [50, 55, 57]. Intravenous acetaminophen was shown to be effective in the treatment of moderate pain in neonates, with a lower pain score noted 30 minutes after administration of the first dose [53]. Intravenous acetaminophen given for 48 hours following surgery in neonates and infants was associated with a decrease in the total morphine dose required when compared with the use of morphine alone [59]. This decrease in total morphine exposure was not replicated in patients using rectal acetaminophen, which is thought to be due to the highly variable acetaminophen levels seen with the rectal formulations [55, 60–62].

Generally, acetaminophen is considered to be a safe medication with mild adverse effects. One of the severe adverse effects is hepatotoxicity. Although the risk is lower in neonates, it can still occur due to high doses (both administration errors and elevated doses given for an extended period of time). Hepatotoxicity can also occur when acetaminophen is given in patients with concurrent hepatic dysfunction; however, there is currently no recommended dose adjustment in these patients [49]. Some studies have suggested patients with direct hyperbilirubinemia have decreased drug clearance and therefore should have their doses reduced, intervals extended, or have the medication withheld [55, 56].

Nonsteroidal Anti-Inflammatory Drugs (NSAIDs)

Nonsteroidal anti-inflammatory drugs (NSAIDs) are a class of medications that exhibit analgesic, anti-inflammatory, and antipyretic properties. Common members of this class include aspirin, ibuprofen, indomethacin, and ketorolac among others [53]. While aspirin and indomethacin are used in neonates for thrombosis prophylaxis after cardiac surgery and patent ductus arteriosus (PDA) closure, respectively, they are not currently recommended for the treatment of pain [53].

Ibuprofen and ketorolac are currently approved by the FDA in patients 6 months and older for analgesic purpose [63, 64]. NSAIDs are renally cleared, and in patients under 6 months, that clearance is delayed. This delay in clearance can lead to serious adverse effects such as acute kidney injury and gastrointestinal bleeding [53, 65, 66].

Gabapentin

Gabapentin is an anticonvulsant marketed for the treatment of partial seizures and neuropathic pain; however, over the past few years, its use in neonates has been documented for the treatment of pain and agitation refractory to conventional treatments [67, 68]. Currently, the exact mechanism for effects on neuropathic pain is unknown. Although gabapentin is structurally similar to gamma-aminobutyric acid (GABA), there is currently no evidence to suggest it binds to $GABA_A$ or $GABA_B$ receptors or influences the uptake or release of GABA [69]. Gabapentin's preferred binding sites have been identified in the brain and associated with presynaptic voltage-gated calcium channels. It is thought that the activation of these channels potentiates the release of excitatory neurotransmitters, which would decrease nociception [69, 70].

Pharmacokinetic studies have been performed in patients as young as 1 month; however, there is currently no neonatal dosing available with all doses extrapolated from pediatric data [67, 70, 71]. In pediatric patients, gabapentin has a half-life of 4.7 hours with an onset of action of 2–3 hours. This medication is excreted renally as unchanged drug with the rate of clearance directly proportional to the creatinine clearance [70]. The published literature currently consists of case reports and an observational study that used gabapentin as an adjunct to opioids and benzodiazepines for the treatment of pain and agitation. Doses commonly started around 5 mg/kg every 8–24 hours. Doses were gradually titrated every few days to effect with the maximum dose ranging from 5 to 10 mg/kg every 8–12 hours [67, 68, 70, 71]. One study suggested that preterm infants should be dosed every 8 hours due to their increased clearance [67]. In both term and preterm infants, decreased agitation and irritability was seen in over 70% with many having an effect in the first 72 hours. Some patients were able to be weaned off of opioids and/or benzodiazepines during the course of gabapentin treatment [67, 68]. Three preterm infants were initiated on gabapentin due to feeding intolerance caused by intestinal hyperalgesia. After starting gabapentin, they were all able to tolerate full enteral feedings [67].

Ketamine

Ketamine is a dissociative anesthetic that is used for anesthesia, including procedural sedation, analgesia, and sedation; we will focus on its use as an analgesic and sedative in this section [72]. There is limited evidence for ketamine's use in the neonatal population. Epidemiological studies have suggested children who have received ketamine had higher rates of cognitive delays and learning disabilities [72–74]. Studies have suggested that the neurobehavioral effects are more common with repeat exposures to ketamine. A study of 49 infants less than 24 months of age who were exposed to ketamine for laser surgery showed decreases in mental and psychomotor development in those who had three or more exposures [73, 74]. The American College of Emergency Physicians has deemed patients less than 3 months to be an absolute contraindication for the use of ketamine due to an increased risk of airway complications such as airway obstruction, laryngospasm, and apnea [75].

Opioid Analgesia

Opioids currently have a large role in the treatment of pain in neonates due to the limited options and limited evidence associated with non-opioid agents [56]. However, over the past few years, minimizing opioids in this population has been encouraged due to the potential long-term negative effects on the developing brain (see next section). Despite these concerns, opioids still have a role in neonatal pain management.

Opioid analgesics work by binding to the endogenous opioid receptors. Opioid receptors are distributed throughout the body, with high levels concentrated in the central nervous system, peripheral nervous system, and gastrointestinal track [76]. There are three main opioid receptors: mu, kappa, and delta. Mu receptors are primarily responsible for pain signal transmission, and in the neonate these receptors have the affinity and distribution similar to that of an adult [76, 77]. The activation of opioid receptors inhibits the formation of adenyl cyclase and ultimately cyclic AMP, and this lack of cyclic AMP prevents the transmission of the pain response. However, the longer the receptors are stimulated, the number of receptors is thought to increase and the level of inhibition of adenyl cyclase decreases which leads to opioid tolerance. The decreased inhibition of adenyl cyclase can be overcome by increasing the dose of opioid or potentially switching agents [76, 77].

Opioids as a class have a wide range of adverse effects that vary in severity. Adverse effects include sedation, constipation, urinary retention, hypotension, and respiratory depression [56, 78–80]. Although most adverse effects will decrease in severity over time, constipation will not improve and may require pharmaceutical intervention to correct. Respiratory depression/apnea is an indication of high levels of circulating opioids. Depending on the severity, decreasing or holding the dose may be enough to reverse this effect. In cases of severe respiratory depression, the opioid antagonist naloxone may be required [56, 81].

While there are many different opioids available today, this section will focus on the three most utilized and most studied in neonates: morphine, fentanyl, and methadone. Please refer to Table 8.4 for medication-specific dosing regimens. Of note, higher doses than those listed may be required in patients with a prolonged exposure to opioids due to tolerance [78, 79].

Morphine

Morphine is an opioid agonist and one of the more studied opioids in the neonatal population. Pharmacokinetic models have been developed in neonates as young as 23 weeks' gestation. Studies demonstrate that morphine clearance increases with age which is represented in the ranges of drug half-life seen across varying gestational ages. Premature infants have an extended half-life of 10–20 hours, while term neonates have an average half-life of 7.5 hours [57, 61, 82, 83]. Regardless of age, morphine has an onset of action of 5–10 minutes for IV and 30 minutes for oral formulations.

Morphine is primarily metabolized by the liver to active metabolites which are excreted in the urine. In patients with renal dysfunction, the active metabolites can accumulate and lead to respiratory depression and hypotension [83]. Although there are no specific recommendations for renal dosing in neonates, caution should be used in patients with any renal dysfunction; a dose reduction or using a different agent should be considered [45].

Due to the decreased absorption of oral morphine, oral doses are usually two to three times higher than those given intravenously [82, 83]. Intravenous/intramuscular morphine doses range from 0.05 to 0.1 mg/kg/dose with frequencies ranging from every 4 to 8 hours, while oral morphine dosing begins at 0.08 mg/kg/dose every 4–6 hours. Continuous infusions typically begin at 0.01 mg/kg/hour and are titrated to effect. The maximum recommended dose is 0.03 mg/kg/hour; however, higher doses have been reported due to tolerance [83, 84] (see Table 8.4).

Fentanyl

Fentanyl is a synthetic opioid and approximately 100 times more potent than morphine. There are a few studies examining the pharmacokinetics of fentanyl in neonates, with one study showing that during continuous infusions of fentanyl, clearance decreased as postnatal age increased. The half-life of fentanyl varies but is considered to be under 2 hours, and the duration of action of a bolus dose is between 30 minutes and 1 hour [79, 85]. Fentanyl is primarily metabolized hepatically to inactive metabolites. Due to fentanyl being metabolized to inactive compounds, it is considered one of the safer opioids to use in patients with renal dysfunction since there is minimal concern for accumulation [79, 85].

Fentanyl comes in a variety of formulations; however, only injectable fentanyl is recommended for use in neonates. Typical intermittent dosing ranges from 1 to 2 mcg/kg every 1–4 hours. Due to the short duration of action of fentanyl, frequent intermittent doses may be needed for adequate pain control. Dosing for continuous infusions typically range from 1 to 5 mcg/kg/hour with ranges up to 20 mcg/kg/hour reported in special circumstances (i.e., ECMO) [79, 85].

One of the major safety concerns associated with fentanyl is chest wall rigidity. This phenomenon has been reported in all age groups but may be more pronounced in younger children. In neonates, the incidence of chest wall rigidity has been reported to be as high as 9% [79, 86]. While the exact cause of this is unknown, it is thought to be due to the highly lipophilic nature of fentanyl and its effect on the central nervous system. Currently, there is no universally agreed upon method to prevent chest wall rigidity from occurring, but some institutions administer intermittent doses over a prolonged period of time, while others dilute the fentanyl to lower concentrations [79, 86].

Methadone

Methadone is a long-acting, synthetic opioid that is commonly used in the treatment of chronic pain and treating neonatal abstinence syndrome [77, 87]. Pharmacokinetic studies have been performed in neonates with a PMA of more than 33 weeks. It is estimated that the half-life of methadone in neonates is similar to that of older children, with a range of 12–20 hours [87–89]. Due to the long half-life, some institutions will dose methadone more frequently in the first 24–72 hours of treatment in order to achieve steady state faster. Methadone is primarily metabolized hepatically to inactive metabolites. It is primarily eliminated by the kidney with up to 10% being unchanged drug; caution should be used in patients with renal dysfunction as accumulation may occur [87, 89].

Methadone is currently available in injectable and oral formulations. The doses of oral formulations are generally double the injectable formulations due to variable oral absorption [87]. Most often methadone is dosed every 6 hours for the first several days to allow drug levels to reach steady state. Once a stable regimen has been reached, the dosing frequency will typically be decreased to every 8 hours with further tapering dependent on the indication.

One of the biggest controversies surrounding methadone is initial dosing, particularly when its use is to allow conversion from a continuous opioid infusion (e.g., morphine) to an oral opioid formulation (methadone) in the setting of chronic opioid use. Multiple methods and equations exist for this conversion and may vary by the institution (Table 8.5) [87, 90]. It is important to note that all opioid conversions are estimations of equivalency and may not be appropriate for all patients.

Risks of Opioid Exposure in Neonates

As previously mentioned, opioids are the most common pharmacologic agents used to treat pain in the NICU. While effective in alleviating pain, they are not without risks. In addition to the short-term adverse effects noted in the prior section, it is important to understand potential long-term effects following exposure to these medications during a critical window of brain development. The potential for opioids to alter brain structure and function, particularly when exposure occurs during early periods of growth and development, has been suggested by both animal and human studies. Indeed, a growing body of evidence raises concern regarding the potential long-lasting effects these medications have in neonates.

Both morphine and fentanyl act on the mu, kappa, and delta opioid receptors, which are present early in the developing brain [91]. Activation of these receptors results in analgesic effects, but is also associated with modulating effects on proliferation, differentiation, and survival of various neuronal cells such as neurons, glia, and stem cells [78, 92]. Rats exposed to opioids during the prenatal and early postnatal periods demonstrate decreased brain volumes and dendritic growth, as well as learning deficits and impaired motor function [93–95]. Certain regions of the brain, such as the cortex and amygdala, appear more susceptible to the detrimental effects of morphine [96]. Apoptosis of human fetal neurons and microglia occurred

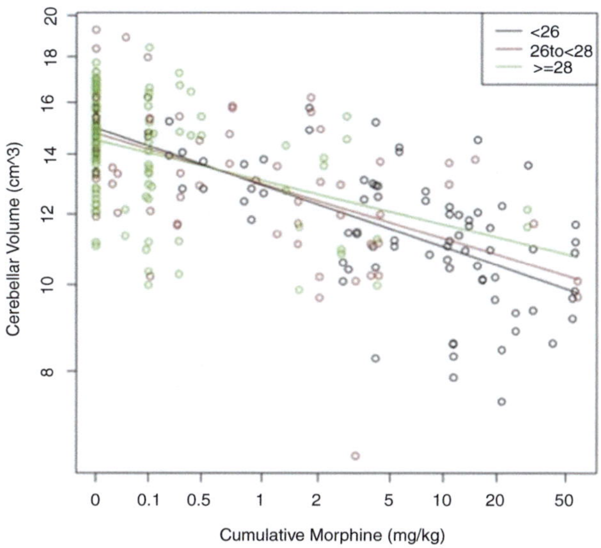

Fig. 8.3 Relationship between cerebellar volumes and morphine exposure stratified by gestational age at birth: < 26 weeks (black), 26 to <28 weeks (red), and ≥ 28 weeks (green) [99]. (Reprinted from the Zwicker et al. [99], © 2016, with permission from Elsevier)

following exposure to morphine in vitro, with escalating doses of morphine resulting in more cell death [97]. In two large randomized controlled trials, the rates of a composite outcome of intraventricular hemorrhage, periventricular leukomalacia, or death were not significantly different in ventilated neonates receiving either a continuous morphine infusion or placebo early in life, suggesting a lack of benefit when used preemptively to treat presumed pain [84, 98]. In a prospective study of 136 preterm infants evaluated at term with MRI, a significant inverse correlation was noted with cerebellar volume and cumulative morphine exposure; a ten-fold increase in morphine exposure was associated with a 5.5% decrease in cerebellar volume (Fig. 8.3) [99].

In preterm neonates, morphine exposure predicts poorer motor and cognitive scores at 18 months' corrected age and is associated with lower visual analysis sub test scores on IQ assessment at 5 years of age [99, 100]. Altogether, these data raise concerns regarding lifelong consequences of opioid exposure in the neonatal period and suggests that a thoughtful approach that weighs benefits and risks is imperative when prescribing opioids in this setting.

Conclusions

It is clear that infants, including those born preterm, have the ability to experience pain, and thus pain assessment is a vital component of their care. Though painful experiences contribute to altered brain development and function, it is not yet clear that treatment of pain eliminates or mitigates this effect. Moreover, common medications used to treat pain, such as opioids, also have potential detrimental effects on the developing brain and thus should be used with caution. Efforts to reduce or altogether avoid painful procedures in neonates are encouraged. When pain is unavoidable, optimizing the use of non-pharmacologic measures to treat pain should be sought and pharmacologic therapy added when deemed necessary by the clinician. Consulting a pharmacist or other specialist in pain management (e.g., palliative care physician, anesthesiologist) can be helpful when pharmacologic therapy is necessary. More research is needed to better understand the interplay between painful experiences and interventions for pain on critical windows of brain development to optimize outcomes. In all infants who are actively dying or receiving a comfort-oriented approach to care for a life-limiting condition, pain and symptom management is standard of care and the infant's comfort supersedes any long-term concerns.

References

1. Lippmann M, Nelson RJ, Emmanouilides GC, Diskin J, Thibeault DW. Ligation of patent ductus arteriosus in premature infants. Br J Anaesth. 1976;48(4):365–9.
2. Anand KJ, Hickey PR. Pain and its effects in the human neonate and fetus. N Engl J Med. 1987;317(21):1321–9.
3. Garland EL. Pain processing in the human nervous system: a selective review of nociceptive and biobehavioral pathways. Prim Care. 2012;39(3):561–71.
4. Humphrey T. Embryology of the central nervous system: with some correlations with functional development. Ala J Med Sci. 1964;1:60–4.
5. Okado N. Onset of synapse formation in the human spinal cord. J Comp Neurol. 1981;201(2):211–9.
6. Rakic P, Goldman-Rakic PS. The development and modifiability of the cerebral cortex. Overview. Neurosci Res Program Bull. 1982;20(4):433–8.
7. Slater R, Cantarella A, Gallella S, Worley A, Boyd S, Meek J, et al. Cortical pain responses in human infants. J Neurosci. 2006;26(14):3662–6.
8. Grunau RE, Holsti L, Haley DW, Oberlander T, Weinberg J, Solimano A, et al. Neonatal procedural pain exposure predicts lower cortisol and behavioral reactivity in preterm infants in the NICU. Pain. 2005;113(3):293–300.
9. Fitzgerald M. The development of nociceptive circuits. Nat Rev Neurosci. 2005;6(7):507–20.
10. Holsti L, Grunau RE, Oberlander TF, Whitfield MF. Prior pain induces heightened motor responses during clustered care in preterm infants in the NICU. Early Hum Dev. 2005;81(3):293–302.
11. Taddio A, Shah V, Gilbert-MacLeod C, Katz J. Conditioning and hyperalgesia in newborns exposed to repeated heel lances. JAMA. 2002;288(7):857–61.
12. Carbajal R, Rousset A, Danan C, Coquery S, Nolent P, Ducrocq S, et al. Epidemiology and treatment of painful procedures in neonates in intensive care units. JAMA. 2008;300(1):60–70.
13. Simons SH, van Dijk M, Anand KS, Roofthooft D, van Lingen RA, Tibboel D. Do we still hurt newborn babies? A prospective study of procedural pain and analgesia in neonates. Arch Pediatr Adolesc Med. 2003;157(11):1058–64.
14. Kesavan K. Neurodevelopmental implications of neonatal pain and morphine exposure. Pediatr Ann. 2015;44(11):e260–4.
15. Brummelte S, Grunau RE, Chau V, Poskitt KJ, Brant R, Vinall J, et al. Procedural pain and brain development in premature newborns. Ann Neurol. 2012;71(3):385–96.
16. Ranger M, Chau CM, Garg A, Woodward TS, Beg MF, Bjornson B, et al. Neonatal pain-related stress predicts cortical thickness at age 7 years in children born very preterm. PLoS One. 2013;8(10):e76702.

17. Hohmeister J, Kroll A, Wollgarten-Hadamek I, Zohsel K, Demirakca S, Flor H, et al. Cerebral processing of pain in school-aged children with neonatal nociceptive input: an exploratory fMRI study. Pain. 2010;150(2):257–67.
18. Grunau RE, Whitfield MF, Petrie-Thomas J, Synnes AR, Cepeda IL, Keidar A, et al. Neonatal pain, parenting stress and interaction, in relation to cognitive and motor development at 8 and 18 months in preterm infants. Pain. 2009;143(1–2):138–46.
19. Doesburg SM, Chau CM, Cheung TP, Moiseev A, Ribary U, Herdman AT, et al. Neonatal pain-related stress, functional cortical activity and visual-perceptual abilities in school-age children born at extremely low gestational age. Pain. 2013;154(10):1946–52.
20. Ranger M, Synnes AR, Vinall J, Grunau RE. Internalizing behaviours in school-age children born very preterm are predicted by neonatal pain and morphine exposure. Eur J Pain. 2014;18(6):844–52.
21. Vinall J, Miller SP, Synnes AR, Grunau RE. Parent behaviors moderate the relationship between neonatal pain and internalizing behaviors at 18 months corrected age in children born very prematurely. Pain. 2013;154(9):1831–9.
22. Ballantyne M, Stevens B, McAllister M, Dionne K, Jack A. Validation of the premature infant pain profile in the clinical setting. Clin J Pain. 1999;15(4):297–303.
23. Stevens B, Johnston C, Petryshen P, Taddio A. Premature infant pain profile: development and initial validation. Clin J Pain. 1996;12(1):13–22.
24. Holsti L, Grunau RE. Initial validation of the behavioral indicators of infant pain (BIIP). Pain. 2007;132(3):264–72.
25. Grunau RE, Oberlander T, Holsti L, Whitfield MF. Bedside application of the neonatal facial coding system in pain assessment of premature neonates. Pain. 1998;76(3):277–86.
26. Hummel P, Lawlor-Klean P, Weiss MG. Validity and reliability of the N-PASS assessment tool with acute pain. J Perinatol. 2010;30(7):474–8.
27. Hummel P, Puchalski M, Creech SD, Weiss MG. Clinical reliability and validity of the N-PASS: neonatal pain, agitation and sedation scale with prolonged pain. J Perinatol. 2008;28(1):55–60.
28. Jonsdottir RB, Kristjansdottir G. The sensitivity of the premature infant pain profile – PIPP to measure pain in hospitalized neonates. J Eval Clin Pract. 2005;11(6):598–605.
29. Committee On F, Newborn, Section On A, Pain M. Prevention and management of procedural pain in the neonate: an update. Pediatrics. 2016;137(2):e20154271.
30. Lago P, Garetti E, Bellieni CV, Merazzi D, Savant Levet P, Ancora G, et al. Systematic review of nonpharmacological analgesic interventions for common needle-related procedure in newborn infants and development of evidence-based clinical guidelines. Acta Paediatr. 2017;106(6):864–70.
31. Witt N, Coynor S, Edwards C, Bradshaw H. A guide to pain assessment and management in the neonate. Curr Emerg Hosp Med Rep. 2016;4:1–10.
32. Kenner C, McGrath J. Developmental care of newborns and infants: a guide for health professionals. 2nd ed. Glenview, IL: National Association of Neonatal Nurses; 2010.
33. Kenner C, McGrath JM, editors. Developmental care of newborns & infants: a guide for health professionals. St. Louis, MO: Mosby; 2004.
34. Benoit B, Martin-Misener R, Latimer M, Campbell-Yeo M. Breast-feeding analgesia in infants: an update on the current state of evidence. J Perinat Neonatal Nurs. 2017;31(2):145–59.
35. Shah PS, Aliwalas LI, Shah V. Breastfeeding or breast milk for procedural pain in neonates. Cochrane Database Syst Rev. 2006;3:CD004950.
36. Hartley KA, Miller CS, Gephart SM. Facilitated tucking to reduce pain in neonates: evidence for best practice. Adv Neonatal Care. 2015;15(3):201–8.
37. Akcan E, Yigit R, Atici A. The effect of kangaroo care on pain in premature infants during invasive procedures. Turk J Pediatr. 2009;51(1):14–8.
38. Alinejad-Naeini M, Mohagheghi P, Peyrovi H, Mehran A. The effect of facilitated tucking during endotracheal suctioning on procedural pain in preterm neonates: a randomized controlled crossover study. Glob J Health Sci. 2014;6(4):278–84.

39. Axelin A, Salantera S, Lehtonen L. 'Facilitated tucking by parents' in pain management of preterm infants-a randomized crossover trial. Early Hum Dev. 2006;82(4):241–7.
40. Bellieni CV, Tei M, Coccina F, Buonocore G. Sensorial saturation for infants' pain. J Matern Fetal Neonatal Med. 2012;25(Suppl 1):79–81.
41. McGinnis K, Murray E, Cherven B, McCracken C, Travers C. Effect of vibration on pain response to heel lance: a pilot randomized control trial. Adv Neonatal Care. 2016;16(6):439–48.
42. Anderson DE, Patel AD. Infants born preterm, stress, and neurodevelopment in the neonatal intensive care unit: might music have an impact? Dev Med Child Neurol. 2018;60(3):256–66.
43. Gooding L. Using music therapy protocols in the treatment of premature infants: an introduction to current practices. Arts Psychother. 2010;37:211–4.
44. van der Heijden MJ, Oliai Araghi S, Jeekel J, Reiss IK, Hunink MG, van Dijk M. Do hospitalized premature infants benefit from music interventions? A systematic review of randomized controlled trials. PLoS One. 2016;11(9):e0161848.
45. De Lima J, Carmo KB. Practical pain management in the neonate. Best Pract Res Clin Anaesthesiol. 2010;24(3):291–307.
46. Robertson RC, Darsey E, Fortenberry JD, Pettignano R, Hartley G. Evaluation of an opiate-weaning protocol using methadone in pediatric intensive care unit patients. Pediatr Crit Care Med. 2000;1(2):119–23.
47. Zempsky WT. Pharmacologic approaches for reducing venous access pain in children. Pediatrics. 2008;122(Suppl 3):S140–53.
48. Gunter JB. Benefit and risks of local anesthetics in infants and children. Paediatr Drugs. 2002;4(10):649–72.
49. Lexi-Comp Online. Acetaminophen (Pediatric and neonatal lexi-drugs). Hudson, Ohio; 2018. Updated 21 May 2018.
50. Ohlsson A, Shah PS. Paracetamol (acetaminophen) for prevention or treatment of pain in newborns. Cochrane Database Syst Rev. 2016;10:CD011219.
51. Graham GG, Scott KF. Mechanism of action of paracetamol. Am J Ther. 2005;12(1):46–55.
52. Cook SF, Stockmann C, Samiee-Zafarghandy S, King AD, Deutsch N, Williams EF, et al. Neonatal maturation of paracetamol (acetaminophen) glucuronidation, sulfation, and oxidation based on a parent-metabolite population pharmacokinetic model. Clin Pharmacokinet. 2016;55(11):1395–411.
53. Jacqz-Aigrain E, Anderson BJ. Pain control: non-steroidal anti-inflammatory agents. Semin Fetal Neonatal Med. 2006;11(4):251–9.
54. Yoon E, Babar A, Choudhary M, Kutner M, Pyrsopoulos N. Acetaminophen-induced hepatotoxicity: a comprehensive update. J Clin Transl Hepatol. 2016;4(2):131–42.
55. Pacifici GM, Allegaert K. Clinical pharmacology of paracetamol in neonates: a review. Curr Ther Res Clin Exp. 2015;77:24–30.
56. Walker SM. Neonatal pain. Paediatr Anaesth. 2014;24(1):39–48.
57. Allegaert K, Tibboel D, van den Anker J. Pharmacological treatment of neonatal pain: in search of a new equipoise. Semin Fetal Neonatal Med. 2013;18(1):42–7.
58. Shah V, Taddio A, Ohlsson A. Randomized controlled trial of paracetamol for heel prick pain in neonates. Arch Dis Child Fetal Neonatal Ed. 1998;79:F209–F11.
59. Ceelie I, de Wildt SN, van Dijk M, van den Berg MM, van den Bosch GE, Duivenvoorden HJ, et al. Effect of intravenous paracetamol on postoperative morphine requirements in neonates and infants undergoing major noncardiac surgery: a randomized controlled trial. JAMA. 2013;309(2):149–54.
60. Harma A, Aikio O, Hallman M, Saarela T. Intravenous paracetamol decreases requirements of morphine in very preterm infants. J Pediatr. 2016;168:36–40.
61. van den Anker JN, Allegaert K. Treating pain in preterm infants: moving from opioids to acetaminophen. J Pediatr. 2016;168:13–5.
62. van der Marel CD, Peters JW, Bouwmeester NJ, Jacqz-Aigrain E, van den Anker JN, Tibboel D. Rectal acetaminophen does not reduce morphine consumption after major surgery in young infants. Br J Anaesth. 2007;98(3):372–9.

63. Lexi-Comp Online. Ibuprofen (Pediatric and neonatal lexi-drugs). Hudson, Ohio; 2018. Updated 18 May 2018.
64. Lexi-Comp Online. Ketorolac (Pediatric and neonatal lexi-drugs). Hudson, Ohio; 2018. Updated 22 May 2018.
65. Aranda JV, Salomone F, Valencia GB, Beharry KD. Non-steroidal anti-inflammatory drugs in newborns and infants. Pediatr Clin N Am. 2017;64(6):1327–40.
66. Ohlsson A, Walia R, Shah SS. Ibuprofen for the treatment of patent ductus arteriosus in preterm or low birth weight (or both) infants. Cochrane Database Syst Rev. 2015;(2):CD003481.
67. Edwards L, DeMeo S, Hornik CD, Cotten CM, Smith PB, Pizoli C, et al. Gabapentin use in the neonatal intensive care unit. J Pediatr. 2016;169:310–2.
68. Sacha GLFM, Kyllonen K, Rodriguez RJ. The use of gabapentin for pain and agitation in neonates and infants in a neonatal ICU. J Pediatr Pharmacol Ther. 2017;22(3):201–11.
69. Kukkar A, Bali A, Singh N, Jaggi AS. Implications and mechanism of action of gabapentin in neuropathic pain. Arch Pharm Res. 2013;36(3):237–51.
70. Lexi-Comp Online. Gabapentin (Pediatric and neonatal lexi-drugs). Hudson, Ohio; 2018. Updated 21 May 2018.
71. Ouellet D, Bockbrader HN, Wesche DL, Shapiro DY, Garofalo E. Population pharmacokinetics of gabapentin in infants and children. Epilepsy Res. 2001;47:229–41.
72. Lexi-Comp Online. Ketamine (Pediatric and neonatal lexi-drugs). Hudson, Ohio; 2018. Updated 21 May 2018.
73. Bhutta AT. Ketamine: a controversial drug for neonates. Semin Perinatol. 2007;31(5):303–8.
74. Hall RW, Shbarou RM. Drugs of choice for sedation and analgesia in the neonatal ICU. Clin Perinatol. 2009;36(2):215–26, vii
75. Green SM, Roback MG, Kennedy RM, Krauss B. Clinical practice guideline for emergency department ketamine dissociative sedation: 2011 update. Ann Emerg Med. 2011;57(5):449–61.
76. Kocherlakota P. Neonatal abstinence syndrome. Pediatrics. 2014;134(2):e547–61.
77. McQueen K, Murphy-Oikonen J. Neonatal abstinence syndrome. N Engl J Med. 2016;375(25):2468–79.
78. Durrmeyer X, Vutskits L, Anand KJ, Rimensberger PC. Use of analagesic and sedative drugs in the NICU: integrating clinical trials and laboratory data. Pediatr Res. 2010;67(2):117–27.
79. Pacifici GM. Clinical pharmacology of fentanyl in preterm infants. A review. Pediatr Neonatol. 2015;56(3):143–8.
80. Terrie YC. An overview of opioids. [Internet]. Cranbury, NJ: Pharmacy Times; 2011 [Cited 12 Nov 2018]. Available from https://www.pharmacytimes.com/publications/issue/2011/june2011/an-overview-of-opioids
81. Maitra S, Baidya DK, Khanna P, Ray BR, Panda SS, Bajpai M. Acute perioperative pain in neonates: an evidence-based review of neurophysiology and management. Acta Anaesthesiol Taiwanica. 2014;52(1):30–7.
82. Anand KJ, Anderson BJ, Holford NH, Hall RW, Young T, Shephard B, et al. Morphine pharmacokinetics and pharmacodynamics in preterm and term neonates: secondary results from the NEOPAIN trial. Br J Anaesth. 2008;101(5):680–9.
83. Lexi-Comp Online. Morphine (Pediatric and neonatal lexi-drugs). Hudson, Ohio; 2018. Updated 11 May 2018.
84. Anand KJS, Hall RW, Desai N, Shephard B, Bergqvist LL, Young TE, et al. Effects of morphine analgesia in ventilated preterm neonates: primary outcomes from the NEOPAIN randomised trial. Lancet. 2004;363(9422):1673–82.
85. Lexi-Comp Online. Fentanyl (Pediatric and neonatal lexi-Drugs). Hudson, Ohio; 2018. Updated 21 May 2018.
86. Coruh B, Tonelli MR, Park DR. Fentanyl-induced chest wall rigidity. Chest. 2013;143(4):1145–6.
87. Lexi-Comp Online. Methadone (Pediatric and neonatal lexi-drugs). Hudson, Ohio; 2018. Updated 12 May 2018.

88. Ward RM, Drover DR, Hammer GB, Stemland CJ, Kern S, Tristani-Firouzi M, et al. The pharmacokinetics of methadone and its metabolites in neonates, infants, and children. Paediatr Anaesth. 2014;24(6):591–601.
89. Wiles JR, Isemann B, Mizuno T, Tabangin ME, Ward LP, Akinbi H, et al. Pharmacokinetics of oral methadone in the treatment of neonatal abstinence syndrome: a pilot study. J Pediatr. 2015;167(6):1214–20. e3.
90. Hudak ML, Tan RC, Committee On D, Committee On F, Newborn, American Academy of P. Neonatal drug withdrawal. Pediatrics. 2012;129(2):e540–60.
91. Zhu Y, Hsu MS, Pintar JE. Developmental expression of the mu, kappa, and delta opioid receptor mRNAs in mouse. J Neurosci. 1998;18(7):2538–49.
92. Tegeder I, Geisslinger G. Opioids as modulators of cell death and survival--unraveling mechanisms and revealing new indications. Pharmacol Rev. 2004;56(3):351–69.
93. Seatriz JV, Hammer RP Jr. Effects of opiates on neuronal development in the rat cerebral cortex. Brain Res Bull. 1993;30(5–6):523–7.
94. Zagon IS, McLaughlin PJ. Motor activity and learning ability in rats perinatally exposed to methadone. NIDA Res Monogr. 1979;27:121–7.
95. Zagon IS, McLaughlin PJ, Thompson CI. Learning ability in adult female rats perinatally exposed to methadone. Pharmacol Biochem Behav. 1979;10(6):889–94.
96. Bajic D, Commons KG, Soriano SG. Morphine-enhanced apoptosis in selective brain regions of neonatal rats. Int J Dev Neurosci. 2013;31(4):258–66.
97. Hu S, Sheng WS, Lokensgard JR, Peterson PK. Morphine induces apoptosis of human microglia and neurons. Neuropharmacology. 2002;42(6):829–36.
98. Simons SH, van Dijk M, van Lingen RA, Roofthooft D, Duivenvoorden HJ, Jongeneel N, et al. Routine morphine infusion in preterm newborns who received ventilatory support: a randomized controlled trial. JAMA. 2003;290(18):2419–27.
99. Zwicker JG, Miller SP, Grunau RE, Chau V, Brant R, Studholme C, et al. Smaller cerebellar growth and poorer neurodevelopmental outcomes in very preterm infants exposed to neonatal morphine. J Pediatr 2016;172:81–7 e2.
100. de Graaf J, van Lingen RA, Simons SH, Anand KJ, Duivenvoorden HJ, Weisglas-Kuperus N, et al. Long-term effects of routine morphine infusion in mechanically ventilated neonates on children's functioning: five-year follow-up of a randomized controlled trial. Pain. 2011;152(6):1391–7.

9 Non-pain Symptom Management

Patrick Hopkins, Jonna Marret, Rhonda Rusinko, Andrew S. Decker, and Rita Dadiz

Abbreviations

COX	Cyclooxygenase
GABA	Gamma-aminobutyric acid
LLFND	Life-limiting fetal or neonatal disorder
LTFD	Life-threatening fetal disorder
NICU	Neonatal intensive care unit
NMDA	N-Methyl-D-aspartate
NSAID	Nonsteroidal anti-inflammatory drug

What Are "Non-pain" Symptoms?

Infants who have life-limiting fetal or neonatal conditions (LLFNCs) such as prenatally diagnosed conditions, extreme prematurity, or other neonatal conditions often experience multiple types of symptoms that impact their comfort and emotional state. As discussed in Chap. 8, nociceptive pain describes the unpleasant sensations

P. Hopkins · R. Rusinko · R. Dadiz (✉)
Golisano Children's Hospital, University of Rochester Medical Center, Department of Pediatrics, Rochester, NY, USA
e-mail: rita_dadiz@urmc.rochester.edu

J. Marret
Golisano Children's Hospital, University of Rochester Medical Center, Department of Pediatrics, Rochester, NY, USA

Baptist Healthcare Systems, Little Rock, AR, USA

A. S. Decker
Department of Pharmacy, University of Rochester Medical Center, Golisano Children's Hospital, Rochester, NY, USA

E. M. Denney-Koelsch, D. Côté-Arsenault (eds.), *Perinatal Palliative Care*,
https://doi.org/10.1007/978-3-030-34751-2_9

that results from the stimulation of nerves when injury or an inflammatory process occurs in the body [1]. However, infants may also experience discomfort, agitation, stress, and distress due to symptoms that may or may not be a result of nociceptive pain. These symptoms are not typically caused by injury and may include: respiratory distress, hunger, vomiting, diarrhea, constipation, overstimulation or sleep disturbances, fever, and delirium. In many situations, distinguishing between pain and "non-pain" symptoms can be difficult, because the physiologic and behavioral responses that infants exhibit in response to distress of any kind may manifest in a similar fashion. In addition, infants' state of comfort may be conceptualized as a spectrum of experiences, with complete comfort and the absence of pain on one end, suffering from pain or other causes on the opposite end, and varying degrees of discomfort and distress in between the two extremes. In this chapter, the authors will focus discussion on the causes of "non-pain" symptoms (as defined above), their clinical presentation, and general concepts of assessment and management.

Case 9.1, Part 1

You have been caring for Chase, a 1-month-old male infant who was born at 23 weeks' gestational age with a birth weight of 480 grams. He was delivered via *emergency cesarean section due to placental abruption and non-reassuring fetal heart tracings. After birth, he required cardiopulmonary resuscitation that included positive pressure ventilation, chest compressions, epinephrine, and a blood transfusion. His Apgar scores were 1, 3, and 6 at 1, 5, and 10 minutes of age, respectively.*

During his first week of life, Chase had an unstable course in the neonatal intensive care unit. He required surfactant and significant ventilatory support for respiratory distress syndrome. He also received intravenous fluid boluses, dopamine, and hydrocortisone to treat hypovolemic shock. After the first week, his blood pressures normalized, and he began to receive breast milk feeds via a nasogastric tube. At 1 month of age, Chase remains on mechanical ventilation because of significant lung disease. He has several bradycardia and desaturation episodes on a daily basis. Chase also has feeding intolerance, with periods of abdominal distention and spitting that are associated with dilated intestinal bowel loops on abdominal radiographs. During these occasions, his feeds are held until he improves.

While taking care of Chase today, you feel that he seems more irritable than usual. Based on Chase's current medical history:

1. *What may be potential causes of his irritability?*
2. *How may you differentiate between pain and discomfort symptoms?*

Assessment of Non-pain Symptoms

The assessment of symptoms that cause discomfort and distress follows similar concepts as for nociceptive pain. Because infants are unable to use words to communicate the symptoms they are experiencing, caregivers and healthcare professionals must be cognizant of the types of behaviors that infants may exhibit to better assess their states of comfort. Research to better characterize and understand infants' perception and response to pain are ongoing. Unfortunately, studies on infant pain show that caregivers and healthcare professionals underestimate the degree of pain that infants experience, because pain has an emotional component that is hard to quantify [2, 3]. Infants who are not stressed (as noted by normal cortisol and catecholamine levels) experience pain that correlates with an increase in brain activity and changes in facial expressions. In contrast, in infants who are stressed (with an increase in cortisol and catecholamine levels), there is a greater increase in brain activity without a similar degree of change in the infants' behavioral response, indicating that stressed infants may not show outward signs of distress and need more careful monitoring [2–5]. In addition, when compared with term infants, preterm infants have a lower pain threshold and appear to be more sensitive to sensory stimulation, which may further accentuate pain-related stress [2, 3, 6].

These cited studies underscore the importance of monitoring infants' discomfort levels along the comfort-to-pain spectrum. Inadequate symptom management often results from a decreased awareness of underlying conditions that may cause infant discomfort and pain and misunderstanding of what infants are able to perceive, along with a decreased appreciation for the importance of promoting infant comfort [4]. With awareness, caregivers and healthcare professionals are better informed to perform proper assessments to guide environmental, non-pharmacologic, and/or pharmacologic interventions to mitigate or alleviate symptoms.

The use of validated tools to assess symptoms that cause distress and discomfort are extrapolated from the pain literature. While there is no recommended universal approach to pain assessment, the American Academy of Pediatrics advocates the use of pain scales to monitor pain [7]. These pain scales have varying degrees of clinical sensitivity, and one scale, NPASS, is appropriate for assessing infant agitation and sedation (see Chap. 8, Table 8.2). These pain scales assess for behavioral responses (e.g., changes in facial expressions, muscle tone, consolability), with or without the assessment of physiologic responses (e.g., changes in the heart rate and blood pressure) [7, 8]. Among behavioral indices, changes in facial expression are the most reliable [9–11]. Pain scales that use a combination of physiologic and behavioral assessments may better estimate infant pain and non-pain symptoms.

Discussion of Case 9.1 Part 1

For Chase, his irritability is caused by many factors related to his chronic lung disease and feeding intolerance. He likely experiences discomfort from mechanical ventilation, with an endotracheal tube in place and the need for intermittent oropharyngeal and tracheal suctioning to clear secretions. Because he is intubated and connected via tubing to a ventilator, healthcare professionals and caregivers may not be able to hold and/or place him into different positions easily. In addition, it may be difficult to clothe or swaddle him with a blanket, because healthcare professionals may want the ability to readily assess him for any signs of respiratory distress. Chase's feeding intolerance, manifested by vomiting, abdominal gaseous distention, and periods of feeds being held, is another source of irritability, with discomfort, pain, and the sensation of hunger (despite being given nutrition via intravenous fluids). Because Chase experiences various types of unpleasant sensations, it may be difficult for healthcare professionals to differentiate between discomfort and pain. General principles of assessment are underscored by the need by healthcare professionals to identify the potential underlying causes of Chase's irritability. Afterwards, healthcare professionals may use tools, such as NPASS, to rate the levels of Chase's agitation and pain to better assess whether non-pharmacologic and pharmacologic interventions should be employed to help Chase achieve comfort.

Case 9.1 Part 2

Chase has been in the NICU for 14 weeks and is now 37 weeks' corrected gestational age. He remains intubated with moderate ventilatory and oxygen support. Prior to ligation of a patent ductus arteriosus 3 weeks ago, he had a double-lumen percutaneously inserted central catheter (PICC) placed for intravenous nutrition and pain/sedation management. Chase has resumed full enteral feeds via a nasogastric tube, but his PICC remains in place for ongoing pain and sedation. Breast milk is no longer available, and he is receiving a high-calorie formula. He continues to have frequent spitting and difficulty stooling, and he is made NPO intermittently for episodes of feeding intolerance.

Chase becomes agitated periodically throughout your shift with restlessness, tachycardia (heart rate of 200–225 bpm), diaphoresis, and hyperthermia (temperature of > 38.5 ˙˙ °C). Many sepsis evaluations have been performed with negative results.

Chase has a calming response to keeping his room dark and the door closed to minimize noise. He becomes calmer and is soothed when a white noise machine is on at his bedside.

1. *What are some other non-pharmacologic measures you could initiate?*
2. *How could you involve a parent or caregiver?*

Management of Non-pain Symptoms

Non-pharmacologic Management

Whenever possible and appropriate, non-pharmacologic management of non-pain symptoms should be considered and trialed before pharmacologic interventions are initiated. Non-pharmacologic therapies include: kangaroo care, nonnutritive sucking, the five Ss (swaddle, side or stomach position, shush, swing, suck), facilitated tucking, music therapy, massage therapy, environmental management, and acupuncture. Also, if developmentally appropriate, the use of swings, mobiles, motion/vibrating chairs, crib aquariums, and noise machines can be employed. The strategies described in this section may be used in combination and individualized as appropriate for infants, depending on their clinical situation. In addition, many of these interventions can be used for pain management as well.

Kangaroo Care

First described over 30 years ago in Bogota, Colombia, kangaroo care is skin-to-skin contact between infants and their parents/guardians. While wearing only a diaper, infants are positioned upright and prone on their caregiver's bare chest [12]. They are then covered with their caregiver's clothing and, if needed, a blanket and hat. A kangaroo care session typically lasts 1–3 hours with continuous monitoring of vital signs. During kangaroo care, infants experience their caregiver's warmth, heart sounds, and rhythmic breathing, which gently stimulate their auditory, tactile, vestibular, and thermal sensory systems. Altogether, these aid in improving the perception of pain [12]. Skin-to-skin contact has been shown to increase the length and quality of sleep, resulting in infants who are more alert and less irritable. No adverse effects on physiologic stability have been found in infants as young as 25 weeks, including those who are on ventilator support [13].

The Five Ss (Swaddle, Side/Stomach Position, Shush, Swing, Suck) [14]

Swaddle

Swaddling infants is the cornerstone of calming and soothing a fussy or agitated infant. Swaddling mimics the boundaries infants experienced in the uterus. Many irritable infants resist wrapping. However, it is a mistake to think this resistance is because they want their hands free; because fussy/agitated infants lack the coordination to control their arms, they may become upset and agitated when their arms are unwrapped. To swaddle correctly, wrap their arms snugly (usually with a blanket) either flexed or straight at their sides, but let their hips be loose and flexed [15] (Fig. 9.1). Always check that swaddled infants do not overheat while wrapped. To maintain a "safe sleep" environment, never let infants sleep in a bed with loose blankets.

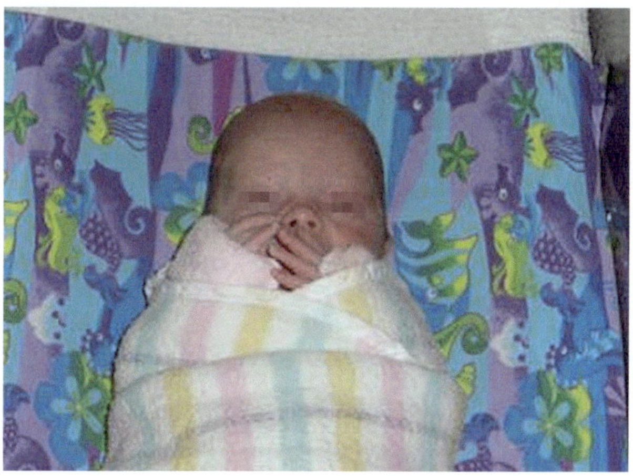

Fig. 9.1. Example of how to position infants for swaddling. Swaddling may be used to calm an agitated infant by wrapping their arms snugly under a blanket, either positioned flexed or straight at their sides, as shown in the photo. The infant's hip and legs should not be tightly restrained to allow for some movement. (Photo courtesy of Royal Prince Alfred Hospital Newborn Care. https://www.slhd.nsw.gov.au/rpa/neonatal/nursing_guidelines.html [15])

Side and Stomach Positions

Positioning fussy/agitated infants on their side or stomach soothes infants by preventing the Moro reflex (and the associated panicked sensation of falling). Laying infants on their backs is the only safe position for sleeping [16], but it can be difficult for calming fussy infants. If needed, positioning infants on their side or stomach should be a temporary intervention with the infant monitored. Caregivers should be educated on the risk of sudden infant death syndrome associated with prone positioning.

Shushing

Contrary to myth, infants do not need total silence to sleep. In the uterus, blood flow is a shush sound (70–91 db) that is similar or greater in decibels than that of a vacuum cleaner (70–80 db) [17]. Shushing comforts by mimicking the whooshing noise blood makes as it flows through the arteries of the placenta. Caregivers may make soft "shushing" noises approximately 2–4 inches from infants' ears and gradually increase the intensity of "shushing" to match the loudness of crying. Instinctively, caregivers and healthcare professionals may feel that loud and harsh shushing is inappropriate. However, they should be instructed to soften their shushing gradually as their infant is in a calmer state or falls asleep.

Swinging

Fetuses are exposed to continuous maternal movements in utero. Because of this, providing infants with a rhythmic, monotonous, jiggling movement is a common method to calm fussy/agitated infants. Some common rhythmic movements include: rocking, dancing, swinging, vibrating (in an infant bouncer), and rhythmic patting on the back or buttocks. Caregivers and healthcare professionals should initiate these types of movements gently with a fast pace and slow down as infants calm down. Infants' heads should be allowed to jiggle slightly (while always supporting the head/neck in a midline position), as this triggers the calming reflex by switching on motion detectors in the head [14]. Infants may also be positioned side-lying on the caregiver's lap with the head/neck supported while implementing small rhythmic up-and-down movements with shushing near infants' ears until they calm down. Infants can then transition to a swing if needed.

Sucking (Nonnutritive)

Nonnutritive sucking in infants is nearly universal, is considered normal, and usually consists of infants sucking on a pacifier or their fingers. Sucking is one of the first types of coordinated and self-regulated behaviors that fetuses and infants begin to exhibit at around 24 weeks' gestation [18]. Nonnutritive sucking is followed by the ability to suck and swallow at approximately 26 weeks, and then for most infants, suck and swallow become fully coordinated around 32–34 weeks' gestation [18]. Encouraging infants to engage in nonnutritive sucking is a benign strategy to calm and soothe infants. Although the mechanism is not completely understood, nonnutritive sucking appears to work by increasing endogenous endorphins. It is effective in lowering pain scores and has a synergistic effect when augmented with breast milk and other non-pharmacologic measures discussed in this chapter [19].

An effective way to soothe fussy/agitated infants is to allow them to suck on a pacifier or caregiver's gloved finger. If appropriate, the pacifier or gloved finger may be dipped in maternal breast milk or formula to help infants initiate sucking.

Facilitated Tucking

Facilitated tucking can be used when infants are too preterm, medically unstable, or too hot to be swaddled. It is accomplished by flexing infants' arms and legs closely to their torsos using blanket rolls, commercially available products, and/or their caregiver's hands to restrict movement while still allowing them to control their bodies (Fig. 9.2) [15]. Research has found that use of facilitated tucking results in decreased crying and overall improved self-regulation, especially when it is paired with other non-pharmacological approaches [20, 21].

Massage Therapy

Massage therapy involves the application of either the caregiver's or healthcare professional's hands on the infant's skin to provide skin-to-skin manipulation. It is most effective when using moderate pressure. It is considered a safe practice when done by caregivers and healthcare professionals who have received training. Massage therapy stimulates infants' circulatory and gastrointestinal systems, which leads to improved weight gain and less fluctuations in vital signs and oxygen requirement. It is also associated with improved sleep, neurologic and neuromotor development, and bonding between caregivers and their infants [22, 23]. Massage therapy can be provided with or without oils such as coconut, safflower, sunflower, and mineral [22, 23].

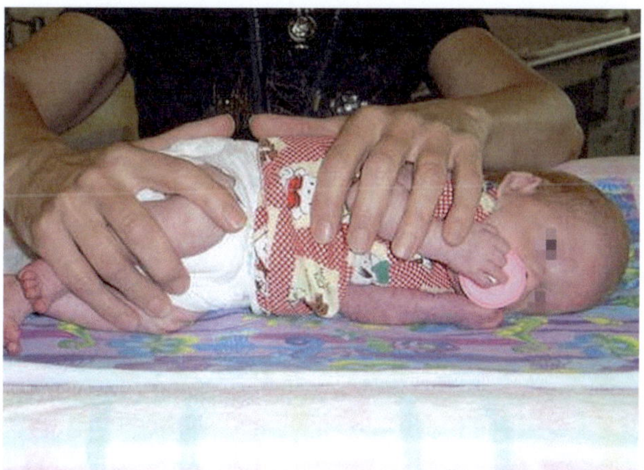

Fig. 9.2. Facilitated tucking. For infants who are too preterm, too hot, or medically unstable to be swaddled, facilitated tucking may be used to calm infants by positioning their arms and legs flexed, closely to their bodies. This photo shows an infant who is being positioned using the caregiver's hands. The caregiver may also use blanket rolls and/or commercially available products to help maintain positioning in a safe manner. (Photo courtesy of Royal Prince Alfred Hospital Newborn Care. https://www.slhd.nsw.gov.au/rpa/neonatal/nursing_guidelines.html [15])

Music Therapy

Using voice and/or instruments, music therapy is a structured intervention that delivers pleasing harmonies, tones, and rhythms in a variety of tempos and volumes to help improve infants' clinical condition. Researchers have found that live music provided by a certified music therapist can increase infants' ability to feed, sleep, and self-regulate [24, 25]. In contrast, some environmental noises, in the forms of alarms, machines, and loud conversations, can have a negative impact on growth and development [24, 25]. Music therapy – in particular, the use of live, entrained (i.e., matched with the infant's breathing rate) breaths and heartbeat sounds – and preferred lullabies can enhance infants' vital signs and provide opportunities for bonding [24, 25].

Environmental Management

Environmental management includes interventions such as dimming the lights, pulling down window shades, keeping doors closed, answering alarms quickly, using soft voices when talking, and maintaining a comfortable temperature in the room. In addition, the bed should be checked for the uncomfortable placement of wires, cords, blankets, or other objects.

Other Non-pharmacologic Methods

As infants grow and develop, a variety of developmentally supportive objects can be introduced, such as swings, mobiles, crib aquariums, sound machines, and motion/vibrating chairs. The use of these items is dependent on infants' gestational ages and physical sizes, medical instability, the developmental appropriateness of the intervention, and infants' acuity and ability to tolerate the intervention.

There will be instances of critically ill infants where many of the above interventions are not appropriate to be implemented fully. Adaptations to several types of interventions can be made by caregivers/families to promote the infant's comfort and are listed in Table 9.1 (Special Considerations of Challenging Conditions) and will be discussed later in the chapter.

Discussion of Case 9.1, Part 2

Infants like Chase, who have multiorgan medical conditions with complex hospitalizations, can have negative responses to medical assessments and interventions performed by healthcare professionals. Grouping routine tasks (e.g., taking Chase's temperature, changing his diaper) and interventions (e.g., suctioning, invasive procedures) would allow Chase to have as much undisturbed quiet time between care activities as possible. This requires regular communication between caregivers to facilitate "resting times" for him.

There are many non-pharmacologic strategies that can be initiated to mitigate signs and symptoms of agitation. For Chase's feeding intolerance, feedings that are ordered every 3–4 hours may be infused via a nasogastric tube over 1–2 hours or even continuously to relieve gastric upset and decrease spitting. Providing feeds continuously via a nasoduodenal tube is another option to support nutrition

Table 9.1 Special considerations for symptom management of common challenging neonatal conditions

Condition	Common symptoms and issues	General approaches and principles	Caregiver involvement
Infant with extreme prematurity	Overstimulation	Cover isolette to promote dark environment for rest Bundle infant care activities (obtaining vital signs, examining infant, changing diaper, etc.) so that infant is not disturbed constantly Surround infant with blanket rolls and positioning aids to promote facilitated tucking Position head with gel and other types of cushioning so that head is not hyperflexed/extended and to prevent dolichocephaly and other abnormal head shapes	Apply a firm touch, rather than stroke infant Cradle infant's head with one hand and buttocks/legs with other hand Provide kangaroo care after infant has improved skin maturity and does not require a dewette to prevent evaporative heat loss from the skin Provide oral swabs with colostrum/breast milk
	Skin breakdown	Apply tape and adhesives to the skin only as needed Consult a skin or wound team for suggestions on the use of skin barrier creams	
	Respiratory distress	Place infant on respiratory support and adjust settings as needed Suction oropharynx or endotracheal tube (if intubated) when there are secretions Use increased FiO2 during suctioning/infant's care as needed	
	Abdominal distention from feeding intolerance	Adjust feeding volumes or types of feeds (if feeding formula) as tolerated Monitor for constipation and provide a glycerin "shave" to promote regular stooling If there is a concern for a pathologic process, obtain an abdominal radiograph to evaluate Consider holding feeds for bowel rest Consider placing a nasogastric tube or replogle to suction for gastric/bowel decompression	

(continued)

Table 9.1 (continued)

Condition	Common symptoms and issues	General approaches and principles	Caregiver involvement
Infant on extracorporeal membrane oxygenation	Agitation	Promote minimal sensory stimulation with dim lighting and a quiet environment (e.g., soft voices and music) Provide medication(s) to alleviate pain and agitation as needed	Read softly to infant at bedside Provide breast milk swabs to oral cavity Apply firm touch, rather than stroking infant Assist with facilitated tucking during care
	Thick secretions	Place a replogle with its tip positioned in the stomach to low intermittent suction; suction the oral cavity gently as needed; provide low-dose glycopyrrolate cautiously if there are copious sections	
	Anasarca from prolonged limited-to-no mobility	Work with the occupational therapist to position/reposition the head and body with gel and other types of cushioning intermittently; to perform gentle range of motion movements to limbs	
Infant with inability to feed enterally for prolonged periods (e.g., esophageal atresia, necrotizing enterocolitis)	Agitation	Place the infant in a swing or vibrating chair Place a visual aid in front of the infant (e.g., crib mobiles, aquariums, and mirrors) Provide music therapy	Provide kangaroo care or hold the infant Engage volunteers ("cuddlers") when caregivers are not available to help keep the infant calm or engaged in an activity (e.g., reading to older infants who have prolonged hospitalization)
	Hunger	Allow nonnutritive sucking on a pacifier	

Infant with severe feeding intolerance or short gut syndrome	Emesis	Consider holding or reducing the volume of feeds Trial a promotilic agent such as metoclopramide or erythromycin, or place a nasoduodenal tube for feeds if vomiting is due to decreased gastric emptying/motility	Offer breast milk swabs to oral cavity
	Hunger	Allow nonnutritive sucking on a pacifier	
	Constipation	Trial polyethylene glycol in preterm infants or pear/prune juice in late preterm/term infants	
	Diarrhea	Trial loperamide	
	Abdominal distention from gas or functional intestinal obstruction	Place a nasogastric tube to gravity or replogle to suction to compress the abdomen if there is intestinal obstruction Trial simethicone drops if there is no intestinal obstruction	
	Oral aversion from frequent suctioning after emesis or frequent, chronic encouragement of oral feedings	Suction gently only as needed Hold or limit oral feeds based on the infant's feeding cues, rather than encouraging the infant to finish feeds orally; provide feeds via a nasogastric tube as needed Work with the occupational or speech therapist to develop and implement strategies for pleasant oral experiences	
	Skin irritation from gastrostomy tube or ostomy bag	Apply tape and adhesives to skin only as needed Consult a skin or wound team for suggestions on the use of skin barrier creams	
Infant with hypoxic ischemic encephalopathy on whole body cooling	Agitation	Surround infant with blanket rolls and positioning aids to promote facilitated tucking Promote minimal sensory stimulation with dim lighting, quiet environment (e.g., soft voices and music) Provide medication(s) to alleviate pain and agitation as needed	Touch, rather than stroke infant Cradle infant's head with one hand and buttocks/legs with other hand Talk or read softly to infant
	Hunger	Allow nonnutritive sucking on pacifier	
	Secretions	Suction gently as needed Consider administering glycopyrrolate	
	Seizures	Provide antiepileptic medication(s) to control seizures	

(continued)

Table 9.1 (continued)

Condition	Common symptoms and issues	General approaches and principles	Caregiver involvement
Older infant on prolonged ventilation (e.g., severe bronchopulmonary dysplasia or chronic pulmonary hypertension)	Agitation	Surround infant with blanket rolls and positioning aids to promote facilitated tucking Provide medication(s) to alleviate pain and agitation as needed If anticipate chronic mechanical ventilation, consider a tracheostomy to allow for the increased ability for caregivers to hold and provide developmentally appropriate interactions	Touch, rather than stroke infant Cradle infant's head with one hand and buttocks/legs with other hand Provide kangaroo care or hold infant Engage volunteers ("cuddlers") when caregivers are not available to help keep infant calm
	Secretions	Suction gently as needed Consider administering glycopyrrolate	
	Oral aversion due to noxious stimuli (e.g., suctioning of oral cavity, placement of nasogastric tube, intubation and reintubation)	Consider tracheostomy if anticipated need for chronic mechanical ventilation Limit noxious oral stimuli to prevent the development of oral aversion	
	Respiratory distress	Adjust respiratory support settings as needed Suction the endotracheal tube or tracheostomy when there are secretions	
	Discomfort secondary to skin irritation from respiratory support (e.g., endotracheal tube, tracheostomy)	Apply tape and adhesives to skin only as needed Consult a skin or wound team for suggestions on the use of skin barrier creams	
	Neonatal abstinence	Promote minimal sensory stimulation with dim lighting and a quiet environment (e.g., soft voices and music) Swaddle infant or provide facilitated tucking Allow nonnutritive a sucking on pacifier Place the infant in a swing or vibrating chair Place on an opioid +/– adjuvant therapy and wean dose slowly using a withdrawal scale	

if he has persistent, excessive spitting because of delayed gastric emptying or poor gastrointestinal motility. Even though Chase is receiving appropriate pharmacological sedation and pain management, non-pharmacological interventions such as applying a cool, moist cloth to his forehead, removing excess clothing/blankets, leaving him clothed in just a diaper, and using a fan to better circulate air in the room may be helpful strategies to mitigate symptoms of hyperthermia and diaphoresis from agitation. In addition, providing music therapy and allowing nonnutritive sucking with an appropriately sized pacifier can help soothe him. Chase's caregivers can be involved by reading or singing softly, using facilitated tucking as a calming measure, or holding him via kangaroo care for as long as he tolerates it and remains medically stable. Healthcare providers and caregivers may need to implement several different non-pharmacological interventions before Chase is calmed and soothed.

Case 9.1 Part 3

Chase is now 49 weeks' corrected gestational age. Due to his continued need for moderate ventilatory/oxygen support, he underwent tracheostomy placement 4 days ago. Chase returned to the NICU heavily sedated and has remained NPO with titratable pain and sedation infusions. The team plans to continue these medications for up to 1 week to reduce the risk of dislodging the tracheostomy prior to the first tracheostomy change.

Today, Chase has been experiencing periodic episodes of grimacing, tachypnea, and tachycardia that have been minimally responsive to escalation in pain management and non-pharmacologic calming techniques. In addition, you note increased thin white secretions that have required suctioning every hour. Chase responds well to a one-time bolus of versed and glycopyrrolate.

1. *When is it appropriate to consider additional pharmacologic management due to his symptoms?*
2. *What other pharmacologic options might you consider for Chase?*

Pharmacologic Management

Pharmacologic management may be required when discomfort and distress are unable to be relieved with non-pharmacologic interventions alone. The management of pain and other symptoms may utilize many of the same medications. This section will focus on how these similar medications can target the relief of different types of symptoms.

Many of the medications below are discussed in their off-label use in the neonatal population, and the studies used to support these applications have been taken or extrapolated from pediatric literature. In addition, this is not an exhaustive list of available medications. Please refer to Table 9.2 for details on dosing and

Table 9.2 Medications for discomfort, distress, and other symptoms

Medication	Route(s)	Gestational age	Starting dose	Frequency	Maximum dose
Acetaminophen [26–29]	Oral	28–32 weeks[a]	12–15 mg/kg	Every 6, 8, or 12 hours	40 mg/kg/day
		33–37 weeks[a]	12–15 mg/kg	Every 6–8 hours	60 mg/kg/day
		38 weeks and greater[a]	10–15 mg/kg	Every 4–6 hours	75 mg/kg/day
	IV	28–32 weeks[b]	10 mg/kg	Every 12 hours	22.5 mg/kg/day
			7.5 mg/kg	Every 8 hours	
		32–36 weeks[b]	7.5–10 mg/kg	Every 6–8 hours	40 mg/kg/day
		37 weeks and greater[b]	10 mg/kg	Every 6 hours	50 mg/kg/day
	Rectal	28–32 weeks	12–20 mg/kg	Every 12 hours	40 mg/kg/day
		33–38 weeks	12–20 mg/kg	Every 8 hours	50–60 mg/kg/day
Albuterol [30, 31]	Nebulization	Not specified	0.1–0.3 mg/kg	Every 2–8 hours	0.5 mg/kg (2.5 mg)
Atropine 0.05% ophthalmic drop[c] [32, 33]	Sublingual	Not specified	1 drop	Every 6–24 hours	2 drops
Clonidine [34, 35]	Oral	35 weeks and older[f]	0.5 μg/kg	Every 4–6 hours	4 μg/kg
Dexmedetomidine [36, 37]	IV infusion	26 weeks and greater	0.05–0.3 μg/kg/hour[g]	Continuous	1.5 μg/kg/hour
Erythromycin [38, 39]	Oral	32 weeks and greater	1.5–5 mg/kg	Every 6 hours	10 mg/kg[h]
Gabapentin [40–42]	Oral	23 weeks and greater	5–10 mg/kg	Every 8–24 hours	35 mg/kg/day
Glycerin [43]	Rectal – pediatric suppository	Not specified[i]	0.25 suppository or small chip	Every 12–24 hours	0.25 suppository or small chip
	Rectal – liquid		0.2 mL	Every 12–24 hours	0.5 mL/kg[j]
Glycopyrrolate[c] [44, 45]	Oral	Not specified	40 μg/kg	Every 6–8 hours	100 μg/kg
	IV		4 μg/kg		10 μg/kg
Haloperidol[c] [46]	IV/IM (lactate)	Term infants	0.05 mg/kg/day	Every 8–12 hours	0.5 mg/kg/day
Ibuprofen[c] [28, 47–49]	Oral/IV	See footnote[k]	5 mg/kg	Every 8–24 hours	10 mg/kg
Loperamide[d] [50, 51]	Oral	38 weeks and greater[e]	0.08 mg/kg/day	Every 8–12 hours	0.2 mg/kg/day
Lorazepam [52, 53]	IV/IM/oral	Not specified	0.05	Every 4–6 hours	0.1 mg/kg[l]
Melatonin[c] [54]	Oral	Not specified	1 mg	Nightly	3 mg

Methadone [55–57]	Oral	34 weeks and greater	0.05–0.1 mg/kg	Every 6 hours	0.3 mg/kg[l]
	IV		0.25–0.05		0.15 mg/kg[l]
Metoclopramide [58, 59]	IV/oral	31 weeks and greater	0.1 mg/kg	Every 6–8 hours	0.15 mg/kg
Midazolam [60, 61]	IV/IM	Not specified	0.05–0.1 mg/kg	Every 1–4 hours	0.15 mg/kg[l]
	IV infusion	32 weeks and less	0.03 mg/kg/hour	Continuous	0.2 mg/kg/hour[l]
		Greater than 32 weeks	0.06 mg/kg/min		
	Oral	Not specified	0.25 mg/kg	Every 4–8 hours	0.5 mg/kg[l]
Morphine [62–64]	IV/IM	Not specified	0.05–0.1 mg/kg	Every 4–6 hours	0.2 mg/kg/dose[l]
	Oral	Not specified	0.08 mg/kg	Every 4–6 hours	0.08 mg/kg/dose[l]
	IV infusion	Not specified	0.01–0.02 mg/kg/hour	Continuous	0.03 µg/kg/hour[l]
Pentobarbital [65]	IV infusion	Not specified	1 mg/kg/hour	Continuous	6 mg/kg/hour
Phenobarbital [66, 67]	Oral/IV	Not specified	3–5 mg/kg/day	Every 12–24 hours	8 mg/kg/day
Polyethylene glycol [68]	Oral	Not specified	0.2–1 g/kg	Every 8–24 hours	1 g/kg
Quetiapine[m] [69–71]	Oral	Term infants	0.5 mg/kg	Every 8 hours	0.5 mg/kg
Risperidone [72, 73]	Oral	Term infants	0.01 mg/kg	Every 12–24 hours	0.02 mg/kg

Notes:

[a]May load with 20–25 mg/kg once

[b]May load with 20 mg/kg once

[c]Extrapolated from pediatric literature, use with caution. Use lowest dose/frequency as possible to achieve symptom management

[d]Dosing for chronic diarrhea in patients with short gut syndrome

[e]Minimal information on patients under 38 weeks

[f]Limited information in patients under 35 weeks

[g]Optional loading dose of 0.1–0.5 µg/kg given over 20 minutes

[h]Dose 10 mg/kg or higher in first 14 days of life have been associated with increased risk of hypertrophic pyloric stenosis

[i]Studied in premature infants (no CGA noted)

[j]Used as enema

[k]Has been studied 24 weeks' corrected gestational age and above for patent ductus arteriosus closure. Use as an analgesic not recommended in patients under 6 months CGA

[l]May exceed due to developed tolerance

[m]Limited data available

administration. Healthcare professionals should strongly consider consultation of pharmaceutical, pain, and/or palliative care specialists when using these medications to manage different types of symptoms.

Cyclooxygenase Inhibitors

Acetaminophen

Acetaminophen, or paracetamol, is a nonspecific cyclooxygenase inhibitor. In addition to pain, it is used for fever management, which is one of the most common causes of discomfort in chronically ill and end-of-life patients. Fever is associated with tachycardia, tachypnea, and distress [74]. The inhibition of cyclooxygenase in the central nervous system causes a decrease in the production of prostaglandins that cause fever when increased. Adverse effects of acetaminophen include slowed neonatal clearance, hepatotoxicity, and nephrotoxicity [75].

Nonsteroidal Anti-inflammatory Drugs (NSAIDs)

NSAIDs, such as ibuprofen and ketorolac, are also nonspecific cyclooxygenase inhibitors. They decrease the production of prostaglandins and are therefore helpful in the reduction of discomfort associated with fever. Caution must be used with the administration of NSAIDs, as insufficient evidence exists to support or oppose their use in infants less than 6 months of age. Potential adverse effects in all age groups include gastrointestinal injury, nephrotoxicity, patent ductus arteriosus closure, and impaired platelet aggregation [76].

Opioids

Morphine

Morphine is an opioid analgesic. Due to its poor lipid solubility, morphine has a relatively slow onset of action and long duration of action. It exercises its primary action at the mu-opioid receptor by mitigating ascending neuronal signals [77]. Morphine exerts both analgesic and sedative properties before it is metabolized in the liver to morphine-3-glucuronide and morphine-6-glucuronide [78].

Morphine is currently used as a first-line agent in the pharmacologic management of neonatal abstinence syndrome (NAS). Morphine reduces or improves symptoms such as irritability, agitation, tremors, tachypnea, feeding difficulty, sleep cycle disturbance, diarrhea, and seizures. However, the use of morphine for NAS should be weaned using a withdrawal scale for guidance, as it has been shown to cause an increase in hospital stay [79, 80].

Morphine is also frequently used during palliative, end-of-life, and withdrawal-of-life support care. In the authors' clinical experience, it can be administered sublingually (starting at 0.1 mg/kg) in neonates who have no parenteral access, such as a newborn who is receiving comfort care. This is because of morphine's dual action in the relief of pain and discomfort. Morphine's sedative effect promotes anxiolysis, comfort, decreased cough, alleviation of dyspnea, diminished perception of air hunger, attenuated respiratory feedback to hypercapnia, and reduced oxygen consumption [81, 82]. When given appropriately, it is generally felt that morphine can lead to adequate relaxation without accelerating death [8]. Adverse effects include decreased gastrointestinal motility, bronchospasm, hypotension, seizure, and respiratory depression [8, 75, 77]. In addition, morphine should not be used in patients with renal dysfunction or patients receiving dialysis due to the buildup of glucuronide metabolites [83].

Methadone

Like morphine, methadone is an opioid analgesic that acts primarily at the mu-opioid receptor. However, unlike morphine, methadone is manufactured synthetically, exhibits a longer duration of action, and has inhibitory activity at N-methyl-D-aspartate (NMDA) receptors. Inhibition of NMDA receptors in the central nervous system mitigates neuronal hyperstimulation and is thought to relieve neuropathic pain. However, there is limited information on methadone's effectiveness and safety profile for this use. A double-blind randomized controlled trial in Canada (NCT01205516) is currently investigating the effect of methadone on treating neuropathic pain. Activation of the NMDA receptor is also advantageous as it helps to reduce opioid tachyphylaxis [84].

Methadone is also commonly used as one of the first-line medications for treatment of NAS and NAS-related non-pain symptoms. Due to its long half-life, safety in renal dysfunction, and decreased propensity toward opioid tachyphylaxis, methadone can be particularly helpful in weaning infants exposed to chronic opioid therapy [84, 85]. Adverse effects of methadone include respiratory depression, constipation, and withdrawal with sudden cessation of use [86] (see also Chap. 8, Table 8.5 for conversions).

Loperamide

Loperamide is a long-acting synthetic opioid agonist active at the mu-opioid receptors in the large intestine. Loperamide is used as an antidiarrheal and has been shown to decrease motility, stool volume, and loss of gastrointestinal fluid. It also increases stool viscosity, density, and gastrointestinal transit time. Chronic diarrhea and excessive ostomy output can lead to dehydration, electrolyte abnormalities, failure to thrive, agitation, irritability, and skin excoriation and breakdown.

Loperamide is extensively metabolized via the first pass mechanism making its systemic availability extremely low at ~0.3%. However, caution must be used in those with hepatic dysfunction due to impairment of the first pass mechanism. Adverse effects include abdominal pain, constipation, drowsiness, and rash [87].

Benzodiazepines

Midazolam and Lorazepam

Benzodiazepines, such as midazolam and lorazepam, stimulate gamma-aminobutyric acid (GABA) A inhibitory receptors in the central nervous system. This causes sedation and reduces agitation and anxiety [8]. Midazolam is active as a parent compound and after metabolism in the liver to 1-hydroxymidazolam [77]. Midazolam is water soluble and short acting. It has the advantage of being a strong anxiolytic while also producing amnesia and muscle relaxation [78]. Lorazepam acts as a primary compound without active metabolites. It has a longer duration of action than midazolam. It can be used to decrease anxiety, seizure activity, and insomnia [88]. In the authors' clinical experience, it can be administered sublingually (0.1 mg/kg) in neonates who have no parenteral access, such as a newborn who is receiving comfort care. Adverse effects of benzodiazepines include myoclonic jerks, respiratory depression, hypotension, and bradycardia [8, 78]. In addition, midazolam should be used with caution in preterm infants, in which early and/or prolonged exposure has been linked to neuroapoptosis, reduced neurogenesis, mitigated hippocampal growth, and worsened neurodevelopmental outcomes [89, 90].

Alpha-2 Agonists

Clonidine

Clonidine is a mixed agonist of inhibitory alpha-2 adrenergic receptors that is utilized as a mild sedative and anxiolytic. When given orally, clonidine reaches its peak concentration within 1.5 hours and is metabolized in the liver. Clonidine has a wide variety of possible uses due to its ability to sedate without depressing the respiratory drive. It can be given as needed for preprocedural and operative agitation. It can be given as a scheduled medication in the treatment of spasticity and drug withdrawal. Clonidine has also been shown to decrease the use of opioids and benzodiazepines when added to the medication regimen. Adverse effects include rebound hypertension, orthostatic hypotension, bradycardia, somnolence, and dry mouth [91].

Dexmedetomidine

Dexmedetomidine is a predominantly selective agonist of alpha-2 adrenergic receptors in the central nervous system. It exhibits a short half-life and is metabolized through cytochrome p450 enzymes. Dexmedetomidine delivers a powerful sedative, anxiolytic, and analgesic effect while also allowing the patient to be aroused when stimulated. In addition, it has been shown to have little influence on pulmonary function or gastrointestinal motility [76].

Dexmedetomidine is frequently used as an additional medication in patients who have reached the maximum benefit of, or are experiencing side effects from, other forms of medications used to control pain and discomfort. In this role, it has been shown to achieve improved relief of discomfort while also decreasing the need for other medications [92]. Adverse effects include bradycardia and hypotension that are especially pronounced when administered in bolus form [8, 76, 78, 92]. In addition, it is important to consider medication compatibility prior to initiating continuous drips due to intravenous access restrictions in infant patients.

GABA Action

Gabapentin

Gabapentin is a GABA analog that is generally well tolerated and has a long half-life. Gabapentin is used for a variety conditions including seizures, pain, and other symptoms such as chronic irritability, hypertonia, and gastrointestinal dysfunction or discomfort. Its precise mode of action is unknown; however, it is thought to inhibit central nervous system voltage-gated calcium ion channels and N-methyl-D-aspartate (NMDA) receptors, leading to a halt in centralized hyperstimulation. Centralized hyperstimulation is speculated to be the cause of neuropathic pain and visceral hyperalgesia experienced in infants and children with neurologic impairment [42, 93].

Gabapentin can be used as an independent treatment, or as an additional medication, when relief of discomfort/distress has not been achieved non-pharmacologically or with reasonable optimization of more traditional medications. Several case series have shown improvement in irritability, contentment, feeding intolerance, insomnia, and opioid/benzodiazepine use with the initiation of gabapentin [94]. Few adverse effects have been reported, but they include nystagmus and possible autonomic instability with sudden cessation of the medication [42, 94]. In addition, healthcare professionals should consult a pharmacist with regards to decreasing the dose and/or frequency of administration in patients with renal dysfunction.

Barbiturates

Phenobarbital and pentobarbital are barbiturates that induce central nervous system depression through the stimulation of GABA receptors, depression of glutamate depolarization, and inhibition of voltage-gated calcium ion channels [95, 96]. Phenobarbital has a long duration of action, while pentobarbital is shorter acting and more potent. Due to its improved side effect profile, phenobarbital is more widely used in the pediatric population; however, both are strong anticonvulsants that can be used in the treatment of seizure activity. In addition, both have sedative properties that can be used for the treatment of agitation, irritability, and insomnia. Due to the availability of medications with similar durations of action, but less adverse effects, pentobarbital has seen little use for the treatment of these types of symptoms. However, phenobarbital has been successful as an adjunctive medication in treating symptoms that are not controlled despite reasonable doses of opioid and benzodiazepines [97]. Phenobarbital has also been used in the treatment of withdrawal from benzodiazepines. Barbiturates have little to no analgesic activity.

Barbiturates' influence on the metabolic clearance of other medications, such as corticosteroids and anticoagulants, via the cytochrome P450 pathway should be considered when administering these drugs concomitantly. It should also be noted that pentobarbital has previously been used in euthanasia protocols; therefore, care should be taken to avoid this implication through discussion with the family about reasons for its use [8]. Additional adverse effects include respiratory depression and hepatotoxicity [96].

Antipsychotics

Haloperidol

Haloperidol is a typical antipsychotic that exerts its action by competitively blocking dopamine (D2) receptors in the brain. It is primarily metabolized by the liver and used in the treatment of acute delirium, specifically hyperactive delirium. Although awareness is increasing, infant delirium is classically underdiagnosed and undertreated. Delirium is characterized by changes in arousal and cognition. Chronic and critically ill infants are at increased risk for delirium due to their underlying illness, ongoing medical care, and pharmacologic needs. In particular, opioids, benzodiazepines, and steroids are frequent offending agents. Infant delirium can often be recognized in a patient that remains uncomfortable and agitated despite non-pharmacologic therapy and/or adequate elevation in analgesics and anxiolytics. Currently, case studies have shown that when delirium is recognized and adequately treated, these difficult to sedate patients show an increase in comfort and a decreased need for sedation [70]. Adverse effects include prolonged QTC, tachycardia, anticholinergic effects, extrapyramidal effects, agitation or sedation, hyperglycemia, hyperlipidemia, seizure, and hepatotoxicity [70, 98].

Risperidone and Quetiapine

Risperidone and quetiapine are second-generation atypical antipsychotics that are metabolized by hepatic cytochrome p450 enzymes. Risperidone exerts its antipsychotic effects by antagonizing dopamine, serotonin, and histamine receptors. Quetiapine blocks dopamine, serotonin, histamine, and alpha-adrenergic receptors. Due to the wide range of receptor blockade, these atypical antipsychotics may be better equipped to treat the mixed and hypoactive subtypes of delirium. They share a similar side effect profile with haloperidol [98].

Anticholinergics

Glycopyrrolate and Atropine

Glycopyrrolate and atropine are synthetic inhibitors of acetylcholine (i.e., anticholinergic medications) that block acetylcholine activity nonspecifically at muscarinic receptors. These medications may be particularly helpful in the reduction of copious oral and tracheal secretions in patients experiencing neurologic devastation, cerebral palsy, prolonged intubation, or tracheostomy [99]. Chronic sialorrhea can lead to skin breakdown, aspiration, and excessive insensible fluid losses [33]. In addition, glycopyrrolate induces smooth muscle relaxation that may mitigate discomfort from gastrointestinal and genitourinary spasms. Adverse effects are similar to other anticholinergic medications and include tachycardia, dry mouth, dilated pupils, rash, constipation, urinary retention, somnolence, and elevated temperature. Glycopyrrolate has the additional potential adverse effect of hepatotoxicity [100, 101].

Osmotic Laxatives

Glycerin Suppository

Glycerin suppositories are osmotic laxatives given to aid in the passage of meconium and stool. Infants may experience impaction and chronic constipation as a result of diet, hydration, and/or medications [102]. Impaction and chronic constipation can lead to symptoms of discomfort, irritability, abdominal distention, feeding intolerance, failure to thrive, encopresis, anal fissures, and vagal nerve stimulation causing bradycardia [103]. Prior to the use of pharmacologic management, organic causes of constipation should be investigated [104]. Adverse effects include diarrhea and anal trauma [103].

Polyethylene Glycol

Polyethylene glycol is an osmotic laxative also used in the treatment of chronic constipation to improve stooling regularity and soften consistency. Polyethylene glycol shows efficacy in achieving initial disimpaction and in the continuation of maintenance therapy for chronic constipation [104]. Adverse effects include diarrhea, which resolves with decreased dosing or discontinuation of the medication [104].

Gastroprokinetic Agents

Metoclopramide

Metoclopramide is a dopamine (D2) receptor antagonist. In the gastrointestinal system, dopamine allows smooth muscle relaxation. However, when blocked by metoclopramide, the smooth muscle becomes more susceptible to cholinergic action. This mechanism causes improved gastric emptying, peristalsis, and reduced emesis. Infants with chronic feeding intolerance, reflux, or gastroparesis leading to failure to thrive may benefit from treatment with metoclopramide. However, it is important to discuss the possible benefits and risks of this medication with parents or guardians and rule out gastrointestinal obstruction prior to use. Adverse effects include extrapyramidal reactions, tardive dyskinesia, hepatotoxicity, restlessness or drowsiness, diarrhea or constipation, hypersensitivity reactions, visual disturbances, and edema. In addition, use with caution in patients with seizure disorders and renal dysfunction [105].

Erythromycin

Erythromycin is a macrolide antibiotic that, like metoclopramide, can also be used as a prokinetic agent in the treatment of gastrointestinal dysmotility. It achieves this by acting as a competitive agonist at the motilin receptor, increasing the quantity of endogenous motilin, and activating cholinergic nerves. Erythromycin is given via the oral route only for this indication due to increased adverse effects when used in intravenous form. Adverse effects include abdominal pain, diarrhea, prolonged QT syndrome, sensorineural hearing loss, hypersensitivity reactions, hypertrophic pyloric stenosis, and hepatotoxicity [106, 107].

Other Medications

Albuterol

Albuterol is a β-adrenergic agonist and is used via aerosolized treatments. It was originally utilized for the management and prevention of bronchospasm in children and adults with asthma and chronic obstructive pulmonary disease. However, due to its ability to decrease airway resistance and increase bronchial airflow, it may also be useful in the short-term relief of dyspnea, shortness of breath, and air hunger related to airflow obstruction. Adverse effects include tachycardia, tremulousness, and possible tachyphylaxis [108].

Melatonin

Melatonin is a hormone secreted in a circadian pattern by the pineal gland that promotes the sleep-wake cycle by binding to melatonin receptors in the hypothalamus [109]. When taken, synthetic melatonin reaches its peak action within an hour after ingestion.

Sleep cycle disturbance is common in both inpatient and outpatient settings, with neurodevelopmentally delayed children bearing the largest burden. Specifically, in the neonatal intensive care unit (NICU), infants may be prone to sleeping in short bursts or sleep-wake inversion. Over time this sleep dysregulation can lead to irritability, anxiety, depression, poor feeding, and difficulty performing and learning tasks. Although reports of effectiveness vary, melatonin can reduce the time of sleep onset and increase the duration of total sleep hours [109]. Adverse effects include somnolence, increased immune system reactivity, and hypothalamic-gonadal axis depression [110].

Discussion of Case, 9.1 Part 3

In our case, Chase exhibits symptoms of pain or irritability 4 days after his tracheostomy placement. With an assessment of the potential factors causing his agitation, the healthcare team identifies that Chase may be experiencing discomfort secondary to frequent suctioning; inability to be repositioned, held, or swaddled with a new tracheostomy; and hunger due to his NPO status. The team initiates non-pharmacologic calming techniques; however, these yield little improvement. When faced with a patient such as Chase, who is at risk for agitation and distress that has not responded to non-pharmacologic methods, it is appropriate to consider medications for his symptoms. In this scenario, the team chooses to use midazolam for anxiolysis and glycopyrrolate to decrease oral secretions and the need for frequent suctioning.

Chase responds positively to these interventions. However, if Chase's symptoms of irritability and distress return within a few hours after the initial midazolam dose, the team may consider providing midazolam as needed versus beginning a continuous infusion. If Chase requires multiple doses of midazolam within a short period of time, then a continuous infusion of midazolam may be required. Using a validated assessment tool can help quantify both his pain/agitation symptoms and response to medications as new medications are started and titrated to a desired effect (see Chap. 8, Table 8.2).

Occasionally, infants like Chase reach the maximum benefit of their first-line analgesic/anxiolytic intravenous infusions, such as morphine and midazolam, and require additional intravenous support as a bridge before weaning these medications. The addition of dexmedetomidine may be considered as it has been associated with improved sedation and reduced need for other medications [92]. Chase is also at risk for sleep-wake cycle disturbances due to frequent need for suctioning secretions and the heavy burden of pain and sedation medications. The team may consider initiating melatonin as it has been shown to decrease the time to sleep and increase the duration of total sleep time [109]. Lastly, atropine ophthalmic drops given sublingually can be considered as an alternative to glycopyrrolate.

Case 9.1 Part 4

Chase is now 5 months old and is at home with his family. His tracheostomy is still in place, and he requires mechanical ventilation at night. Before discharge home, a gastrostomy tube (GT) was also placed. He is offered small amounts of food orally. However, his major source of caloric intake is via *GT feeds at night. Recently, his weight decreased below his growth curve because of increased work of breathing after weaning his ventilatory support to increase daytime mobility. The caloric density of his feeds was subsequently increased.*

Chase's parents and members of his care team tell you that he does not seem as comfortable as he was before. He is grimacing, appears to be straining, and has periods where he is inconsolable.

1. *What are potential causes of Chase's increased discomfort and distress?*
2. *What strategies may be helpful in relieving this discomfort and distress?*

Management of Specific Symptoms

Infants with LLFNDs may exhibit various symptoms that include, but are not limited to, increased work of breathing, seizures, feeding/nutritional issues, constipation, and delirium. In addition, infants who are exposed to chronic opioid use for pain control may experience symptoms of withdrawal if the opioid is stopped abruptly. Symptoms that may be distressing to infants can be even more distressing to their caregivers [111]. Remarkably, a recent survey on United States Neonatal End-of-Life Comfort Care Guidelines documented that most guidelines do not address secretions, gastrointestinal distress, or anxiety [112]. There are limited studies on infants' experiences of discomfort and scant high-level evidence for best practices. As a result, common sense principles have typically been applied. A number of common clinical situations will be presented to illustrate some of these principles.

Increased Work of Breathing

Difficulty breathing and dyspnea are distressing for older children and adults to experience. The literature suggests that infants can also experience dyspnea [113]. For some infants, this symptom may be a part of an evolving disease process, such as prematurity-related bronchopulmonary dysplasia, congenital diaphragmatic hernia, or pulmonary hypertension. Strategies to decrease respiratory distress should be discussed with families as a part of any goals of care conversation. For some infants, strategies may include supplemental oxygen, noninvasive respiratory support (e.g., nasal cannula, continuous positive airway pressure), intubation, or a tracheostomy with mechanical ventilation. Infants with LLFNCs may not be able to handle their own secretions, and gentle frequent oral, nasal, or tracheal suctioning may be required. Position changes may help relieve mechanical obstructions, improve chest expansion, and permit easier removal or drainage of secretions. Holding and comforting an infant in a more upright position may decrease oxygen demand sufficiently to relieve distress. This intervention, whenever possible, should be offered to families to engage them in active care delivery, promote the ongoing bond with their child, and provide them the opportunity to carry out normal parental activities. Should these strategies be ineffective, pharmacological management, if not already employed, should be considered. Medications such as albuterol, caffeine, and/or diuretics may be helpful in reducing the infants' work of breathing. If infants continue to experience dyspnea or air hunger, consider obtaining a pulmonology consult and the appropriateness of trialing opioids. Opioids for significant increased work of breathing would be very appropriate at end of life. As described earlier, morphine for air hunger and lorazepam for anxiety or agitation in the setting of respiratory distress can be administered sublingually in very small volumes to an infant receiving comfort care.

Seizures

A seizure is an abnormal electrical discharge in the brain. If the discharge is localized, the expression of the seizure will reflect the area of the brain that is affected (focal seizures). If the discharge spreads to both hemispheres, the physical expression of the seizure will be widespread (generalized seizures). If it is determined that an infant may be experiencing seizure activity, the team should obtain an electroencephalogram and consult a neurologist for possible pharmacologic management. Similar to respiratory distress, seizures can be distressing to watch. Families may have little knowledge about seizures, their cause, and/or treatment, and they may never have seen someone seize. Clear explanations at an appropriate level to families' emotional states and educational level should be provided, including any interventions that may be helpful. For example, it is fine to talk to their child as this is happening. If the seizures are not being treated or are intractable, families should be told about what they might expect during a seizure (e.g., body movements, worsening oxygen saturations, and monitor alarms that may be triggered), what they can do to help their child, and what they can do to decrease their own anxiety. The presence of other family members or care providers may be reassuring and comforting. For healthcare professionals, it is important that antecedent events be noted and any triggers that may precipitate seizures be removed or addressed. Additionally, particular care will be needed if it is deemed acceptable to orally feed infants who have a history of seizure activity, because the potential for aspiration exists.

Feeding and Nutrition

A natural human response is to comfort, care for, and provide nutrition to infants. Infants may breast, bottle, or gavage feed with the goal of providing nutrition and/or comfort. Occasionally, a gastrostomy tube or intravenous line may need to be placed. This should be done after evaluating the risks and benefits in terms of infants' physical needs and comfort and the families' ongoing goals of care wishes [114]. Withholding food and fluids may be an option some families choose when their infant has a severe or lethal condition. Whenever ethically justifiable, families should be supported by the healthcare team in their choices. Requests may be denied when they fall outside of accepted, reasonable treatment. If there are any conflicts, healthcare professionals should consult their institution's ethics committee (see Chap. 3).

For infants who are feeding, but with difficulty, a speech language pathologist evaluation and a swallow study may be helpful. These can help inform the ongoing care surrounding oral nutrition. Even infants with diagnosed poor oral coordination may sometimes be fed using thickened feedings. Care must be taken not to provide food and fluids to an infant who cannot protect their own airway. However, feedings that provide comfort may be determined to ethically outweigh the risk of aspiration should the family wish to offer feeds. Care providers need to be aware that should infants experience an acute life-threatening event during a feed, families may believe that they caused the demise of their child. Support and explanations should be provided, and opportunities for ongoing exploration and clarification of evolving parental goals of care should be provided.

Oral and Eye Care

Infants who are not feeding or receiving fluids would benefit from various comfort measures. As infants become more dehydrated, their mucus membranes will become dry and may crack. Providing frequent eye drops and oral lubricants may alleviate some discomfort and permit blinking and swallowing. Swabs of colostrum, breast milk, or formula can also be used to keep the mouth moist. This is a task in which many families may appreciate participating.

Constipation

Dehydration can affect the gastrointestinal tract by causing inspissated stools. In addition, infants with LLFNDs may require opioids and anticonvulsants for treatment and comfort, and these medications are associated with constipation as a side effect. If infants are feeding, increasing the caloric density of feeds can also be associated with constipation. Because infants have limited physiologic reserve, providing feeds along with other activities may be associated with an increased energy demand and result in increased heart rate, increased respiratory rate, and/or desaturations. Stooling may also elicit a vagal nerve response associated with a slowing of the heart rate. If constipation causes discomfort, oral prune or pear juice may be given to promote stooling. Glycerin suppositories and saline enemas may also be used to help evacuate stool. For small infants, a pediatric suppository is too large a dose for administration. Using scissors or a relatively blunt blade, a sliver, or "shave" of the length of the suppository can be "cut" off and given to infants. Caregivers should smoothen the edges of the glycerin shave to prevent any irritation or trauma to the skin and tissues upon insertion.

Agitation and Delirium

Agitation may occur when infants are experiencing pain and/or delirium. If agitation is being caused by pain, healthcare professionals should determine the potential cause of pain, manage the pain symptoms, and then reassess whether there is improvement of the infant's agitation. If agitation persists despite appropriate pain management, then delirium should be considered.

Delirium occurs acutely as fluctuating changes in awareness and cognition in the setting of serious medical illness [115]. It tends to wax and wane in response to both physiologic and environmental factors. While delirium has been recognized in both adult and pediatric patients, infants also likely experience delirium. However, delirium in infants is often not recognized or is underdiagnosed, because healthcare professionals lack awareness of this condition and usually do not consider it as a reason for continuing distress despite the use of sedative or analgesic agents. In addition to delirium, infants likely experience sundowning, where sundowning relates to the onset or increase in behavioral disturbances as dusk or darkness falls. No standard definition for sundowning exists [116].

Delirium is difficult to assess in nonverbal patients. The European Society for Paediatric and Neonatal Intensive (ESPNIC) published a position statement that provides clinical recommendations regarding the assessment of pain, sedation, withdrawal, and delirium [117]. This group also provided suggestions related to the assessment of interventions for treatment. The majority of tools exist for older children and adults. However, the Cornell Assessment of Pediatric Delirium (CAPD) scale, which contains behavioral evaluations of infant interactions, movements, and consolability, may be used for infants from birth to age 18 [70, 118]. Scores of 9 or greater (out of a highest possible score of 32) correlate strongly with a psychiatric diagnosis of delirium.

Evidence about the treatment of delirium in infants is scant but continues to emerge. Like pain, non-pharmacologic strategies should be used first. These strategies may include changes in lighting or swaddling and comforting affected infants. More research is needed to determine which interventions provide the greatest benefit. Case reports have suggested the off-label use of atypical antipsychotics like risperidone or quetiapine to treat unconsolable infants with altered sleep-wake cycles. Groves et al. report three cases of delirium, of which the CAPD scale was used in two cases [70, 118]. These infants showed an improvement in symptoms, and sedatives and narcotics were weaned. It is important to note that the medications used in the management of delirium have been associated with prolonged QT syndrome, and electrocardiograms should be followed.

Neonatal Abstinence Syndrome

Some infants with long NICU hospitalizations are exposed to chronic opioid or benzodiazepine use for pain relief, sedation, or another indication. Stopping these medications abruptly may precipitate withdrawal, and in the case of narcotics, the infant may develop neonatal abstinence syndrome. Withdrawal symptoms may be denoted by the mnemonic "withdrawal" and include excessive *w*akefulness, *i*rritability, *t*remulousness, *h*yperactivity or high-pitched cry, *d*iarrhea, *r*espiratory distress, *a*pnea, *w*eight loss, respiratory *a*lkalosis, and *l*acrimation [119]. The severity of symptoms may be evaluated by using various scoring tools. The most commonly used tool in the United States is the modified Finnegan Score® [120]. This tool uses both subjective (e.g., irritability, high-pitched crying, poor feeding, poor suck, increased muscle tone, tremors, watery stools) and objective (e.g., fever, respiratory rate, duration of sleep) data. However, other scoring scales are used, including the Lipsitz Neonatal Drug-Withdrawal Scoring System, the Neonatal Withdrawal Inventory, and the Neonatal Narcotic Withdrawal Index [121–123].

Infants who exhibit withdrawal symptoms may be very irritable. The first line of management should employ environmental strategies to decrease stimulation, promote restful sleep, and provide a soothing milieu that may decrease symptoms of withdrawal. The five Ss have been applied with varying success [14]. Often in healthcare settings and homes, various electronic devices are available to provide ambient soothing sounds or rocking motions to help calm irritable infants. Any equipment should only be used for its intended purpose following all the manufacturer's recommendations.

If environmental measures are not successful, then the treatment of withdrawal hinges around reintroducing the medication or similar medications that are no longer required, and then slowly, over the course of days to weeks, weaning these medications to the point of discontinuation. The agents used to help infants with neonatal abstinence syndrome vary from institution to institution and on the preferences of the healthcare team. Many institutions standardize the weaning process with protocols that are developed to reflect the types of medications from which infants are withdrawing. Medications such as morphine or methadone may be used, starting with a dose that abates withdrawal symptoms and then weaning the dose by 10–20% every 1–5 days by using a withdrawal scale for guidance on the frequency of weans [80, 124]. If healthcare professionals find that an infant's withdrawal symptoms are severe enough that weaning is not possible or is slower than anticipated with therapy, adjunctive use of other medications such as phenobarbital and clonidine may be helpful to reduce withdrawal symptoms [80]. Healthcare professionals should consult their pharmacists and palliative care specialists who have expertise with pain management regarding dosing and potential weaning regimens in challenging cases.

Discussion of Case 9.1, Part 4

Chase's parents have indicated that he is not as comfortable as he was before. Acknowledging the parents' concerns and listening to their assessment can be helpful in developing a plan to achieve greater comfort. Chase's grimacing, straining, and periods when he is inconsolable may be related to many things. He has developed increased work of breathing after his ventilator settings were weaned and has not been gaining weight, suggesting that he has increased metabolic demands. Could this distress be from air hunger and anxiety associated with difficulty breathing? If this is the case, then moving Chase to a quieter area with minimal stimulation may help. If his increased work of breathing persists, then his ventilator settings may need to be readjusted. Another likely cause for Chase's irritability is constipation related to the use of an increased caloric density formula to promote weight gain. It would be important to ask his family about the timing of his last bowel movement and the frequency and consistency of his stools. If his stools are infrequent and hard, then giving Chase a glycerin suppository and starting prune juice or a laxative to help him stool may help him achieve a more comfortable state. Positioning his knees to his chest may be help him evacuate stool.

How Caregivers May Provide Support

Family Inclusion

Families' input is essential in their child's care, because they are a part of the caregiving team as the parents/guardians. As recently as the 1970s, parents were excluded from providing care for their sick child in hospital settings [125]. The counterculture movement and the rise of feminism led to mothers demanding to be present at their child's bedside. Currently there is an emphasis on providing patient- and family-centered care [126]. Many children's units now consist of single-family rooms. These children's units were designed, often incorporating parental input, with the intent to provide a more holistic, inclusive, homelike environment without compromise to care. Parents are no longer conceptualized as visitors, but rather as co-providers of care. However, parents still report that they are not permitted to be involved in the care of their child and feel unwelcome [127]. In this qualitative study, the authors explored parental perspectives of neonatal intensive care at the end-of-life. Themes emerged surrounding access to their child, being listened to, and being able to be present at the bedside and during rounds. Families desired involvement in decision-making and care delivery. Other issues that were raised included the need to receive clear and timely information, delivered in a compassionate manner. Families wanted to discuss goals of care, "do not resuscitate" (DNR) status, and anticipatory guidance for what might be ahead. For families who know that their infant has an LLFND and who wish to spend as much time with their infant as possible, especially in the setting of comfort care, they should be offered the option of having their infant room-in with them at all times.

Most caregivers and healthcare professionals are familiar with the idea of the "golden rule"; this may be paraphrased to, "Do not do something to someone that you would not want them to do to you." Applying this principle whenever possible may inform the use of some environmental strategies to promote comfort and mitigate distress. These environmental interventions should take into account family wishes. Participants benefit from a quiet and warm room with lighting, heating controls, and amenities to provide care similar to a home. Space should be provided where the family can personalize the room with pictures, decorations, and other meaningful objects. This environment should be modulated to provide optimal space for the infant's medical care, balancing attention to ensure that families' ongoing activities of daily living are promoted. The ability for families to mark celebrations and participate in rituals, spiritual practices, and supportive care that is in line with families' belief structures is also desirable [128].

The Interdisciplinary Healthcare Team

Perinatal and pediatric palliative care stresses symptom management for the patient and family, provides interdisciplinary interventions to maximize the quality of life, and attempts to maximize health and treat suffering, including existential suffering [129]. This care can be provided in multiple settings including the infants' home, skilled nursing facilities, and hospital units. Von Gunten describes basic palliative care skills that all members of the palliative care should possess. These teams are usually interdisciplinary and may be comprised of various members including: nurses, advanced practice nurses, physicians, speech language therapists, chaplains, respiratory therapists, occupational and physical therapists, social workers, lactation consultants, child life specialists, and volunteers [130]. Healthcare professionals should be skilled in communicating with empathy, identifying families' goals of care, providing symptom management, and collaborating with other members of the healthcare team.

Three major barriers have been identified that may impede the optimal approach to palliative care: the delivery of health professions education in silos, inadequate communication skills training, and curricula with minimal to absent content about palliative care [131]. Healthcare providers who work independently of one another sometimes provide conflicting information to families. This inconsistency can add unnecessary stress to families and caregivers. The perinatal palliative care team should present as a unified team with explicit and shared goals for each patient and family.

Patient and family experiences are paramount to individualized care planning. A team-based, family-centered approach should be used for the assessment of families' needs, intervention planning, and communication of information. With appropriate exposure and education, multidisciplinary healthcare teams can perform the work of a palliative care team, paying attention to families' goals of care, interpreting medical information, managing complex symptoms, and providing support and anticipatory guidance. Interprofessional team meetings to discuss infants' current status and symptoms and to develop ongoing care plans should also include a review of families' level of understanding of the situation and to relay potential outcomes (for more information, see Chap. 15).

Preparing for Discharge

Some families may be able to take their infants home from the hospital or other type of healthcare facility. Discharge may result after overcoming challenges associated with the infants' LLFND and demonstrating a period of stability. For other infants, discharge enables transition to the home environment for continuing palliative care. Whatever the reason, discharge planning may cause families and caregivers to experience anxiety, especially if caregivers experience stress when their infants have symptoms of discomfort or distress and/or need to go home with medical equipment. In these instances, healthcare professionals should help families and caregivers prepare by educating and involving them in different aspects of their infants' care over time, as soon as families are ready. Should infants need to go home on respiratory or feeding equipment, the healthcare team may provide education to families by simulating the home environment and involving families in simulations of potential issues and emergencies that they may encounter at home [132] (see also Chaps. 13 and 14).

Special Considerations for Challenging Conditions

Infants with complex medical conditions pose special challenges to the healthcare team, because they often experience multiple types of symptoms that can confound the team's ability to alleviate their distress or discomfort (Table 9.1). In addition, in some situations when infants must remain immobile or have limited mobility, such as with infants on extracorporeal membrane oxygenation (ECMO) or infants who have many critical lines and tubes, the usual strategies to provide comfort (e.g., kangaroo care, the five Ss, alternative positioning) may not be possible. During these challenging situations, caregivers may feel helpless, because they feel that they are not able to nurture their child by helping to alleviate distress. While strategies to provide comfort may be limited in these situations, caregivers and healthcare professionals should always work together to collectively identify the infants' key stressors, which would enable them to focus on developing strategies to address them. In addition, healthcare teams should elicit the help of child life specialists, palliative care specialists, and other professionals who have expertise in providing medical and supportive care to chronic infants with special needs. Collaboration across multidisciplinary teams often results in viable solutions.

Special Considerations During End-of-Life Care

Caring for a dying infant takes particular sensitivity to parents' coping process and the infant's symptom management. Comfort may be the focus of care from the moment of birth when families choose a comfort-oriented plan of care after delivery or after attempts at life-saving measures are unsuccessful or felt to be overly burdensome. In some cases, the end-of-life may come during aggressive resuscitation measures such as chest compressions. As soon as it is clear that the infant is approaching the final minutes, hours, or days of life, symptom management should be entirely focused on the infant's comfort.

Signs and Symptoms of the Dying Process

Regardless of the timing, infants who are at the end-of-life will undergo physiologic and behavioral changes and require careful symptom assessment that is tailored to their individual needs. They will show changes in their level of consciousness, breathing pattern, heart rate, blood pressure, muscle tone, temperature, and color that can elicit feelings of alarm and distress from both family members and healthcare professionals. Families and healthcare professionals who have not experienced end-of-life care should be counseled so that they understand and better anticipate that these symptoms may occur as part of the natural process. Symptoms related to changes in circulation and infants' hemodynamic status, such as bradycardia, hypotension, hypothermia, cyanosis, and mottling, do not need treatment. Respiratory symptoms, such as increased work of breathing, agonal breathing, and intermittent apnea, may also occur and can be difficult for families to observe. It is important again to provide reassurance that these are normal breathing patterns at the end-of-life and that agonal breathing patterns do not represent infant agony. However, whenever there is an assessment of infant discomfort due to increased work of breathing, administering an analgesic medication such as morphine may alleviate respiratory-related distress. In addition, when infants have increased secretions coupled with respiratory distress, they may exhibit very noisy breathing. Gentle suctioning along with the administration of analgesia and/or anticholinergic drying agents can provide at least partial relief and allay distress from caregivers and healthcare professionals.

Comfort Care in the Delivery Room

When comfort care is the plan of care from the moment of delivery, the infant remains in the mother's room if possible. Normal warming, drying, and swaddling or skin-to-skin positioning can be performed. The subsequent management will be entirely based on the individual infant's underlying disease process and signs and symptoms of distress. A baby with anencephaly, for example, may have no specific signs of distress, but may later show tachypnea or secretions. In contrast, an infant with pulmonary hypoplasia from renal agenesis or a large congenital diaphragmatic hernia will likely have significant respiratory distress from the moment of birth, and the infant should receive administration of morphine and lorazepam sublingually as soon as possible, with repeat doses every 20–30 minutes if symptoms are not controlled. It may be helpful to order the medication in a "shadow chart" (for the infant prior to delivery) so that the medication can be readily available in the delivery room.

Withdrawal of Life-Sustaining Treatment

When an infant is being removed from life-sustaining therapy (e.g., withdrawal from a ventilator or ECMO), special management is required. To avoid air hunger, pain, or anxiety, premedication with an opioid (typically morphine or fentanyl) and a benzodiazepine (typically midazolam) bolus with concurrent initiation of a continuous infusion should be initiated. In many situations, the infant will already be on some combinations of these medications, in which case the bolus should be approximately double the baseline rate. The bolus should be given approximately 5 minutes prior to withdrawal of support. A provider should be at the bedside to assess for distress until the infant is stable or has died. The opioid and benzodiazepine can be re-dosed every 5 minutes until the distress resolves. Before or after the ventilator is stopped, the infant can be held by family. Other symptoms such as respiratory secretions should be managed. When suspicion is high that there will be copious secretions, premedication with an anticholinergic medication such as glycopyrrolate can be helpful [3].

To help ease some of the distress that infants and families may experience during end-of-life care and to facilitate a peaceful environment, healthcare professionals should limit excess environmental stimulation that may heighten families' emotions and stress, such as unnecessary noise and bright, harsh lighting. If infants are connected to a cardiorespiratory monitor, then the volume of alarms signaling bradycardia, hypotension, and poor oxygen saturations may be minimized or inactivated. Families may be positioned so that they are facing away from cardiorespiratory monitors, or the monitors may be turned to face a different direction. If not needed, then monitors may also be turned off. If in a private room, the door should be closed to provide privacy and eliminate noise from outside of the room. If the infant is in a room shared with other infants, then privacy screens should be placed around the infant's bedside space. Alternatively, if possible, the other infants in the room should be moved to another location. Thoughtful, small changes in the environmental milieu usually help decrease unnecessary stressors that families experience at the end-of-life.

Summary

Although not as extensively studied as pain, the assessment and management of infant "non-pain" symptoms are emerging as an increasingly important area to improve patient well-being and quality of life. The clinical presentation of symptoms of discomfort and distress are sometimes difficult to distinguish from pain. However, increased awareness of potential causes of these symptoms would aid caregivers and healthcare professionals in the recognition of infant distress and discomfort. With better recognition, non-pharmacologic, environmental, and pharmacologic interventions may be implemented based on infants' individual needs. Specific conditions should be evaluated and addressed with particular attention to incorporating caregivers in their infants' care with the support of the multidisciplinary healthcare team. Because providing chronic and/or end-of-life care is usually an emotional experience and can be challenging, it is essential that the healthcare team have basic palliative care knowledge, work together collaboratively to include caregiver goals in the management of infant discomfort, communicate effectively with all individuals involved, and, if needed, discuss the transition to end-of-life care in a hospital or home setting.

References

1. American Academy of Pediatrics, Committee on Psychosocial Aspects of Child and Family Health, American Pain Society, Task Force on Pain in Infants, Children, and Adolescents. The assessment and management of acute pain in infants, children, and adolescents. Pediatrics. 2001;108(3):793–7.
2. Jones L, Fabrizi L, Laudiano-Dray M, Whitehead K, Meek J, Verriotis M, Fitzgerald M. Nociceptive cortical activity is dissociated from nociceptive behavior in newborn human infants under stress. Curr Biol. 2017;27(24):3846–51.
3. Jones L. The mystery of how babies experience pain. The Conversation. 2017. Accessed 21 May 2018 at: https://theconversation.com/the-mystery-of-how-babies-experience-pain-88714
4. Mathew PJ, Mathew JL. Assessment and management of pain in infants. Postgrad Med J. 2003;79:438–43.

5. Holsti L, Grunau RE, Oberlander TF, Whitfield MF. Specific newborn individualized developmental care and assessment program movements are associated with acute pain in preterm infants in the neonatal intensive care unit. Pediatrics. 2004;114(1):65–72.
6. Oberlander TF, Grunau RE, Whitfield MF, Fitzgerald C, Pitfiled S, Saul JP. Biobehavioral responses in former extremely low birthweight infants at four months' corrected age. Pediatrics. 2000;105(1):1–10.
7. American Academy of Pediatrics, Committee on Fetus and Newborn and Section on Anesthesiology and Pain Medicine. Prevention and management of procedural pain in the neonate: an update. Pediatrics. 2016;137:1–13.
8. Carter BS, Brunkhorst J. Neonatal pain management. Semin Perinatol. 2017;41(2):111–6.
9. Craig KD. The facial display of pain in infants and children. Pain Res Manage. 1998;10: 103–21.
10. Harrison D, Evans C, Johnston L, et al. Bedside assessment of heel lance pain in the hospitalized infant. J Obstet Gynecol Neonatal Nurs. 2002;31:551–7.
11. Hadjistavropoulos HD, Craig KD, Grunau RE, Whitfield MF. Judging pain in infants: behavioural, contextual, and developmental determinants. Pain. 1997;73(3):319–24.
12. Whitelaw A, Sleath K. Myth of marsupial mother: home care for very low birth weight infants in Bogota, Colombia. Lancet. 1985;1:1206–8.
13. Jefferies AL. Kangaroo care for the preterm infant and family. Paediatr Child Health. 2012;17(3):141–3.
14. Karp H. The happiest baby on the block – the new way to calm crying and help your baby sleep longer. New York: Bantam Dell; 2002.
15. Royal Prince Alfred Hospital Newborn Care. Comfort care. Royal Prince Alfred Newborn Care Nursing Guidelines. Accessed 28 Sept 2018 at: https://www.slhd.nsw.gov.au/rpa/neonatal/nursing_guidelines.html
16. American Academy of Pediatrics Task Force on Sudden Infant Death Syndrome. SIDS and other sleep-related infant deaths: updated 2016 recommendations for a safe infant sleeping environment. Pediatrics. 2016;138(5):1–12.
17. Kruger C, Horesh E, Crossland BA. Safe sound exposure in the fetus and preterm infant. J Obstet Gynecol Neonatal Nurs. 2012;42(2):166–70.
18. Pillai Riddel RR, Racine NM, Turcotte K, et al. Non-pharmacological management of infant and young child procedural pain. Cochrane Database Syst Rev. 2011;10:CD006275.
19. Shah PS, Aliwalas LI, Shah V. Breastfeeding or breast milk for procedural pain in neonates. Cochrane Database Syst Rev. 2006;3:CD004950.
20. Liaw JJ, Yang L, Katherine Wang KW, Chen CM, Chang YC, Yin T. Non-nutritive sucking and facilitated tucking relieve preterm infant pain during heelstick procedures. Int J Nurs Stud. 2012;49(3):300–9.
21. Hall RW, Anand KJ. Pain management in newborns. Clin Perinatol. 2014;41(4):895–924.
22. Kulkarni A, Kaushik JS, Gupta P, Sharma H, Agrawal RK. Massage and touch therapy in neonates: the current evidence. Indian Pediatr. 2010;47(9):771–6.
23. Field T, Diego M, Hernandez-Reif M. Preterm infant massage therapy research: a review. Infant Behav Dev. 2010;33(2):115–24.
24. Allen KA. Music therapy in the NICU: is there enough evidence to support integration for procedural support? Adv Neonatal Care. 2013;13(5):349–52.
25. Loewy J, Stewart K, Dassler AM, Telsey A, Homel P. The effects of music therapy on vital signs, feeding, and sleep in premature infants. Pediatrics. 2013;131(5):902–18.
26. Lexi-comp Online. Acetaminophen (Pediatric and neonatal lexi-drugs) Hudson; 2018. Updated periodically. Accessed Nov 2018.
27. Micromedex Healthcare Series. Acetaminophen (NeoFax) Greenwood Village; Thompson Micromedex. Updated periodically.
28. Ohlsson A, Shah PS. Paracetamol (acetaminophen) for prevention or treatment of pain in newborns. Cochrane Database Syst Rev. 2016;(10):CD011219.
29. Ohlsson A, Walia R, Shah SS. Ibuprofen for the treatment of patent ductus arteriosus in preterm or low birth weight (or both) infants. Cochrane Database Syst Rev. 2015;(2):CD003481.

30. Lexi-comp Online. Albuterol (Pediatric and neonatal lexi-drugs) Hudson; 2018. Updated periodically. https://online.lexi.com/lco/action/doc/retrieve/docid/pdh_f/130001. Accessed 2 Nov 2018.
31. Albuterol. In: Neofax [database on the internet]. Greenwood Village: Truven Health Analytics; 2018 [cited 2018 Nov 3]. Available from: www.micromedexsolutions.com. Subscription required to view.
32. Norderyd J, Graf J, Marcusson A, et al. Sublingual administration of atropine eyedrops in children with excessive drooling – a pilot study. Int J Paediatr Dent. 2017;27:22–9.
33. Rapoport A. Sublingual atropine drops for the treatment of pediatric sialorrhea. J Pain Symptom Manage. 2010;40(5):783–8.
34. Lexi-comp Online. Clonidine (Pediatric and neonatal lexi-drugs) Hudson; 2018. Updated periodically. Accessed 2 Nov 2018.
35. Clonidine. In: Neofax [database on the internet]. Greenwood Village: Truven Health Analytics; 2018 [cited 2018 Nov 3]. Available from: www.micromedexsolutions.com. Subscription required to view.
36. Lexi-comp Online. Dexmedetomidine (Pediatric and neonatal lexi-drugs) Hudson; 2018. Updated periodically. Accessed 2 Nov 2018.
37. Dexmedetomidine. In: Neofax [database on the internet]. Greenwood Village: Truven Health Analytics; 2018 [cited 2018 Nov 3] Available from: www.micromedexsolutions.com. Subscription required to view.
38. Lexi-comp Online. Erythromycin (Pediatric and neonatal lexi-drugs) Hudson; 2018. Updated periodically. Accessed 2 Nov 2018.
39. Erythromycin. In: Neofax [database on the internet]. Greenwood Village: Truven Health Analytics; 2018 [cited 2018 Nov 3] Available from: www.micromedexsolutions.com. Subscription required to view.
40. Lexi-comp Online. Gabapentin (Pediatric and neonatal lexi-drugs) Hudson; 2018. Updated periodically. Accessed 2 Nov 2018.
41. Gabapentin. In: Neofax [database on the internet]. Greenwood Village: Truven Health Analytics; 2018 [cited 2018 Nov 3] Available from: www.micromedexsolutions.com. Subscription required to view.
42. Edwards L, DeMeo S, Hornik CD, Cotten CM, Smith PB, Pizoli C, Hauer JM, Bidegain M. Gabapentin use in the neonatal intensive care unit. J Pediatr. 2016;169:310–2.
43. Lexi-comp Online. Glycerin (Pediatric and neonatal lexi-drugs) Hudson; 2018. Updated periodically. Accessed 2 Nov 2018.
44. Lexi-comp Online. Glycopyrrolate (Pediatric and neonatal lexi-drugs) Hudson; 2018. Updated periodically. Accessed 2 Nov 2018.
45. Glycropyrollate. In: Neofax [database on the internet]. Greenwood Village: Truven Health Analytics; 2018 [cited 2018 Nov 3] Available from: www.micromedexsolutions.com. Subscription required to view.
46. Lexi-comp Online. Haloperidol (Pediatric and neonatal lexi-drugs) Hudson; 2018. Updated periodically. Accessed 2 Nov 2018.
47. Lexi-comp Online. Ibuprofen (Pediatric and neonatal lexi-drugs) Hudson; 2018. Updated periodically. Accessed 2 Nov 2018.
48. Ibuprofen. In: Neofax [database on the internet]. Greenwood Village: Truven Health Analytics, 2018 [cited 2018 Nov 3] Available from: www.micromedexsolutions.com. Subscription required to view.
49. Jacqz-Aigrain E, Anderson BJ. Pain control: non-steroidal anti-inflammatory agents. Semin Fetal Neonatal Med. 2006;11(4):251–9.
50. Lexi-comp Online. Loperamide (Pediatric and neonatal lexi-drugs) Hudson; 2018. Updated periodically. Accessed 2 Nov 2018.
51. Li ST, Grossman DC, Cummings P. Loperamide therapy for acute diarrhea in children. PLoS Med. 2007;4(3):e98.
52. Lexi-comp Online. Lorazepam (Pediatric and neonatal lexi-drugs) Hudson; 2018. Updated periodically. Accessed 2 Nov 2018.

53. Lorazepam. In: Neofax [database on the internet]. Greenwood Village: Truven Health Analytics; 2018 [cited 2018 Nov 3] Available from: www.micromedexsolutions.com. Subscription required to view.
54. Lexi-comp Online. Melatonin (Pediatric and neonatal lexi-drugs) Hudson; 2018. Updated periodically. Accessed 2 Nov 2018.
55. Lexi-comp Online. Methadone (Pediatric and neonatal lexi-drugs) Hudson; 2018. Updated periodically. Accessed 2 Nov 2018.
56. Methadone. In: Neofax [database on the internet]. Greenwood Village: Truven Health Analytics; 2018 [cited 2018 Nov 3] Available from: www.micromedexsolutions.com. Subscription required to view.
57. Ward RM, Drover DR, Hammer GB, Stemland CJ, Kern S, Tristani-Firouzi M, et al. The pharmacokinetics of methadone and its metabolites in neonates, infants, and children. Paediatr Anaesth. 2014;24(6):591–601.
58. Lexi-comp Online. Metoclopramide (Pediatric and neonatal lexi-drugs) Hudson; 2018. Updated periodically. Accessed 2 Nov 2018.
59. Metoclopramide. In: Neofax [database on the internet]. Greenwood Village: Truven Health Analytics; 2018 [cited 2018 Nov 3] Available from: www.micromedexsolutions.com. Subscription required to view.
60. Lexi-comp Online. Midazolam (Pediatric and neonatal lexi-drugs) Hudson; 2018. Updated periodically. Accessed 2 Nov 2018.
61. Midazolam. In: Neofax [database on the internet]. Greenwood Village: Truven Health Analytics; 2018 [cited 2018 Nov 3]. Available from: www.micromedexsolutions.com. Subscription required to view.
62. Lexi-comp Online. Morphine (Pediatric and neonatal lexi-drugs) Hudson; 2018. Updated periodically. Accessed 2 Nov 2018.
63. Morphine. In: Neofax [database on the internet]. Greenwood Village: Truven Health Analytics; 2018 [cited 2018 Nov 3]. Available from: www.micromedexsolutions.com. Subscription required to view.
64. Anand KJ, Anderson BJ, Holford NH, Hall RW, Young T, Shephard B, et al. Morphine pharmacokinetics and pharmacodynamics in preterm and term neonates: secondary results from the NEOPAIN trial. Br J Anaesth. 2008;101(5):680–9.
65. Lexi-comp Online. Pentobarbital (Pediatric and neonatal lexi-drugs) Hudson; 2018. Updated periodically. Accessed 2 Nov 2018.
66. Lexi-comp Online. Phenobarbital (Pediatric and neonatal lexi-drugs) Hudson; 2018. Updated periodically. Accessed 2 Nov 2018.
67. Phenobarbital. In: Neofax [database on the internet]. Greenwood Village: Truven Health Analytics; 2018 [cited 2018 Nov 3]. Available from: www.micromedexsolutions.com. Subscription required to view.
68. Lexi-comp Online. Polyethylene glycol (Pediatric and neonatal lexi-drugs) Hudson; 2018. Updated periodically. Accessed 2 Nov 2018.
69. Lexi-comp Online. Quetiapine (Pediatric and neonatal lexi-drugs) Hudson. Updated periodically. Accessed 2 Nov 2018.
70. Groves A, Traube C, Silver G. Detection and management of delirium in the neonatal unit: a case series. Pediatrics. 2016;137(3):e1–4.
71. Brahmbhatt K, Whitgob E. Diagnosis and management of delirium in critically ill infants. Pediatrics. 2016;137(3):e1–5.
72. Lexi-comp Online. Risperidone (Pediatric and neonatal lexi-drugs) Hudson; 2018. Updated periodically. Accessed 2 Nov 2018.
73. Edwards LE, Hutchinson LB, Hornik CD, Smith PB, Cotton CM, Bidegain M. A case if infant delirium in the neonatal intensive care unit. J Neonatal-Perinatal Med. 2017;10:119–23.
74. Aronoff DM, Neilson EG. Antipyretics: mechanisms of action and clinical use in fever suppression. Am J Med. 2001;111(4):304–15.
75. Witt N, Coynor S, Edwards C, Bradshaw H. A guide to pain assessment and management in the neonate. Curr Emerg Hosp Med Rep. 2016;4:1–10.

76. Mayock DE, Gleason CA. Pain and sedation in the NICU. NeoReviews. 2013;14(1): e22–33.
77. McPherson C. Sedation and analgesia in mechanically ventilated preterm neonates: continue standard of care or experiment? J Pediatr Pharmacol Ther. 2012;17(4):351–64.
78. Anand KJS. Pharmacological approaches to the management of pain in the neonatal intensive care unit. J Perinatol. 2007;27:S4–11.
79. Siu A, Robinson CA. Neonatal abstinence syndrome: essentials for the practitioner. J Pediatr Pharmacol Ther. 2014;19(3):147–55.
80. Kocherlakota P. Neonatal abstinence syndrome. Pediatrics. 2014;134(2):e547–61.
81. Hauer JM. Treating dyspnea with morphine sulfate in nonverbal children with neurological impairment. Pediatr Pulmonol. 2015;50:E9–12.
82. Peiffer C. Morphine-induced relief of dyspnea: what are the mechanisms? Am J Respir Crit Care Med. 2011;184(8):867–9.
83. Dean M. Opioids in renal failure and dialysis patients. J Pain Symptom Manag. 2014;28(5):497–504.
84. Manfredonia JF. Prescribing methadone for pain management in end-of-life care. J Am Osteopath Assoc. 2005;105(3):18S–21S.
85. Johnson MR, Nash DR, Laird MR, Kiley RC, Martinez MA. Development and implementation of a pharmacist-managed, neonatal and pediatric, opioid-weaning protocol. J Pediatr Pharmacol Ther. 2014;19(3):165–73.
86. McNicol ED, Ferguson MC, Schumann R. Methadone for neuropathic pain in adults. Cochrane Database Syst Rev. 2017;5:CD012499.
87. National Center for Biotechnology Information. Compound summary for CID 3955. PubChem Compound Database. Accessed 9 Sept 2018 at: https://pubchem.ncbi.nlm.nih.gov/compound/3955
88. National Center for Biotechnology Information. Compound summary for CID 3958. PubChem Compound Database. Accessed 24 Feb 2018 at: https://pubchem.ncbi.nlm.nih.gov/compound/3958
89. McPherson C, Grunau RE. Neonatal pain control and neurologic effects of anesthetics and sedatives in preterm infants. Clin Perinatol. 2014;41(1):209–27.
90. Duerden EG, Guo T, Dodbiba L, et al. Midazolam dose correlates with abnormal hippocampal growth and neurodevelopmental outcome in preterm infants. Ann Neurol. 2016;79(4):548–59.
91. Basker S, Singh G, Jacob R. Clonidine in paediatrics – a review. Indian J Anaesth. 2009;53(3):270–80.
92. Gertler R, Brown HC, Mitchell DH, Silvius EN. Dexmedetomidine: a novel sedative-analgesic agent. Proc (Bayl Univ Med Cent). 2001;14(1):13–21.
93. Rose MA, Kam PCA. Gabapentin: pharmacology and its use in pain management. Anaesthesia. 2002;57(5):451–62.
94. Hauer JM, Wical BS, Chamas L. Gabapentin successfully manages chronic unexplained irritability in children with severe neurologic impairment. Pediatrics. 2007;119(2):e519–22.
95. National Center for Biotechnology Information. Compound summary for CID 4763. PubChem Compound Database. Accessed 25 Feb 2018 at: https://pubchem.ncbi.nlm.nih.gov/compound/4763
96. National Center for Biotechnology Information. Compound summary for CID 4737. PubChem Compound Database. Accessed 12 Feb 2018 at: https://pubchem.ncbi.nlm.nih.gov/compound/4737
97. Fraser GL, Riker R. Phenobarbital provides effective sedation for a select cohort of adult ICU patients intolerant of standard treatment: a brief report. Hosp Pharm. 2006;41:17–23.
98. Silver GH, Kearney JA, Kutko MC, Bartell AS. Infant delirium in pediatric critical care settings. Am J Psychiatry. 2010;167(10):1172–7.
99. Buck ML. Glycopyrrolate use in children. Pediatr Pharmacother. 2010;16(12):1–4.
100. National Center for Biotechnology Information. Compound summary for CID 11693. PubChem Compound Database. Accessed 24 Feb 2018 at: https://pubchem.ncbi.nlm.nih.gov/compound/11693

101. National Center for Biotechnology Information. Compound summary for CID 174174. PubChem Compound Database. Accessed 10 Sept 2018 at: https://pubchem.ncbi.nlm.nih.gov/compound/174174
102. Shah V, Chirinian N, Lee S, EPIQ Evidence Review Group. Does the use of glycerin laxatives decrease feeding intolerance in preterm infants? Paediatr Child Health. 2011;16(9):e68–70.
103. Biggs WS, Dery WH. Evaluation and treatment of constipation in infants and children. Am Fam Physician. 2016;73(3):469–77.
104. Ahmed M, Pai B, Reynolds T. Use of polyethylene glycol in children less than 3 years of age. J Coll Physicians Surg Pak. 2012;22(4):267–8.
105. National Center for Biotechnology Information. Compound summary for CID 4168. PubChem Compound Database. Accessed 9 Sept 2018 at: https://pubchem.ncbi.nlm.nih.gov/compound/4168
106. Curry JI, Lander TD, Stringer MD. Review article: erythromycin as a prokinetic agent in infants and children. Aliment Pharmacol Ther. 2001;15:595–603.
107. Patole S, Rao S, Doherty D. Erythromycin as a prokinetic agent in preterm neonates: a systematic review. Arch Dis Child Fetal Neonatal Ed. 2005;90:F301–6.
108. Slaughter JL, Stenger MR, Reagan PB, Jadcherla SR. Inhaled bronchodilator use for infants with bronchopulmonary dysplasia. J Perinatol. 2015;35(1):61–6.
109. Omar SH, Nabi S. Melatonin, receptors, mechanism, and uses. Syst Rev Pharm. 2010;1(2):158–71.
110. Janjua I, Goldman RD. Sleep-related melatonin use in healthy children. Can Fam Physician. 2016;62(4):315–6.
111. Cole JCM, Moldenhauer JS, Jones TR, Shaughnessy EA, Zarrin HE, Coursey AL, Munson D. A proposed model for perinatal palliative care. J Obstet Gynecol Neonatal Nurs. 2017;46:904–11.
112. Haug S, Farooqi S, Wilson CG, Hopper A, Oei G, Carter B. Survey on neonatal end-of-life comfort care guidelines across America. J Pain Symptom Manag. 2018;55(3):979–84.
113. Wolfe J, Grier HE, Klar N, Levin SB, Ellenbogen JM, Salem-Schatz S, Emanuel EJ, Weeks JC. Symptoms and suffering at the end of life in children with cancer. N Engl J Med. 2000;342:326–33.
114. Parravicini E, Lorenz JM. Neonatal outcomes of fetuses diagnosed with life-limiting conditions when individualized comfort measures are proposed. J Perinatol. 2014;34(6):483–7.
115. American Psychiatric Association. Diagnostic and statistical manual of mental disorders. 5th ed. Arlington, VA: American Psychiatric Publishing; 2013.
116. Canevelli M, Valletta M, Trebbastoni A, Sarli G, D'Antonio F, Tariciotti L, et al. Sundowning in dementia: clinical relevance, pathophysiological determinants and therapeutic approaches. Front Med. 2016;3:73.
117. Harris J, Ramelet AS, van Dijk M, Pokorna P, Wielenga J, Tume L, et al. Clinical recommendations for pain, sedation, withdrawal and delirium assessment in critically ill infants and children: an ESPNIC position statement for healthcare professionals. Intensive Care Med. 2016;42:972–86.
118. Traube C, Silver G, Kearney J, Patel A, Atkinson TM, Yoon MJ, et al. Cornell assessment of pediatric delirium: a valid, rapid, observational tool for screening delirium in the PICU. Crit Care Med. 2014;42(3):656–63.
119. Finnegan LP, Connaughton JF Jr, Kron RE, Emich JP. Neonatal abstinence syndrome: assessment and management. Addict Dis. 1975;2(1–2):141–58.
120. Finnegan LP, Kaltenbach K. Neonatal abstinence syndrome. In: Hoekelman R, Nelson NM, editors. Primary pediatric care. 2nd ed. St Louis, MO: Mosby; 1992. p. 1367–78.
121. Lipsitz PJ. A proposed narcotic withdrawal score for use with newborn infants: a programmatic evaluation of its efficacy. Clin Pediatr. 1975;14(6):592–4.
122. Zahorodny W, Rom C, Whitney W, Giddens S, Samuel M, Maichuk G, Marshall R. The neonatal withdrawal inventory: a simplified score of newborn withdrawal. J Dev Behav Pediatr. 1998;19(2):89–93.

123. Green M, Suffet F. The neonatal narcotic withdrawal index: a device for the improvement of care in the abstinence syndrome. Am J Drug Alcohol Abuse. 1981;8(2):203–13.
124. Hudak ML, Tan RC. Neonatal drug withdrawal. Pediatrics. 2012;129(2):e540–60.
125. Ahmann E, Abraham MR, Johnson BH. Changing the concept of families as visitors: supporting family presence and participation. Bethesda, MD: Institute for Family Centered Care; 2003.
126. Hill C, Knafl KA, Santacroce SJ. Family-centered care from the perspective of parents of children cared for in a pediatric intensive care unit: an integrative review. J Pediatr Nurs. 2017;41:22–33.
127. Currie ER, Christian BJ, Hinds PS, Perna SJ, Robinson C, Day S, Meneses K. Parent perspectives of neonatal care at the end-of-life. J Pediatr Nurs. 2016;31:478–9.
128. Carter B. More than medication: perinatal palliative care. Acta Pediatrica. 2016;105:1255–6.
129. Johnson L, Snama JM, Cupt MC, Baker JN. End of life care for hospitalized children. Pediatr Clin N Am. 2014;61:835–54.
130. VonGunten CF. Secondary and tertiary palliative care in US hospitals. J Am Med Assoc. 2002;287(7):875–81.
131. Marc-Aurele KL, English NK. Primary palliative care in neonatal intensive care. Semin Perinatol. 2017;41:133–9.
132. Arnold J, Diaz MC. Simulation training for primary caregivers in the neonatal intensive care unit. Semin Perinatol. 2016;40(7):466–72.

The Role of the Palliative Care Specialist in Perinatal Care

10

Rachel E. Diamond, Barbra L. Murante, and David N. Korones

Perinatal palliative care (PPC) has evolved remarkably over the last several decades from a neonatal symptom management service to a multidimensional model of care including comprehensive family-centered antenatal consultation and preparation, postnatal pain and symptom management, and even ongoing bereavement support for families [1]. Palliative care physicians are especially well-suited for their role in this field as they all must complete specified and intensive Accreditation Council for Graduate Medical Education (ACGME) fellowship programs to develop expertise in the fields of symptom management, directing difficult conversations and fostering optimal communication, as well as providing holistic care and support for the entire family unit. Nurses and nurse practitioners also can provide many of the same expertise and have palliative care-specific training opportunities (see Chap. 17 for details).

When a serious medical condition is diagnosed in the prenatal or neonatal period, involvement of a PPC specialist can be helpful to families for general support, to help them review and better understand diagnosis and prognosis, and to establish and reevaluate goals of care. A palliative care specialist can also be of help in treating troublesome symptoms a baby might experience, or manage comfort medications at end-of-life. This integrated model of care allows for a fluid coexistence of curative or life-prolonging treatments along with comfort-oriented care, with the ability to adjust focus and goals depending upon the clinical course of the infant [2]. Palliative care specialists working within such a model may function as consultant, advocate for the infant and family, or even primary caregiver depending on the status of the fetus or infant, location of care, and the goals of the family.

R. E. Diamond (✉)
University of Rochester Medical Center, Department of Pediatric Palliative Care, Rochester, NY, USA
e-mail: rachel_diamond@urmc.rochester.edu

B. L. Murante · D. N. Korones
Department of Pediatrics, University of Rochester Medical Center, Rochester, NY, USA

E. M. Denney-Koelsch, D. Côté-Arsenault (eds.), *Perinatal Palliative Care*,
https://doi.org/10.1007/978-3-030-34751-2_10

When and How to Involve the Perinatal Palliative Care Team

Ideally PPC specialists should be involved with such families early and as often as needed. A key to early involvement of the PPC team is awareness of this service and an appreciation on the part of the obstetrician and/or neonatologist of how the team can support the baby and family. A good working relationship with obstetricians and neonatologists is essential for this to work: it takes mutual respect, respect for the primary relationship between the specialists and the family, and respect for the boundaries and limits of the palliative care team's discussion with families particularly as it pertains to goals of care. This does not mean such discussions should not be broached; only that what is discussed should be mutually agreed upon by all the medical teams involved.

If possible, the relationship between a family and palliative care specialist begins prenatally when a fetal ultrasound or other antenatal testing reveals a significant medical problem such as a hypoplastic left ventricle or trisomy 18. There are multiple opportunities for the palliative care team to meet the family: in the inpatient setting if the mother is hospitalized for a complication of pregnancy, as a standalone outpatient visit, or a visit coordinated with an obstetric or other visit. One particularly attractive setting is a family meeting with other subspecialists such as maternal-fetal-medicine specialists (high-risk obstetricians), neonatologists, genetic specialists, a social worker, and a care coordinator [3]. Such a meeting provides a family the opportunity to hear from everyone together, thus ensuring consistency of care and communication. It also gives the palliative care specialist the opportunity to make sure that the family understands not only the dizzying morass of medical information they are hearing, but that they grasp the "big picture." The palliative care specialist can pose questions a family might be reluctant to ask and subspecialists might be reluctant to bring up, such as, "Is my baby going to be OK?" "What is the prognosis?" "Is this too much to put a baby through?" "Do the decisions we are thinking of fit with our family and faith values?" Such questions provide an opportunity for the family to digest all relevant information they have been given, explore options and goals of care, and take time to make decisions. If a baby survives delivery, the palliative care specialist remains involved to reassess goals in light of new information as well as provide symptom relief for the infant, even in the setting of concurrent life-prolonging treatment.

Case 10.1

William's parents happily assumed they were carrying a healthy pregnancy until their anatomic ultrasound at 19 weeks when multiple fetal anomalies were discovered. These anomalies included a small open neural tube defect with brain abnormalities, facial dysmorphisms, a small omphalocele, clenched hands, and multiple cardiac malformations. Subsequent amniocentesis performed over the following weeks confirmed the diagnosis of trisomy 18. William's parents read extensively about trisomy 18 in both scientific literature and on Internet blog sites, largely written by parents of children with trisomy 18. They also had a very strong faith that supported and drove many of their decisions in life. Their faith, as well as their own personal values, precluded termination of the pregnancy as an option. They did, however, recognize the life-limiting nature of William's diagnosis and wanted to place the central focus of care on his comfort while still opting for some life-prolonging measures that would not result in undue suffering. With the help of a multidisciplinary team led by perinatal palliative care specialists, they were able to take part in frequent family meetings both pre- and postnatally to discuss possible outcomes and options for William that aligned with their values and goals for him and their family. The perinatal palliative care specialists were able to guide the family in making appropriate decisions in light of the medical information provided that was in line with their own system of beliefs and hopes, and the team was then able to communicate and advocate on the parents' behalf to the rest of the medical teams involved. The team was also able at each stage of their journey to facilitate enjoyment, allowing the family to make the most of their time with the baby.

Family Meeting

For most couples, pregnancy and childbirth are an exciting and happy life event. However, for the estimated 2–3% of couples who receive a life-limiting or lethal fetal diagnosis, the joy of a normal, healthy pregnancy is suddenly snatched away from them [4, 5]. Some families will choose to terminate their pregnancy. However, 40% will decide to carry the pregnancy to term [6]. Instead of just "letting nature take its course," families can develop a plan with a shared goal for how they would like to see events unfold. That might range from maximally aggressive care to simple medical care with no heroic interventions to purely comfort-oriented care (see also Chap. 4, Fig. 4.2). How a family decides is complex and depends on many factors such as the underlying disease, the nature of interventions and medical supports required to keep the baby alive, and the values and faith of the family. The PPC team can meet with families early in their pregnancy, take the time to get to know the family, and allow the family to develop comfort with the team. Using their training in conducting such meetings, the PPC team can help translate a family's values into a more concrete plan of care for their baby. Eventually from such meetings (ideally in conjunction with medical subspecialists), a plan of care emerges that can allow for comprehensive support to be provided from the time of diagnosis through the baby's birth, life, and death.

Arranging an initial meeting is often done with the assistance of the obstetrician or nurse midwife. Indications for such a meeting may include general introductions of the team to a family, information-sharing, decision-making, resolving communication challenges, discussing a change in the status of a pregnancy or infant's clinical course, or for general support. This meeting can take place in the hospital or office setting or even in the home, depending upon the family, the medical team, and resources available within a community. There is not a specific or ideal gestational age at which to initiate the prenatal palliative care meeting. The timing can vary amongst different families based upon their personal needs and the diagnosis of their infant. Ideally, the initial meeting will occur after there has been adequate testing and imaging to have an accurate diagnosis. Sometimes a precise diagnosis cannot be arrived at antenatally. Involvement of a palliative care team should be considered in this situation, particularly if a serious problem is suspected and/or there is uncertainty regarding diagnosis and prognosis. Involvement of a PPC team can be a scary proposal for some families as they may incorrectly associate such involvement with hospice or being terminally ill. Proposing the integration of the team into standard care can be suggested in a very matter-of-fact, nonthreatening way by providing the facts about their services and expertise in helping families navigate unexpected diagnoses, complex and confusing medical options, and psychologically stressful situations. It can be very helpful to tell families that a role of the palliative care team is to "make sure everyone is on the same page" and to be "an extra layer of support."

Oftentimes, a meeting with the palliative care team takes place in the hospital or clinic setting. Hospital-based meetings allow for families to meet some of the people with whom they may interact after the birth of their child (e.g., the neonatologist, a geneticist, a pediatric cardiologist, a social worker), as well as tour the different areas their baby may be in (e.g., labor and delivery, the neonatal or pediatric intensive care units). Attempting to coordinate this meeting to occur on the same day as another appointment can be helpful for expectant parents, particularly if they travel a long way for the visit. However, it can also be overwhelming and exhausting. When community-based palliative care programs are available, a home visit offers a convenient and comfortable alternative setting for families. It also provides a more natural environment for expectant parents to invite other supports to be present (see also Chap. 14).

Preparing for a Family Meeting

Group meetings can be intimidating for some families. Parents may be young and many are not medically savvy. Sitting at a table with a large group of white-coated, older physicians, nurse practitioners, nurses, and other team members, coupled with the raw emotion of having a baby with a potentially life-limiting illness, can be overwhelming for a young couple. Prior to such a meeting, it is helpful to "coach" parents, let them know what will be discussed, gently explain to them who will be there, let them know that there will be no surprises, and encourage them to write down questions they might want to ask. This role could be carried out by a care coordinator (usually nurse or social worker) who provide continuity of care. Couples should also be encouraged to bring along close friends or family (e.g., a parent) if they wish. Such advocates can take notes for the family, ask questions a young couple or young single mother might be afraid to ask, and provide emotional support during hard discussions. Similarly, prior to the family meeting, the palliative care team can "coach" the medical specialty teams, asking them what will be covered, and urging them not to spring surprises regarding medical problems or prognosis on the family during the meeting. Bad or unexpected news might be more effectively delivered in more intimate settings at another time. It is also helpful to have a brief huddle with all meeting participants to determine who will lead the meeting and reach consensus on the goal of the meeting.

Conducting the Meeting

Starting with introductions is standard, and parents and other family members should be encouraged to introduce themselves and identify their place in the family. All hospital staff should similarly introduce themselves and their role in the care of the mother and child. Parents will likely have had prior discussions with their obstetrician and other specialists and have some understanding of the diagnosis and prognosis of their fetus. But it is important to hear directly from them just what their understanding of the situation is. Therefore, a good starting point to a meeting is asking the parents what their knowledge is of their infant's diagnosis or problem. Once parents' have had time to share their understanding of what brings them there, the medical specialists and pediatric palliative team can then provide clarification and add any additional details needed.

Conducting family meetings is a skill that comes with time and practice. Excellent communication skills are essential, but it is a slightly different skillset than one-on-one communication. Table 10.1 lists some important aspects of communication to attend to during a family meeting.

The family meeting should also be used as a forum to provide and gather information and its conclusion; the group leader should summarize what was discussed, including the plan moving forward [7]. Once there is a good mutual understanding of the diagnosis, and the parents' questions have been answered, it is time to discuss what the different outcomes may be. Presenting all of the possible scenarios opens up realistic discussions of options that can guide alternative birth plans.

In cases where the diagnosis and prognosis of a condition are specific, families can make informed decisions about goals of care. Some example questions for eliciting the family's goals and values are in Table 10.1. For those conditions in which the diagnosis or prognosis is uncertain, the challenges are greater and call for flexibility on the part of the health care team and recognition of the additional stresses this places on the family. The palliative care team can provide support in this setting, reassuring the family that even in the face of uncertainty, the infant can be cared for and kept comfortable while efforts are undertaken to arrive at a diagnosis.

Table 10.1 Recommendations for facilitating a successful perinatal palliative care family meeting

Recommendation	Comments
Setting	A friendly and comfortable setting should be encouraged If possible, meet in a room with soft lighting, not a workroom Have tissues available Seating arrangement is important and deserving of some thought. It should facilitate support for the family, avoid shouting across the table, and avoid creating "camps" with family on one side of the table and health care team on the other
Choose a facilitator	Identify one person to facilitate the meeting Facilitating a meeting means making sure there is an organized approach to the difficult tasks at hand, listening, assuring that all voices are heard, taking the pulse of emotions in the room, and knowing when it is time to stop. It does not mean dominating the meeting
Include key family members, friends, and health care professionals	Only key health professionals should be present at the meeting Ideally, family should be asked who they want at the meeting
Confirm goals of meeting	Goals of the meeting should be confirmed at the start of the session The family should be invited to add any additional goals
Elicit family's understanding of situation	Start with: "What is your understanding of your baby's condition?" Allows team to know what information they already know, in their own words, and what clarifying explanations they may need Provide written notes explaining medical terms
Share any new information in a clear, honest way	Avoid medical jargon Check for understanding Ask for permission to proceed if they appear overwhelmed
Elicit their goals and values	Once there is a shared medical understanding of the baby's condition, explore their goals and values Example questions: "Based on what you know, what are your goals for your baby? "What are you most worried about?" "Is there anything you would want to avoid?" "What are you hoping for at the time of birth?"
(Sometimes) Make a recommendation	Once you know the family's understanding of their baby's condition, and you have elicited their goals and values, you can make a recommendation for a care plan that fits with these Example: "Based on what I've heard you say and what we know about your baby, would it be OK if I make a recommendation for how we might care for your baby?"
Summary and plan	Set up a follow-up plan Ask for any remaining questions

When the Baby Is Born

The birth of a baby with a complex chronic condition or potentially terminal diagnosis is a bundle of mixed emotions for parents and families. There is the joy and the beauty of a newborn child, particularly poignant when that child might have only a short time to live and/or is quickly whisked off to the intensive care unit for testing and multiple interventions. In addition, there is relief that a significant hurdle has been overcome as the infant makes it to term and survives the delivery process. The birth of a neonate in peril may also be an opportunity to get a better idea of how her physiology will fare outside the womb and to get answers to so many previously unanswered questions. But it may also be a time of intense fear and anxiety for parents and families as the baby no longer has the protective environment of the womb. Uncertainty may be replaced by the certainty of a grim prognosis, or at best, the reality of a long road of intensive medical care ahead [8].

Ideally at this point a palliative care specialist has been involved and knows the family, their values, and how they make medical decisions. Many times the babies are delivered by an obstetrician on call not previously known to the family, and the neonatologist on duty might not have met the family as well. Palliative care presence (the care coordinator or any member of the team who knows the family) at this difficult time can be an important thread of continuity and a welcome familiar face to the family. He or she has likely talked specifically about goals of care for the baby and, knowing the family's wishes, can advocate on their behalf to the neonatologists and other subspecialists. Regarding goals of care, families typically fall into three categories as they decide on courses of medical management for their babies: (1) aggressive intervention without limits to prolonging life (i.e., the "do everything" approach), (2) selective interventions depending on the clinical scenario and risk to benefit ratio (the "wait and see" approach), or (3) very limited interventions to prolong life with a heavy focus on the comfort of the baby (the "comfort care" approach). The specific role of the palliative care specialist after the baby is born will depend on the family's approach to care. But regardless of whether they choose aggressive care or comfort, there is an important role for the palliative care specialist to play.

No Limitations of Medical Care

With the more aggressive approach to care, or the "do everything" model, parents are often hoping to extend the life of their baby by nearly any means possible. They are often driven by the hope that their baby might be in that small percentage of children who exceed their expected prognosis. Sometimes parents may be holding out for a treatment or cure that is not yet available, but if they keep their baby alive long enough, they may gain access to an experimental drug or clinical trial. Usually families with such a mindset choose to deliver in a tertiary medical center where they have access to more sophisticated medical technology, specialists, and experts. Palliative care specialists remain involved with the team in a consultant capacity, providing support and guidance to families as they navigate these complex waters as well as providing recommendations for symptom management for the baby in the process. In addition, if things do not go well for the baby, the parents' goals may change. Hence it is important for the palliative care specialist to maintain a relationship with the family and help guide them in the pros and cons of changing the direction of care.

A Middle Ground

Some parents opt for a more middle-of-the-road approach to their baby's care, or the "wait and see" model. This approach is appropriate when there are unknowns in prognosis and/or diagnosis that often can only be addressed after the baby is born. Parents wait to make firm decisions about goals of care until they see the severity of their particular baby's disease and how much support the baby will require in order to survive. Parents might opt for this approach even when the diagnosis and prognosis are certain, but the parents themselves are not certain about what they want and need more time to figure things out and for the disease to declare itself. Other parents, even with the certainty of diagnosis and a grim prognosis, want neither heroic measures nor pure comfort care, but rather, simple medical interventions that might give them a little more time with their baby. For example, William's parents knew he had trisomy 18 and that his prognosis was very poor. Yet they chose to admit him to the NICU and allow supplemental oxygen and IV fluids hoping these simple interventions might provide comfort and give them a little more time with their baby. Generally, families pursuing a middle ground approach to care choose to deliver in tertiary medical centers where they have the option of more specialized interventions if they choose. This mode of thinking allows for a more fluid model of goal setting. However, it can also leave parents unprepared to make a crucial care decision in the heat of the moment should their baby experience a sudden and unexpected turn for the worse. Palliative care specialists can be helpful in the prenatal setting by anticipating some of these events, exploring with parents in the setting of family meetings what options would be offered and what course of action would make the most sense for them and their baby. This can avoid some of the pressure and stress of making decisions in the moment after the baby is born. That said, many parents' goals for their baby change after the infant is born and parents see him/her alive for the first time. It is not unusual that the more time parents have to bond with their baby, the more attached they become, and their desire to have still more time becomes stronger. In addition, even severely impaired babies (e.g., those with brain malformations or hypoxic ischemic encephalopathy or severe cardiac defects) may look unaffected, making it particularly difficult for a parent to consider limiting care in any way. All this further underscores the importance of a longitudinal relationship of a family with the palliative care team. Such a team can guide parents on difficult decision-making, reminding them to factor in the longer-term impact of the disease on their baby and working with them to clarify their goals of care, which by nature evolve over time and never form in a vacuum [9].

Case 10.2

For William's parents the "wait and see" approach was most in line with their values and hopes as a family. Given that there is a spectrum of clinical severity in patients with trisomy 18 that sometimes cannot be fully predicted prior to birth, his parents were faced with the possibility of several possible outcomes. They consulted with specialists and had multiple family meetings with an interdisciplinary palliative care team including physicians, nurse practitioners, and social workers to establish separate birth and resuscitation plans for varying possible outcomes for William. They thought through plans for a stillbirth, a live birth requiring mild to moderately invasive interventions (stimulation, bag valve mask, CPAP), and a live birth that would require highly invasive interventions (intubation, ECMO). His parents decided they wanted standard resuscitation measures for William when he was born; however, if he was ill enough to require intubation or chest compressions, they wanted to avoid such aggressive interventions and immediately transition to comfort care and hold William for whatever time he had remaining. If he did well after birth, his parents decided they would be okay with temporary intubation for surgical procedures only.

For William's parents the palliative care team planned to remain involved after his birth as consultants to provide support and advocacy as well as aggressive symptom management as he concurrently underwent potentially life-prolonging interventions.

The Comfort Approach

Parents who have opted for a comfort-oriented approach at birth are generally focused solely on treating any symptoms of pain or distress without the goal of prolonging life. Others may transition to a comfort approach after a trial of life-sustaining treatment has failed or is felt to be overly burdensome. This latter scenario is discussed below. In a comfort approach, parents frequently want time and physical closeness with their baby for as long as possible so any interventions that would require the baby to be taken away are less desirable [10]. In such a situation an infant can be delivered at any facility deemed safe for both mother and baby. Some parents may want to deliver at a smaller facility closer to home or even in the home itself. Extending PPC services to smaller and more rural facilities can be a challenge. Most PPC teams are based in tertiary care pediatric hospitals and might not have the resources to provide hands-on care for a baby and family who live hours away. In such instances, it is incumbent upon the PPC team to determine if there are pediatric palliative care or hospice services available in the area and, if not, to work with the obstetrician, local pediatrician, and local hospice service to make sure the family gets good quality end-of-life care for the newborn child. The PPC team can make itself available by phone (or telemedicine) to whichever team assumes care of the child and family. Many families choose to deliver in a tertiary care center. The palliative care team often assumes a more central role in a baby's care in such situations, often serving as the admitting inpatient team when a patient is approaching end-of-life, and the focus of care is symptom management and supporting the family and siblings.

During a woman's pregnancy and after the infant is born, the various approaches should be discussed and weighed in the setting of what is medically realistic and what interventions are appropriate to be offered, in addition to what a family's values are and how they place importance on quantity and quality of life. Once a family's goals and values are known, palliative care specialists as well as other medical specialists should not shy away from providing medical recommendations as to what appropriate interventions might be in a given situation. They possess a medical expertise in knowing likely risks vs benefits of interventions in specific clinical scenarios, and withholding their knowledge would place an undue burden on families to make decisions they are likely not equipped to make [11]. To provide a recommendation is to give guidance and can lift some of the crushing burden of decision-making that is so often thrust on parents. Families should be informed that there is no right or wrong decision, that what is right is what feels right for them and their baby, even if that differs from what we recommend.

Of utmost importance during these critical periods is that medical teams need to be prepared to "meet a family where they're at" in the decision-making process. While recommendations can help, pushing a palliative care agenda, even if that seems like the most appropriate path for the baby, is ill-advised. If time allows, the palliative care specialist should give families space and support to make decisions without an agenda. Certainly there are instances where a baby is in extremis and decisions need to be made urgently, in which case parents should be gently guided through the process with sensitivity.

Transition to a Comfort Approach After Withdrawal of Life-Sustaining Treatment

If life-sustaining treatments such as mechanical ventilation, extracorporeal membrane oxygenation (ECMO), or other prolonged intensive care interventions are not leading to the parents' desired goal, the infant is approaching death despite these interventions, or the interventions are felt to be causing undue burden on the baby without a high likelihood of survival without severe morbidity, parents may elect to withdraw these treatments. In this case, PPC specialists may facilitate the conversation about a transition of care with the parents and the NICU and pediatric intensive care unit (PICU) teams, help clarify goals of care, and provide guidance to parents of what to expect after withdrawal. They may also help manage the care of the infant during and after withdrawal (though this may also be done by the ICU team). Specific pharmaceutical and symptom management is discussed in Chap. 9, section on "Withdrawal of Life-Sustaining Treatment". PPC specialists can be instrumental in supporting parents and staff, providing anticipatory guidance, and helping the ICU team manage the baby's care.

Case 10.3

William was born vaginally per mom's wishes despite some brief periods of fetal bradycardia. He did well after delivery, requiring a few minutes of positive pressure ventilation to help him transition and then remained comfortable on CPAP. Surgery on his abdominal defect was successful and the neurosurgery service was consulted and planned to repair his spinal canal defect the following day. A cardiologist was consulted and performed an echocardiogram that showed abnormalities not seen on prenatal imaging. Over the next 24 hours, William developed increased work of breathing and progressive hypoxia despite maximal support with CPAP. Given William's steady respiratory decline, his parents met at the bedside with the neonatologist and palliative care specialist. They were informed that William's anatomical abnormalities were major contributors to his respiratory distress and that the only way to reverse this was to undergo major surgery, surgery that William would likely not survive. Having thought through many difficult scenarios for William and knowing what they knew about babies with trisomy 18, they decided that they wanted to transition to a purely comfort-based approach to his care. The pediatric palliative care specialists were asked for recommendations for comfort medications although the neonatology team remained the primary team throughout the process. William was started on intravenous morphine as needed for pain and air hunger. His parents elected to hold him and were able to do some memory-making activities such as hand and feet molds as well as family photographs. His CPAP was removed once parents felt ready early in the morning on his second day of life and he died shortly thereafter, peacefully, in their arms. During and after his death, the pediatric palliative care team was frequently present at the bedside, supporting and guiding the family through William's dying process as well as supporting the other medical staff.

Symptom Management

Symptom management of an ill or dying infant is crucial in preserving his or her comfort and quality of life. It is also therapeutic for parents and families to know that their baby is not suffering, and if the baby dies, the grieving process may be much less complicated and the potential for guilt and regret significantly reduced. It is a challenge for busy neonatologists in large and busy NICUs with many critically ill infants to focus on symptom management. Having a palliative care specialist involved to assist with relieving symptoms is a crucial part of the interdisciplinary approach that must be taken with these complex children.

Table 10.2 Target symptoms and comfort medications for neonates at the end of life

Target symptom	Common neonatal comfort medications given in the hospital	Common neonatal comfort medications given in the home
Pain, dyspnea	IV: fentanyl, morphine PO/buccal: morphine, methadone, acetaminophen	PO/buccal: morphine, methadone, acetaminophen
Anxiety, seizures	IV: midazolam, dexmedetomidine PO: lorazepam, clonazepam, clonidine, phenobarbital, gabapentin	PO: lorazepam, clonidine, diazepam
Agitation	PO: gabapentin, clonidine	PO: gabapentin, clonidine
Spasticity	PO: baclofen, clonidine	PO: baclofen, clonidine
Airway secretions	IV: glycopyrrolate PO: glycopyrrolate	PO: glycopyrrolate

For infants who are terminally ill, common symptoms include dyspnea, agitation, and pain. Infants who are more stable may be able to go home if that is something the parents want and they have palliative care services available to them (e.g., from a community-based palliative care team). Most infants who are able to go home can be managed with oral medications, typically an opioid for pain and dyspnea (e.g., morphine) and a benzodiazepine for agitation (e.g., lorazepam) [12]. For the terminally ill infant who is unable to go home due to more severe symptoms of pain, dyspnea, and agitation, opioids and benzodiazepines can be administered intravenously.

In addition, there are many infants in the NICU who are critically ill but not terminally ill. Many of these chronically ill infants are opioid- and benzodiazepine-tolerant and management of their pain, agitation, and dyspnea can be a challenge. As is the case with any baby, it is often hard to be certain what is wrong. Is it pain? Is it air hunger? Is it agitation? Or is it agitation due to pain or air hunger or both? Oftentimes a judicious trial and error approach to symptom management must be taken. Typically this involves empiric escalation of opioids and benzodiazepines, and/or the addition of other medications, such as dexmedetomidine or gabapentin. It is also important to ask the parents and the bedside nurses what in their opinion is most effective for managing their baby's symptoms. Common symptoms and medications to relieve those symptoms are detailed in Table 10.2. More detailed descriptions of pain and symptom management are found in Chaps. 8 and 9.

Conclusion

The death or debility of a fetus or an infant is much greater than just that: It is also the death of a future unrealized and the inherent hope and joy that come along with pregnancy and childbirth. The process is inevitably an emotional one for all involved, often associated with the highest of highs and the lowest of lows. The experience can be tempered by involvement of perinatal palliative care specialists who can guide families through the process most easily while ensuring that their infant endures minimal suffering and has the best quality of life possible throughout the process.

References

1. Balaguer A, Martín-Ancel A, Ortigoza-Escobar D, Escribano J, Argemi J. The model of palliative care in the perinatal setting: a review of the literature. BMC Pediatr. 2012;12:25.
2. Milstein J. A paradigm of integrative care: healing with curing throughout life, "being with" and "doing to". J Perinatol. 2005;25:563–8.
3. Kenner C, Press J, Ryan D. Recommendations for palliative and bereavement care in the NICU: a family-centered integrative approach. J Perinatol. 2015;35(Suppl 1):S19–23.
4. Côté-Arsenault D, Denney-Koelsch E. "Have no regrets": parents' experiences and developmental tasks in pregnancy with a lethal fetal diagnosis. Soc Sci Med. 2016;154:100–9.
5. Rocha Catania T, Bernardes L, Guerra Benute GR, Bento Cicaroni Gibeli MA, Bertolassi do Nascimento N, Aparecida Barbosa TV, et al. When one knows the fetus is expected to die: palliative care in the context of prenatal diagnosis of fetal malformations. J Palliat Med. 2017;20(9):1020–31.
6. Breeze AC, Lees CC, Kumar A, Missfelder-Lobos HH, Murdoch EM. Palliative care for the prenatally diagnosed lethal fetal abnormality. Arch Dis Child Fetal Neonatal Ed. 2007;92(1):F56–8.
7. Hudson P, Quinn K, O'Hanlon B, Aranda S. Family meetings in palliative care: multidisciplinary clinical practice guidelines. BMC Palliat Care. 2008;7(12):1–12.
8. Côté-Arsenault D, Krowchuk H, Wendasah JH, Denney-Koelsch E. We want what's best for our baby: prenatal parenting of babies with lethal conditions. J Prenat Perinat Psychol Health. 2015;29(3):157–76.
9. Naik AD, Martin LA, Moye J, Karel MJ. Health values and treatment goals of older, multimorbid adults facing life-threatening illness. J Am Geriatr Soc. 2016;64(3):625–31.
10. Nelson KE, Rosella LC, Mahant S. Survival and surgical interventions for children with trisomy 13 and 18. JAMA. 2016;316(4):420–8.
11. Entwistle VA, Carter SM, Cribb A, McCaffery K. Supporting patient autonomy: the importance of clinician-patient relationships. J Gen Intern Med. 2010;25(7):741–5.
12. Hall RW, Anand KJS. Pain management in newborns. Clin Perinatol. 2014;41(4):895–924.

11 Spiritual Care in the Perinatal Period

Maurice Hopkins

Key Points

1. Life-limiting illnesses for babies diagnosed in utero cause profound spiritual distress.
2. Although widely recognized, spiritual distress is often undercared for.
3. There is a distinct difference between religious and spiritual care.
4. Chaplains are spiritual specialists but clinicians can be spiritual generalists.
5. Clinicians need to have a certain comfort level to help address spiritual distress.
6. Staff support is especially relevant and necessary in perinatal palliative care.

> I had watched the parents' faces- at first wan, dull, almost otherworldly- sharpen and focus. And as I sat there, I realized that the questions intersecting life, death, and meaning, questions that all people face at some point, usually arise in a medical context. –Paul Kalanithi, *When Breath Becomes Air*

Dr. Paul Kalanithi wrote this in his well-known book *When Breath Becomes Air* [1]. This realization came to him as he listened to an experienced pediatric neurosurgeon explain to a shocked set of parents that their child had a newly diagnosed brain tumor. It was a moment of clarity for a doctor in training in the midst of a chaotic and life-changing moment for that family. Paul realized what many clinicians who work in palliative care already know – that the collision of life, death, and meaning happen after a life-altering diagnosis is given to patient and family. It can be difficult for

M. Hopkins (✉)
Golisano Children's Hospital at University of Rochester Medical Center/CompassionNet, Department of Pediatrics, Rochester, NY, USA
e-mail: maurice_hopkins@urmc.rochester.edu

E. M. Denney-Koelsch, D. Côté-Arsenault (eds.), *Perinatal Palliative Care*,
https://doi.org/10.1007/978-3-030-34751-2_11

clinicians to realize in this sudden urgency for decision-making and determining goals of care that patients and their caretakers rely heavily on their individual spirituality.

In regards to perinatal palliative care (PPC), it is often during midpregnancy that unexpected or unforeseen medical information is delivered to expectant parents. In utero fetal diagnoses of medical complications are wrought with spiritual implications for entire family systems. The mystery surrounding creation of life itself is a spiritual experience under the best of circumstances, but when a sudden unexpected life-limiting or fatal medical diagnosis of the child is added to a pregnancy, the spiritual distress that families can feel is often unparalleled. Clinicians need to recognize this anguish as spiritual distress in order to help alleviate it as much as possible. Unfortunately, spiritual suffering is poorly diagnosed and as a result can often be underaddressed. Practitioners of PPC must be comfortable dealing with these issues as they arise in their everyday work. Many clinicians are generally undertrained and thus uncomfortable having spiritual discussions with their patients. This chapter will attempt to alleviate some of the anxiety and trepidation that many staff feel as they attempt to recognize and address the spiritual and religious support needs of the patients that they serve in perinatal palliative care.

Spirituality and Religion

There are many misconceptions medical clinicians hold in regards to spiritual care. Perhaps the biggest misunderstanding is the distinction between spirituality and religion. At the most basic level, spirituality is a much broader concept of which religion can be a component. In this sense, all people have spirituality but only some express it through their specific religion. All children when they are born and grow are spiritual beings. However, they are not religious until they are taught a particular religious tradition. That is why parents must provide for the religious education of their children if they so choose. Spirituality has a much larger scope than religion and is thus harder to define. There has been much work in the field of medical research to find a unifying definition of spirituality so that it can be measured consistently in relation to evidence-based health outcomes.

Religion is much easier to define and understand but generally causes the most unease amongst clinicians. This unease is due largely to a lack of understanding of religions other than their own and the resultant lack of confidence discussing them. Religion is defined as a set of beliefs shared by a group of people with sacred texts, rituals, and corporate gathering with a moral code of conduct. The Divine, God, Ultimate Truth, and nirvana are examples of objects worshiped in religious organizations. Religions have been developed and passed down over centuries with teachings that have been developed and taught from one generation to the next [2]. Christianity, Islam, Judaism, Buddhism, and Hinduism are the five major world religions, but there are many more. Religious care for patients can be provided for by their specific clergy or by chaplains of the same religion. Religious care does vary greatly and professional clergy should be consulted to provide specific religious customs when possible. Chaplains can often provide for the religious care of patients and families either themselves or through contacts with community clergy, if the family does not have a connection to a local faith community.

Spirituality, on the other hand, is far more vague and, consequently, much harder to identify. There are currently several healthcare professionals who are working to better define spirituality as it relates to overall patient wellness and resiliency. Dr. Christina Puchalski defines spirituality as: "every person's inherent search for ultimate meaning and purpose in life. The meaning can be found in religion but may often be broader than that including a relationship with god/divine figure or transcendence; relationships with others; as well as spirituality found in nature, art, and rational thought" [3].

Drs. Gowri Anandarajah and Ellen Hight defined spirituality as "a complex and multidimensional part of the human experience. It has cognitive, experiential, and behavioral aspects. The cognitive or philosophic aspects of spirituality include the search for meaning, purpose, and truth in life and the beliefs and values by which an individual lives. The experiential and emotional aspects involve feelings of hope, love, connection, inner peace, comfort, and support" [4].

As these two examples illustrate, spirituality is a term that is frequently used but very difficult to concretely explain. Inside spirituality there is a mixture of faith, hope, meaning, purpose, morality, transcendence, theology, nature, cognitive, experiential, and behavioral components which vary with every individual. So in this way spirituality is as varied as the complex human being cared for by perinatal palliative care teams. What one individual finds meaningful in their life may be completely inconsequential for another. It is essential for clinicians, especially palliative care teams, to recognize that in order to truly be holistic and treat the patient biopsychosocially, spiritual care must be addressed.

Case 11.1

Mary and Kim were a same-sex couple who wanted to have children. Kim had previously, through a donor, become pregnant with twins only to lose them during the pregnancy. After years of grief and disappointment, they were able to conceive again with another set of twin boys. After the pain of their previous losses, they were excited, nervous, and daring bravely to dream again. The pregnancy proceeded nicely until the twins were born prematurely at 28 weeks. They were appropriately worried but also suffering as the pain from their previous losses came flooding back.

The first time that I walked into their room and introduced myself as the chaplain, I got a reaction that I had not ever received before. Mary looked directly at me and said "We are lesbians in a relationship. We are not religious and did not ask to see a chaplain." I quickly was able to explain to them that I was part of the team in the NICU and that I was merely checking in on how they and the twins were doing. After some polite small talk, I left the room. A few days later I made a special point to stop and ask them how the twins were doing. This time they were slightly more open as we talked about a topic that we could both agree on, the health of their two sons. I continued to visit occasionally and slowly built a relationship with them. Eventually one day Mary apologized for the way she greeted me the first day. She explained that due to their sexuality, they as a couple had been treated badly by churches in the past. I apologized for how they had been treated in the past. I had slowly gained their trust over time because I did not have any religious agenda and truly shared their love and concern over the health of their sons. They talked about how meaningful having their babies in their lives was. They felt that every day was magical with their newborns as we explored their roles as parents in their lives. In this regard I was able to join them through our shared life experiences and care for their spiritual needs regardless of their prior bad experiences.

The good news is that although spirituality appears very complex in theory, addressing it in practice it is not. Whatever gives a patient's life meaning is their own personal spirituality. It is the conscious things that we use to navigate our everyday lives, but it is also in the unconscious as we make both every day and major life decisions. If clinicians truly empathetically listen to the wishes, goals, and priorities of those under their care, the tenants of their individual spirituality can be seen. It can be challenging to recognize that what someone is sharing is rooted in their own spiritual beliefs. Clinically trained chaplains are experts at listening for spirituality as they sit and talk to patients, but clinicians do not need to be chaplains to recognize it. As people face truly life-altering decisions regarding goals of care for themselves or their child, their spirituality is expressed as they reach conclusions and explain their thought process. The reality is that all interdisciplinary team members provide spiritual care, as seen in Fig. 11.1. Different disciplines have their own specific duties, responsibilities, and expertise but there is always overlap. Chaplains specialize in religious and spiritual care but true spiritual care occurs in the center overlapping area where all disciplines intersect. True spiritual care happens when clinicians treat the whole person, including their spirit, so that they feel supported no matter what care decisions are made.

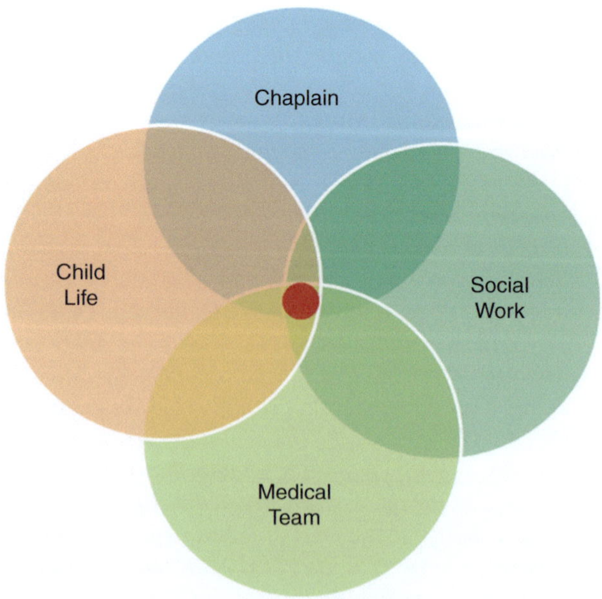

Fig. 11.1 Relationship of chaplain within the interdisciplinary team for true spiritual care

Case 11.2

Mike and Jenny were an "older" couple, both in their late thirties, when they were pleasantly surprised that they were pregnant with their third child. The first two children were teenagers so there was going to be a sizable age gap between their children. They were both Christians who attended church regularly and they saw the pregnancy as a blessing even though it was unexpected. Everything was going along fine until Jenny had her 20-week ultrasound. The baby was diagnosed with a very complex congenital cardiac defect that involved multiple components. Jenny's veteran male obstetrician was very quick to recommend that they terminate the pregnancy due to the severity and lethality of the baby's cardiac defect. Instantly, Mike and Jenny's response was NO! Their religious and spiritual beliefs instantly informed their decision without any debate. Their values, beliefs, and meaning in their lives would not even consider terminating the pregnancy. The obstetrician was adamant that they end the pregnancy. He even expressed to the parents that they were being selfish to bring a child into the world with this cardiac diagnosis which would cause great suffering to the child. Jenny instantly fired the doctor and transferred her care to a larger regional academic children's hospital.

Upon meeting with their new obstetrician, they were given their options for the baby. They were also able to meet with the perinatal palliative care team. Mike and Jenny had three options offered to them: termination, comfort care after birth, or full cardiac surgical interventions once the baby was born. After some time and careful consideration, Mike and Jenny decided to do a combination of the second and third options. They decided to wait for the baby to be born, get a clearer picture of the actual cardiac defect, and then decide how to proceed. With the exception of their first obstetrician, Mike and Jenny were so appreciative of the care and respect they received from the various medical teams.

I got involved as the chaplain on the day of the birth. Mike and Jenny wanted the baby to be blessed. So, I accompanied them from the labor and delivery unit with Jenny in a wheelchair, over to the neonatal intensive care unit and conducted the blessing. As it turned out the baby did not have the multiple serious cardiac defects that were originally diagnosed on ultrasound but only transposition of the great vessels. The baby had the single surgery, recovered, and went home shortly after. Over many follow-up visits with the family throughout their hospitalization, we had many spiritual conversations. The one statement that still stands out is when Jenny was holding the baby and she said "I was told to abort her." The statement jarred me as I looked at the loving mother hold her healthy baby girl.

Fortunately this was a couple that was strong enough to stand up to their doctor for their own religious/spiritual beliefs, but it makes me wonder about those families who are not bold enough. This couple's obstetrician clearly did not recognize or address how their spirituality impacted their medical decision-making. Clinicians who work in perinatal palliative care and support families such as this one may need to advocate for or empower families to let the spiritually informed decisions to be heard and respected by medical providers.

Abstract Versus Tangible

There is another spiritual phenomenon that occurs with expectant families in PPC programs that has to do with the abstract versus tangible aspect of an unborn baby. In many cases, the serious medical issues of the child are diagnosed while the baby is still in utero. Most families say when asked that they were thankful for the diagnosis prior to birth. They generally feel that the earlier knowledge gives them time to process this news, to accept, talk, research, and adjust. This preemptory work of acceptance before the birth relieves the shock and surprise experienced by families with babies that had no advanced diagnosis. Labor and delivery of a baby is hectic and stressful enough without serious medical surprises. These families who have the benefit of early diagnosis also benefit from involvement of the PPC team throughout the remainder of the pregnancy. Birth plans and goals of care can be considered, discussed, and decided upon over time after careful spiritual discernment.

Once the shock lessens, families who receive a fetal diagnosis that warrants perinatal palliative care experience a full gambit of emotions throughout the remainder of the pregnancy. There can be a spiral effect of thoughts and emotions that surface, fade, and then reemerge again. This can include fear, anger, grief, disillusionment, or uncertainty. Through all these stages, the family's spirituality is at work both internally and externally. As a couple comes to terms with the baby's diagnosis through the support of each other, family, friends, and the PPC team, they slowly make their decisions. Clarifying their goals of care and sharing their values is their spirituality in action. They must decide what gives their lives, and consequently their future family's life, meaning. The spiritual and religious beliefs of the family will come to the surface in the quick decisions, as well as in the carefully thought out conclusions. Spirituality is at the heart of the ultimate decision between the three choices that the family must make: termination, comfort measures at birth, aggressive medical care, or something in between.

This is when the abstract versus the tangible then comes into play. Clinicians must understand and accept that during the pregnancy even though the baby is very real, the decisions made by the parents are made in the abstract. The family decides what they think they will do when the baby is born. Once the birth occurs, the newborn becomes very literally a tangible child. It is not uncommon for parents to change their treatment plan decisions once they are able to hold the baby. Changes in plans are usually openly accepted by the care team but not always completely understood. PPC practitioners need to be cognizant of how this concept of abstract vs tangible influences decision-making for families both before and after the birth.

Practical Advice for Clinicians

Spirituality and religion are infused into the very nature of humanity. Each and every person is a physical being with spiritual beliefs. Spirituality and meaning are the largest influences on medical decisions made by individuals every day.

Given this widely accepted understanding of spirituality, it is fair to ask the question: Why are healthcare providers afraid to have spiritual conversations with patients and families? Over time the subjects of religion and spirituality have become too private, personal, or controversial to talk about, especially in the current healthcare climate. A patient's religious or spiritual beliefs are a huge part of who they are and how they understand illness or disease. Given this understanding of the importance of spirituality, it seems negligent to leave it detached from health and wellness discussions. A doctor will examine a patient's entire body and ask questions about the most intimate details of their life in order to best treat them, yet they are hesitant to ask about religious beliefs. In order to fully treat a patient in the biopsychosocial model of medical care, spiritual care must be incorporated as well. The reality is that most clinicians are not trained to discuss spiritual matters, even though they know they exist, and are thus uncomfortable asking patients and families.

Conversely, it is also fair for clinicians to wonder if patients and families want their healthcare providers to inquire about their spiritual beliefs. Studies have shown that a majority of patients actually want their physicians or healthcare providers to address their spiritual or religious needs if they were gravely ill [5]. It is therefore logical that parents facing a severe prenatal diagnosis of their unborn baby would also want to talk about these issues. In surveys of general pediatricians at academic hospitals, 76% agreed that patient and family spiritual/religious concerns were relevant to their practice, but 51% never or rarely asked [6]. These same pediatricians also answered that only 13% received any formal instruction in their medical education on how to have spiritual conversations with their patients. It would be interesting to see the same survey conducted with pediatric and perinatal palliative care doctors, who may be more attuned to these issues. It is clear that the need to address the spiritual and religious beliefs of patients and families is wanted and needed by both the provider and receiver of healthcare, but there has not been sufficient spiritual education and training for healthcare providers.

Spiritual Generalists

Clinicians can be trained how to have spiritual conversations that get to the heart of medical decision-making for patients and families, especially in PPC. One way for clinicians to conceptualize their role in spiritual conversations with patients and families is through the idea of spiritual generalist versus spiritual specialist [7]. Clinicians should learn the basic skills of a spiritual generalist so that they can fully assess a patient. This may take a small amount of training, but it is not a difficult, burdensome, or overly time-consuming task. Basic spiritual conversations do not need to be strictly relegated to chaplains. There is a tendency in healthcare that when a patient mentions any spiritualty, a chaplain is called to have that conversation. Although involving a chaplain in this instance is a great next step, the clinician should not be afraid to have the conversation with the patient to the extent of their comfort and ability. Clinically trained chaplains are spiritual specialists and should be consulted if there are religious needs or if the clinician senses any spiritual distress from the patient or family. Through this concept of generalist and specialist, spirituality can be addressed throughout the spectrum of the relationship from diagnosis to birth and onward in PPC.

Spiritual conversations are not as difficult and scary as most clinicians fear. The common fear is that one must be an expert in religions or have extensive chaplain training to competently have spiritual conversations. The reality is that these conversations truly rely upon deep caring and openness. Clinicians must simply demonstrate spiritual and cultural humility and do not require expert knowledge on religions. Simply by asking genuinely open curious questions about someone's belief system easily initiates spiritual conversations. For example, "Tell me about your faith" or "How does your religion help you during this illness?" This allows the patient to be the expert in their spirituality and understanding of what gives meaning in their own life. Clinicians simply need to change their posture from expert to that of a learner and most patients will open up regarding their beliefs. If patients simply refuse to talk about spirituality, that is perfectly acceptable as well, but it demonstrates that the clinician is open to discussing anything pertinent to their decision-making.

Clinicians, especially chaplains, need to have a comfort with their own beliefs in order to provide genuine spiritual care to patients and families. The mandatory first step in this process is for the care providers to "know" their own beliefs whether spiritual or religious. Once this is worked out, clinicians can provide care from their own firm foundation to assist others who are in spiritual distress. When providers have a strong grasp of their own beliefs, they can truly meet patients and families where they are, especially when decisions are made that conflict with one's own strongly held beliefs. Termination of a pregnancy with a perinatal diagnosis is a very relevant example of a possible conflict for clinicians. Termination is often offered to couples who receive a severe fetal diagnosis and PPC providers must be able to support couples in whatever choices they make. Moral and ethical decisions that conflict with one's own beliefs usually require greater spiritual care than ones we agree with, so caregivers must recognize their own biases. Perinatal spiritual care begins at diagnosis and continues on throughout, regardless of outcome.

Clinically trained chaplains are trained to provide pastoral care across an interfaith spectrum of belief systems in medically complex situations. For this reason, chaplains may be better able to provide spiritual care for couples in their decision-making than their specific clergy. Community clergy belong to and are ordained by specific faiths or denominations that have stringent doctrines that may or may not be accepting of the difficult choices parents inevitably have to make in PPC. Chaplains, and clinicians, must be cognizant of their own beliefs so that they do not impose them on couples in their times of greatest vulnerability. Pastoral malpractice happens when care providers impose their own beliefs on confused and hurting families to influence their decision-making.

Case 11.3

Bill and Ashley are a young married couple in their twenties. They are Christians who attend church regularly. They were overjoyed when they conceived their first child, who they named Austin. Twenty weeks into the pregnancy, they received the diagnosis that Austin had hypoplastic left heart syndrome. The couple was shocked, but after many visits with pediatric cardiologists and surgeons, they felt somewhat more accepting and assured. They were told that his condition would require several surgeries but they were thankful because there was a path forward for Austin. It would be a long road but at least it was a road.

Eventually Austin was born, and after a few days in the NICU, he had his first surgery. Throughout the next several months, Austin had many complications and setbacks. In an effort to help keep Austin healthy, his parents restricted visitors to a bare minimum. This extended time in the hospital put a tremendous strain on Bill and Ashley's marriage as they struggled to cope in the individual ways. Eventually Austin declined to a point that Bill and Ashley decided to remove life support so that he could die peacefully in their arms. On that day before the removal of support, they brought in their home church pastor to baptize Austin. I was able to prepare the pastor ahead of time for what he would see and facilitate the baptism with staff. After the baptism, pictures, and final goodbyes from extended family, Austin died in his parents' arms.

In the ensuing months I was able to follow-up with Bill and Ashley for bereavement care. They expressed so many common emotions and thoughts following the death of Austin. Perhaps their greatest fear centered around having another baby. They feared that if they conceived another child, it may again have a congenital heart anomaly. Bill looked me straight in the eye and said that they could not handle going through the same situation again. They also expressed that they would not want the next baby to suffer like Austin had. Bill said that if the exact diagnosis happened again, "he would like to not be a Christian for a day so that we could abort the baby." This statement really impacted me as I heard it and still today. I realized that a chaplain plays a vital role in situations like this. Bill would not have made that same statement to his pastor. Chaplains play an important role by providing spiritual and religious support without judgement, which is exactly what this couple needed in that moment.

Spiritual and Religious Care

Clinicians are generally hesitant, and even fearful, to have religiously specific conversations with families. This hesitancy usually comes from a false assumption that the family will want to know something specific to their religion that the provider will not have answers for. Rarely is this the case and usually the family member just simply needs to express things aloud. In this circumstance the clinician can rely on their spiritual humility, ask clarifying questions, and allow the parent to be the expert in their own faith. In these types of situations, couples may ask why God has or has not allowed something to happen. These questions are generally rhetorical in nature as the person asking is not looking for a concrete answer. What they are really looking for is an empathetic silence or a sincere heartfelt "I do not know."

Each individual has his or her own theology and understanding about how God works, regardless of their faith or religion. Everyone falls somewhere on a continuum from not believing in God to believing He is involved in everyday life. A life-limiting fetal diagnosis or loss of a baby can seriously shake individuals' faith. They may express that God is punishing them or that they feel abandoned by God. These types of statements can feel scary in the moment but ultimately it is good that these feelings get expressed. This type of spiritual distress does need to be addressed by professional chaplains or the family's specific clergy. Spiritual distress of this type can cause serious issues over time and can be directly correlated to bereavement and grief coping over time [8]. Belief in afterlife or not has significant impact on long-term coping for parents who experience the loss of a child. This is also why it is important to perform requested religious rituals at the time of death so that parents can always feel that they did what was required at the time of death without future regret.

Birth Rituals

There are not many religious customs that are required or requested at the birth of a child that is not expected to live long. The Islamic faith has a custom that involves the father, or family elder, of the child whispering the call to prayer (Adhon) into the ear of the child so that it is the first thing the child hears as it enters the world. In Christian tradition, parents may request a blessing or baptism. The act of baptizing of babies varies greatly inside the spectrum of Christian denominations. In the case of blessing or baptism, any person is permitted to do it in the case of emergency, so it does not have to be a chaplain or clergy person. There is also a delicate balance that must be struck around baptism in settings other than churches. For most Christian denominations, baptism is a community ceremony whereby not just the parents but the entire church commits to help raise the child and support the parents. So if a child is not imminently dying and is expected to go home and the family has their own faith community, they should be encouraged to do the baptism with their home church family. Baptism should be done outside the church only in urgent situations and the family is in great distress. Most other religious customs that normal healthy children go through are done over time as they grow and are not needed if the child only lives for a short period of time.

Death Rituals

Death rituals may need to be honored and understood by clinicians in the event of the death of a child in the perinatal period of life. Christian death rituals may include any combination of baptism before death, blessings, or prayers. In the Islamic faith tradition, the body is washed and shrouded shortly after death. Autopsy or cremations are not done in the Islamic faith and burial should be as soon as possible. Ideally, bodies are not embalmed and buried without a casket, but this varies by the laws of the municipality where the death occurs. Jewish death rituals may include specific prayers. Jewish funerals are usually as soon as possible and as simple as possible. Cremation may be allowed with Jewish deaths depending on how conservative the family's Judaic faith is. These death rituals listed are only typical examples for each faith. A disclaimer must be given that there are many variations of these rituals inside of each faith tradition based on a multitude factors. After death, clinicians must especially let the family lead with the rituals that are meaningful to them, and help in any way possible.

Staff Support

Staff support is another important component of what professional chaplains are able to provide. The chaplain is there to provide support not only for the patient and family, but also the staff (Fig. 11.2). Posttraumatic event or death debriefings are so important for clinical staff. The chaplain's acceptance, tolerance, and appreciation of different belief systems can be an invaluable resource for staff as they debrief difficult situations [9]. It is so important soon after an event to pause and gather together. There is tremendous power in simply talking about feelings aloud without the family present. This helps staff to stop, acknowledge what happened, and provide a safe place to grieve if necessary. Debriefings are so important in helping to reduce staff burnout from the mentally, emotionally, and spiritually

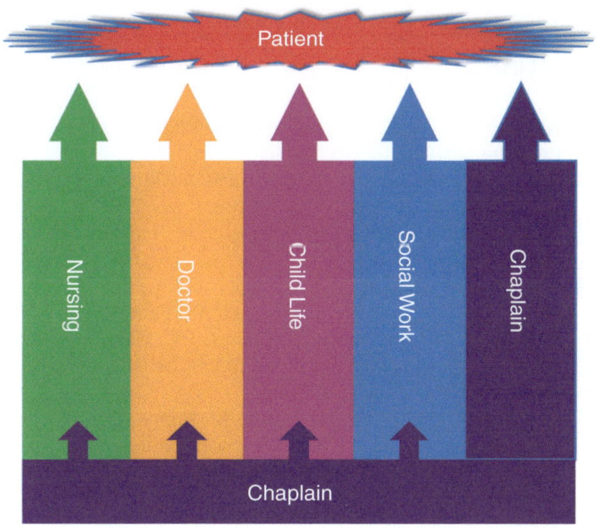

Fig. 11.2 Chaplains provide direct patient care as part of the interdisciplinary team, but also support the entire team's own spiritual needs

draining work that they do in PPC. Clinicians must feel that their emotions are valid and that they are not alone in their suffering. One of the most positive results of a debrief is that employees genuinely feel like the institution truly cares about its employees. This perception contributes positively to employee retention, work satisfaction, and health.

Staff support is especially relevant and necessary in PPC. Infant loss, miscarriage, termination, and fertility issues span all ages and genders of clinicians involved. Even in the medical community, there is still an unspoken wall of silence where pregnancy loss is not openly discussed [10]. Given the prevalence and quantity of pregnancy issues, it is safe to assume that members of the PPC team have had experienced some level of loss in the past or present. Even without a personal connection to loss, clinicians are affected by the loss and grief that permeates infant loss.

Conclusion

In palliative care, especially perinatal, there are spiritual implications for entire family systems. Clinicians need to recognize this anguish as spiritual distress in order to help alleviate it as much as possible. Unfortunately, spiritual suffering is often poorly diagnosed and as a result can often be underaddressed. Although having a professional clinically trained chaplain is ideal for a palliative care team, practitioners of perinatal palliative care must be comfortable dealing with spiritual/religious issues as they arise in their everyday work. Many clinicians are generally undertrained and thus uncomfortable having spiritual/religious discussions with their patients and families. Staff must feel comfortable as a spiritual generalist for when, or if, they do not have access to a spiritual specialist, such as a chaplain.

References

1. Kalanithi P. When breath becomes air. Waterville: Thorndike Press, a part of Gale, Cengage Learning; 2016. p. 69–70.
2. Koenig HG. Medicine, religion, and health: where science and spirituality meet. West Conshohocken: Templeton Foundation Press; 2008. p. 11–6.
3. Puchalski CM. Spirituality and medicine: curricula in medical education. J Cancer Educ. 2006;21(1):14–8.
4. Anandarajah G, Hight E. Spirituality and medical practice: using the HOPE questions as a practical tool for spiritual assessment. Am Fam Physician. 2001;63(1):81–9.
5. Ehman JW, Ott BB, Short TH, Ciampa RC, Hansen-Flaschen J. Do patients want physicians to inquire about their spiritual or religious beliefs if they become gravely ill? Arch Intern Med. 1999;159(15):1803–6.
6. Grossoehme DH, Ragsdale JR, McHenry CL, Thurston C, DeWitt T, VandeCreek L. Pediatrician characteristics associated with attention to spirituality and religion in clinical practice. Pediatrics. 2007;119(1):e117–23.

7. Robinson MR, Thiel MM, Meyer EC. On being a spiritual care generalist. Am J Bioeth. 2007;7(7):24–6.
8. Rosenbaum JL, Smith JR, Zollfrank R. Neonatal end-of-life spiritual support care. J Perinat Neonatal Nurs. 2011;25(1):61–9.
9. Burke SS, Matsumoto AR. Pastoral care for perinatal and neonatal health care providers. J Obstet Gynecol Neonatal Nurs. 1999;28(2):137–41.
10. Cowchock FS, Meador KG, Floyd SE, Swamy GK. Spiritual needs of couples facing pregnancy termination because of fetal anomalies. J Pastoral Care Counsel. 2011;65(1–2):4.1–10.

Perinatal Bereavement Care

12

Ashley Pinkeney

Introduction

If we were to search through the dictionary, we would not find a word that describes someone who has lost a child. If you experience the death of a spouse, you are considered a widow. If you experience the loss of a parent, you're considered an orphan. A parent who has lost a child has no name, perhaps because it is so hard for others to understand this kind of loss. A bereaved parent experiences this loss on a daily basis. It is easy to think of the death of a loved one as one single event, but as many bereaved parents will tell you, they experience this event every day. During a day that seems to be going fine, quiet memories can sneak up and paralyze them with waves of emotion.

We, as providers, should recognize that the loss of a child is inconceivable from so many perspectives. This grief is not like any other grief; the loss of an infant carries many layers of complexity. This chapter will talk about perinatal loss, exploring the anticipatory grief parents experience when their fetus has been given a lethal diagnosis, and the nuanced grief experiences that can occur following an infant loss through miscarriage, stillbirth, or neonatal death.

The Right to Grieve

Perinatal loss has been defined as the death of a baby via ectopic pregnancy, miscarriage, stillbirth, and neonatal or infant death [1]. It is common for the world to minimize a perinatal loss: *disenfranchised grief* occurs when society fails to recognize the significance of a loss in the mourner's life [2]. Because the fetus or infant is

A. Pinkeney (✉)
Department of Pediatric Palliative Care, Golisano Children's Hospital, University of Rochester Medical Center, Rochester, NY, USA
e-mail: apinkeney@thehealingconnectioninc.org

E. M. Denney-Koelsch, D. Côté-Arsenault (eds.), *Perinatal Palliative Care*,
https://doi.org/10.1007/978-3-030-34751-2_12

physically and psychologically absent, this loss also encompasses elements of *ambiguous loss* [1]. Bereaved parents sometimes receive the message from others that the short length of their child's life means that their grief experience should not be as intense as if the child were older. Bereaved parents tell us that this assumption is categorically untrue. The depth and intensity of grief that these parents experience can be devastating. Perinatal loss is not only the loss of a life, it is the loss of hopes and dreams for the future—the loss of a life unfulfilled.

For parents who have struggled with infertility, or cannot have other children because of birth complications, this loss of the future is especially acute. Well-meaning persons can make the situation worse with comments like, "You can always have other children." For most parents, the birth of another child following a perinatal loss does not mean that the child who is deceased is being replaced. Every child is unique, and the parents wanted and love the baby they lost. These parents deserve the space to have their infant's life remembered and honored, without comparison to living children they have or may have in the future.

Whatever the circumstances surrounding a fetal or infant death, parents have the right to grieve the loss of this young life that is a part of their family. They should not have their loss minimized, or their grieving rushed. Many times, when family and friends talk to a bereaved parent about what they "should" feel, or how they are going through the "stages" of grief, they do not understand that a new normal is now in place. Whatever discomfort they are experiencing, support persons should not expect the bereaved parent to get back to "normal" quickly, or perhaps ever.

Grief and Mourning Theories

Perspectives on Grief

This section will provide an overview of several ways to conceptualize grief, loss, and mourning. Grief has been described as "the process of experiencing the psychological, social, and physical reactions of loss" [3]. This definition normalizes that a person may experience a multitude of reactions as they move through their grieving process.

Several scholars and theorists have outlined the progression of grief, loss, and mourning, so clinicians can choose from a variety of theoretical orientations to contextualize the experiences of individuals and families. While the terms grief, mourning, and bereavement are frequently used interchangeably, they each have contextually different meanings. *Bereavement* defines the loss itself: the state of having lost a loved one [3]. *Mourning* is the process of moving through and adapting to the internal and external changes that are continually occurring while the mourner lives with loss every day [4]. The theoretical approach chosen to support these families should take into account the parents' history and life experiences. One particular grief theory is not going to fit every person or couple, so it is important to be knowledgeable about multiple perspectives of bereavement in order to provide the best care for parents and families.

Death and Dying

Psychiatrist Elisabeth Kübler-Ross changed society's perspective on death from "curing" the patient to "caring" for the patient as they approach the end of their life. *On Death and Dying,* first published in 1969, is full of exchanges between Dr. Kübler-Ross and her patients about reactions to their own impending death [5]. Her work helped medical professionals become more aware and sensitive to the needs of the dying. Through a series of interviews with hospice patients, she identified a common set of emotional responses to death and the knowledge of dying. These are known as the five stages of dying: denial, anger, bargaining, depression, and acceptance (Table 12.1). The dying may experience these stages in any order, recurrently, or in combination.

In popular culture, the work of Dr. Kübler-Ross is seen as the "go-to" theory on death and dying, but the author stressed that her book was "not meant to be a textbook on how to manage dying patients," nor is it a "complete study of the psychology of the dying." While this theory does speak about the experiences of the dying, and in the context of this chapter, infants will not be able to move through this process due to their developmental capabilities, it's crucial to recognize that some

Table 12.1 Stages of dying

Denial	"No, not me, it can't be true." the initial and most common response to the knowledge of impending death. It can serve as a defense mechanism to ease anxiety and fear about the inevitability of death. "Denial is usually a temporary defense replaced by partial acceptance"(P. 36)
Anger	"Why me?" this anger, which can be expressed as rage, envy or resentment, is difficult for the family and staff to cope with, especially when the patient's anger is displaced and projected onto others and the environment around them. Rather than taking the anger personally, support persons can help by understanding the patient's anger and helping them to feel respected and understood
Bargaining	Bargaining is "an attempt to postpone, it has to include a prize for 'good behavior' and also sets a self-imposed 'deadline' and it includes an implicit promise that the patient will not ask for more if this one postponement is granted"(P. 73). Most promises are made with God and are usually kept in secret, referenced indirectly or mentioned only in a Chaplain's presence. Promises may be marked with quiet guilt, so they are important to address openly
Depression	Depression is "preparatory grief that a terminally ill patient undergoes in order to prepare for the final separation from this world" (P. 76)
	Reactive depression. The cause of this depression is known and others try to alleviate unrealistic guilt and shame. Once the patient's critical concerns are addressed (e.g., reorganization of household duties), the depression may seem to lift
	Preparatory depression is a "tool for coping with impending loss…. The patient is in the process of losing everything. If he is allowed to express his sorrow, he will find final acceptance easier and he will be grateful to those who can sit with him during this stage without constantly telling him not to be sad" (P. 77)
Acceptance	"If given enough time to work through the other 4 stages, a terminally ill patient can reach a stage where they have mourned their impending loss and contemplate their coming end with a degree of quiet expectation" (P. 99)

Adapted from Kübler-Ross [5]

bereaved families use Kübler-Ross's five stages as a frame of reference as they discuss their grief experiences. If this frame seems less than useful, providers have an opportunity to educate the families about other bereavement theories that may better fit the parent's world view following the loss of their child.

Overview of Bereavement Theories

Several theories of grief are summarized in Table 12.2.

These theories can be used to conceptualize the grief experience. Each perspective can help therapists and care team members as well as educate bereaved parents to know what is normal and how parents may grieve and to normalize their mourning experiences.

Table 12.2 Brief summary of bereavement theories and perspectives

Theory	Perspective
Dual process model of grief // Stroebe and Schut (1999) [6]	The dual process model (DPM) describes loss-oriented and restoration-oriented stressors that are associated with grieving. *Loss-oriented stressors* come from focusing on and processing the loss of the person who has died as well as the relationship with that person. *Restoration-oriented stressors* refer to secondary sources of stress and coping, e.g., feelings of isolation, grief bursts that occur in the presence of baby items or reminders the baby is no longer alive. Stroebe and Schut argue that healthy grieving means engaging in a *dynamic process of oscillating* between loss-oriented and restoration-oriented coping, between confronting the loss and avoiding the loss. In a healthy grief process, we cope with our grief at times and seek respite at other times
Tasks of mourning // J. William Worden (1991) [4]	*Task 1: Accept the reality of the loss*
	Task 2: Work through the pain of the grief
	Task 3: Adjust to an environment in which the deceased is missing: External, internal, and spiritual
	Task 4: Find an enduring connection with the deceased while embarking on a new life
4 phases of grief // Bowlby and Parkes (1970, 2018) [7, 8]	*Shock and numbness.* Emotions that occur as a defense mechanism to cope in the immediate aftermath of the death
	Yearning and searching. The stage where one longs and pines for the deceased. The emotional experience of the mourner may include weeping, anger, anxiety, confusion, and preoccupation. Parents may also experience "heavy arms," a deep desire to hold their baby
	Disorganization and despair. Bereaved persons may isolate themselves from other people and from activities they once enjoyed. In this stage, the emotional experience from the yearning and searching stage may diminish, because the mourner is accepting the reality of the loss. The bereaved may experience apathy, anger, despair, hopelessness, and questioning
	Reorganization and recovery. The grieving person integrates into a "new state of normal." The intensity of sadness and other intense emotions may lessen while positive memories of the deceased increase

Table 12.2 (continued)

Theory	Perspective
Continuing bonds // Klass, Silverman and Nickman (1996) [9]	This paradigm shifts away from previous grief perspectives that portray a linear process of grief that concludes with acceptance of a loss or investment in a new life. Continuing bonds suggest that within the grieving process, a bond is created that will allow the connection with the deceased to exist in various ways throughout the lifetime of the bereaved. This type of bond takes into consideration the natural development of healthy human attachment in relationships, which is extended to the relationship with the deceased. Parents may take on activities that honor their child or make their legacy live on.
Meaning reconstruction // Robert Neimeyer [10]	Significant losses can cause a disruption in the way that the bereaved make sense of all of their life experiences, due to a change in the assumptive world. A bereaved person engages in these 3 efforts as a part of the grieving process to rationalize their grief experience: *Sense making*: To make sense of the loss *Benefit finding*: To find a benefit or "silver lining" from the loss experience *Identity change*: Reorganizing their identity to be perceived as a "survivor"
The 6 R processes of mourning // Therese Rando [11]	The 6 processes of mourning are broken down into three phases of grief and mourning. While they are interrelated and can build upon each other, the processes may also occur concurrently or out of the sequence, which demonstrates how the mourning process fluctuates for the bereaved Avoidance phase 1. Recognize the loss Confrontation phase 2. React to the separation 3. Recollect and re-experience the deceased and the relationship 4. Relinquish the old attachments to the deceased and the old assumptive world Accommodation phase 5. Readjust to move adaptively into the new world 6. Reinvest emotional energy into goals and people that are a part of this new world

Manifestations of Grief

Normal Grief or Uncomplicated Grief

Despite decades of research, questions remain about what constitutes normal, uncomplicated grief reactions and what defines a grief reaction that slips into a complicated, pathological reaction. The general consensus is that when a person is grieving, they feel difficult thoughts, emotions, and memories that are associated with the loss [2]. The mourner experiences a broad range of physical sensations, cognitions, emotional experiences, and behaviors [4]. Helping parents normalize their experiences can provide a frame of reference and comfort in their grieving process. Table 12.3 provides an overview of experiences that are common to the bereaved.

Table 12.3 Common manifestations of grief (Worden) [4]

Physical sensations	**Cognitions**
1. *Feeling tightness* in the throat, chest, or forehead	1. *Disbelief.* This is often the first experience upon hearing of a death
2. *Dry mouth*	2. *Confusion.* Having trouble concentrating, being forgetful, and experiencing confused thinking
3. *Breathlessness*, feeling short of breath	3. *Preoccupation.* Spending time thinking about your child or obsessing about their suffering and dying
4. *Nausea* and/or a hollow feeling in the stomach	4. *Sensing your loved one's presence.* This is most likely to happen shortly after the death
5. *Hypersensitivity to noises*	5. *Hallucinations.* It is a fairly common and a normal symptom of grief to see or hear a loved one, usually within a few weeks after their death
6. *Lack of energy or weakness* in the body.	
7. *Sense of disbelief* or "dream-like state"	
8. *Sense of depersonalization*	
Behavioral characteristics	**Emotional experiences**
1. *Sleep disturbances:* Difficulty sleeping or sleeping too much	1. *Shock*
2. *Appetite disturbances:* Poor appetite or overeating	2. *Numbness*
3. *Forgetfulness or absentmindedness*	3. *Sadness*
4. *Social withdrawal*	4. *Irritability and anger*:
5. *Dreams of the deceased*	(a) Feeling frustrated that the death could not have been prevented
6. *Avoiding reminders of one's child*	(b) Feeling as though you have been "abandoned" by one's loved one
7. *Visiting places or carrying reminders of the baby*	5. *Anxiety*
8. *Crying*	6. *Loneliness*
9. *Sighing*	7. *Fatigue*
10. *Searching or calling out for the baby*	8. *Helplessness*
11. *Restlessness*	9. *Yearning*
12. *Treasuring items that belonged to the deceased*	10. *Guilt*
	11. *Emancipation/relief*

Adapted from Worden [4]

Additional Variants of Grief

Anticipatory Grief

Anticipatory grief is "grieving that occurs prior to the actual loss" [4]. In perinatal palliative care (PPC), anticipatory grief usually occurs when parents are informed, sometime during pregnancy, that their fetus has a life-threatening condition. According to Worden, the mourning process therefore begins early and usually involves Tasks of Mourning (Table 12.2, Bereavement Theories). While working through *Task 1: Accepting the Reality of the Loss*, families may go through a period of anticipation, knowing that as the pregnancy approaches the due date, so does their child's impending death. While parents may hold onto hope while anticipating the loss of their baby, the reality of death is realized in this Task. In *Task 2: Processing the Pain of Grief,* the emotional experience may be similar to that of post death bereavement and the intensity may increase as the length of the anticipatory grief period grows. With *Task 3, Adjust to a World Without the Deceased*, parents may begin to rehearse issues that may come up when the child has died and plan what they will do after the death. This is a coping strategy, as they are trying to make sense of a life without their loved one. It also can lead to useful birth planning.

A clinician should monitor the emotional well-being of families during the anticipatory grief period because their pain may increase as the birth looms nearer. In the case of prenatal diagnoses, parents may prematurely disengage emotionally, especially fathers [12] who do not have the same physical connection with the baby as the mother. This disengagement may be rooted in fear of the pain they will experience emotionally following the death of their baby and the expectation that if they are not emotionally attached, it will not hurt as much when the inevitable occurs.

Rogalla (2018) has discussed the relationship between proactive coping abilities and personal growth in individuals who anticipate the loss of a loved one [13]. She found that anticipatory grief experiences positively correlate with post death mourning experiences and that complications in the anticipatory grief experience may lead to poorer bereavement outcomes following the death.

For families who have been informed of a life-limiting fetal condition (LLFC), anticipatory grief should be monitored as the parents engage in the developmental tasks of pregnancy (see also Chap. 2, Fig. 2.3, Developmental tasks of pregnancy). Clinicians may be able to facilitate "good grief," an experience that reflects joy and honors the life of the deceased, while respecting and supporting those left behind. When handled well, the time of anticipatory grief can be managed in a way that supports a healthy mourning process. Otherwise, bereaved families can be at risk for complicated grief experiences and disenfranchised grief.

Complex Mourning Reactions

As clinicians, it is important to be familiar with the normal experiences of grief, in order to avoid pathologizing the experiences of families. However, the mourning process can be more complex than uncomplicated grief manifestations. As Worden discusses in his book, *Grief Counseling and Grief Therapy* (2018) [4], grief can be categorized into additional subtypes. A *chronic grief reaction* occurs when the grief reaction is prolonged and reaches no satisfactory conclusion. These mourners do not move through the mourning period and typically require therapeutic interventions to assess what points of "stuckness" are present and need resolution. *Delayed grief* occurs when the mourner experienced an emotional reaction at the time of the death, but it may not have felt significant at that time because he/she lacked support, lacked social sanction, needed to be strong for someone else, or felt overwhelmed. Delayed grief can also happen to those who are overwhelmed by multiple losses in a short period of time. The manifestation of *exaggerated grief* resembles normal grief behaviors, but they appear with such intensity that a formal diagnosis from the

Diagnostic and Statistical Manual V (DSM-V) [14] may apply. Understanding the patient's mental health history is important because the experience of grief can be a catalyst for reemergence of formally defined mental health disorders such as major depression, anxiety, phobias, substance abuse, post-traumatic stress disorder, and manic episodes. Finally, *masked grief reactions* may occur when mourners are unaware of unresolved grief surrounding their loss and experience somatic complaints or maladaptive behaviors.

According to the Center for Complicated Grief, founded by Dr. Katherine Shear, *complicated grief* is "a persistent form of intense grief in which maladaptive thoughts and dysfunctional behaviors are present along with continued yearning, longing and sadness and/or preoccupation with thoughts and memories of the person who died. Within the paradigm of this emerging diagnosis, grief continues to dominate life and the future seems bleak and empty. Irrational thoughts that the deceased person might reappear are common and the bereaved person feels lost and alone." In complicated grief, complex mourning can tip into clinical pathology [15].

Grief and Co-morbid Diagnoses

Grief Versus Depression

The DSM-V is used by clinicians and researchers to diagnose and classify mental disorders. The current edition recognizes that grief and major depressive disorder overlap in some of their symptoms and that grief can sometimes trigger a full-blown major depressive episode, especially if one has a history of depression. As in a masked grief reaction, physical health may concurrently decline. Grief and depression differ in that grief tends to decrease over time and occurs in waves that are triggered by thoughts or reminders of the deceased loved one while with depression, the symptomology is more enduring and persistent [16].

For a bereaved individual, depression can also serve as a defense mechanism to mourning. If the individual is able to turn their emotions on themselves, the emotional intensity is deflected away from the deceased and keeps the bereaved from focusing on their loss experiences. Major depressive disorder is diagnosed if there is a loss of self-esteem and feelings of morbid preoccupation with worthlessness and guilt not related to the death. Major depression can also be accompanied by sluggish or hesitant speech, prolonged difficulty in carrying out activities of daily living, hallucinations, and delusions (excluding, however, a "visionary experience" of the deceased). Finally, the strongest indication of depression is thoughts of suicide or self-harm, which is different from thoughts of "joining the deceased" [4].

Grief and Post-traumatic Stress Disorder

The grief experience is typically considered by professionals when assessing the mental health of parents; however, it is difficult to distinguish between naturally occurring grief and the type of psychiatric distress that can be found with post-traumatic stress disorder (PTSD). While there is an overlap of symptomology, they can exist parallel to each other within one's mental health. If PTSD is treated, it is often seen as secondary to grief. Research studies have maintained that the development of PTSD in an individual following an infant loss is based on individual sociodemographic factors, although the diagnosis may be at a slightly higher risk if they have prior losses [17].

In the DSM-V, the diagnosis of any of the depressive disorders can be expanded in the case of peripartum onset. Postpartum PTSD, while not addressed in the DSM-V, can emerge in the peripartum period. According to the DSM-V, diagnosis of PTSD is based on five criteria, all of which must begin after a serious traumatic event(s) [14]:

A. Exposure to actual or threatened death, serious injury, or sexual violence.
B. Presence of intrusion symptoms associated with the traumatic event.
C. Persistent avoidance of stimuli associated with the traumatic event.
D. Negative alterations in cognitions and mood associated with the traumatic event.
E. Marked alterations in arousal and reactivity associated with the traumatic event.

In research on post-traumatic stress disorder (PTSD) after childbirth, Zimmerman (2013) [18] stated that 10.5–30% of women label their labor experiences as traumatic without meeting the full diagnostic criteria for PTSD. The organization Postpartum Support International (PSI) [19] estimates that 9% of women experience PTSD following childbirth. Traumas that may produce PTSD include prolapsed cord, unplanned C-section, use of vacuum extractor or forceps to deliver the baby, baby unexpectedly going to NICU, feelings of powerlessness, poor communication, and/or lack of support and reassurance during the delivery. Women who have experienced a previous trauma, such as rape or sexual abuse, are at a higher risk for experiencing postpartum PTSD, as are women who have experienced a severe physical complication or injury related to pregnancy or childbirth.

The Edinburgh Postnatal Depression Scale (EPDS) is the depression screening tool most frequently used in obstetrical practices. This scale is accurate in screening for depression, but it does not screen for PTSD. Several common inventories that screen for PTSD are available [20] and can be used in conjunction with the EPDS, especially for mothers who had a traumatic birth experience.

The PTSD experience is not limited to birthing mothers. Fathers or partners to the birthing mothers may also experience PTSD. The specific symptomology that qualifies an anticipatory grief event and a perinatal death as a traumatic event has been detailed in the DSM-V [14] under post-traumatic stress disorder criterion: A2 (witnessing in person, the event(s) as it occurs to others) and A3 (learning that a traumatic event occurred to a close family or close friend). In cases of actual or threatened death of a family member or friend, the event(s) must have been violent or accidental, which may qualify the death of an infant, including a prenatal loss, as a traumatic event [17].

In the research of Christiansen, fathers experience PTSD at rates of 5–8.4% from 7 weeks to 18 years post loss of their baby [17]. Although there have been inconsistent findings surrounding the type of infant loss and gestational period of the loss, it should not be concluded that parents with early losses experience less severity in symptomology than those with later losses [17]. In the case of subsequent pregnancies, fathers reported PTSD at rates of 15.6% during the pregnancy and 0% following the birth of a healthy child [17].

While there has been research on gender differences in the PTSD experience, research has shown that fathers can display symptoms following a perinatal loss; however it may be at slightly lower severity and prevalence to the mothers [21]. Additionally, the symptomology that is present may be a less visible form than what is reported by mothers [22]. The difference can be attributed to differing social expectations, measures used that may not fully capture symptomology present in the father and the fact the fathers are less likely to receive professional help [17, 21]. Screening and accurate diagnosis and treatment of PTSD are crucial not only for both parents but for their relationship with any children they have in the future.

With this population, especially with fathers, clinicians may find that clients may drop out from certain types of therapy. Taking a thorough loss/trauma history, utilizing trauma-focused interventions, expressing the importance of having a supportive venue, and providing psychoeducation about the connection between symptoms they are experiencing and their loss may reduce the dropout rate and create an open therapeutic space for the bereaved parents [17].

PTSD teaches us that while birth can be a beautiful thing, it can also be terrifying. There are many things that could go wrong, no matter how much preplanning and education is done. As providers, we need to validate that the delivery may have been a traumatic experience for both parents and follow-up accordingly.

Case Studies: Stories from Bereaved Families

Real Life and Death Narratives

The following stories are taken from informal interviews and therapy sessions with the permission of the families. These families have been candid about their experiences with perinatal loss, and they hope their loss experiences can help to educate others. All names have been changed to protect the privacy of families. These cases will be used throughout the remainder of the chapter.

Case 12.1 Noelle and Martin

These parents were willing to speak about their grief experience as individuals and as a couple, following the loss of their daughter, Melody. Melody was delivered at 23 3/7 weeks of gestation, and died after 14 hours. Prenatal diagnoses of proximal myotonic myopathy (PROMM) and maternal chorioamnionitis (infection) were shared with the parents. Cause of death was septicemia (which Noelle also contracted) and extreme prematurity. Noelle developed septic arthritis as well as a host of other medical complications after birth. One year after Melody's death, Noelle and Martin welcomed a son David and another year later, they welcomed a daughter, Amelia. Noelle's and Martin's experiences will be discussed in relation to maternal bereavement, paternal bereavement, and the needs of bereaved families.

Case 12.2 Cathy and Daniel

Cathy was willing to share the life story of her son Lucas, as well as her experience with motherhood during his brief 11-day life. Cathy and her husband Daniel had been married for 15 years when their firstborn, Lucas, was delivered. Prior to his birth, he was diagnosed with tetralogy of Fallot with pulmonary atresia and confluent pulmonary arteries. Surgeries during his first days of life had gone well and the parents were optimistic about his prognosis. However, on day 10, Cathy and Daniel noticed Lucas was "pale and lethargic" in his crib. Suddenly he coded and was put on extracorporeal membrane oxygenation (ECMO), a treatment that uses a pump to circulate the infant's blood through an artificial lung and back into the baby's bloodstream. After 24 hours of monitoring, it was found that the right side of his heart was not active and Lucas was unlikely to recover. Cathy and Daniel decided to withdraw ECMO support and allow him to die peacefully. At just 11 days old, Lucas lost his fight with congenital heart disease.

Cathy sought bereavement counseling 7 months following her infant loss. She reported an escalation of her grief during this time. She felt that she had been grieving appropriately after Lucas died the previous June, but in August, she became pregnant again and miscarried at 3 months. Since the loss of Lucas, she has experienced 3 miscarriages and still longs to be a mother to a living child.

Case 12.3 Miranda and Jared

This couple came in for support group and bereavement counseling following the loss of Nikolai, who died 8 days after birth complicated by uterine rupture in which both mother and baby nearly died. Miranda awoke from the birth, hours later in the ICU, where her husband then told her about Nikolai's condition and that a hysterectomy was performed to save her life. Nikolai was diagnosed with severe hypoxic ischemic encephalopathy. The parents decided to pursue comfort care after receiving this diagnosis. Miranda and Jared felt completely at peace with his death, as they were able to take him outdoors after he was extubated. He died in his parents arms, under the stars. When the couple first came to the bereavement group, they were experiencing typical grief reactions. They also wanted to address worries about supporting their other two school-aged children, Zach and Micah, wondering if the children's grief reactions were normal.

Paternal Bereavement

> …Everyone goes through their grief in their own way. It's so important to keep communicating with your partner because they lost a child too. Mothers get such emphasis on the loss but fathers need to get attention too. – Noelle

The grief responses and coping styles of bereaved mothers have been extensively studied, but the experiences of bereaved fathers are not well understood, especially in the context of infant loss. Bereaved fathers describe frustration with lack of compassion for their experiences and the limited resources available to help them recover. They describe feeling torn between the need to care for themselves and to care for their families. They are aware that they feel different from mothers following the loss, that others perceive them differently, and that they see the world in a different manner. Many men come to the conclusion that they need to "be tough" and keep pushing forward, to avoid compromising the well-being of those who count on them.

Martin spoke of his experience following the death of Melody (Case 12.1):

> I'm more open about talking about her than Noelle is, and it comes out in conversations with other people but it's still a secret club no one wants to be a part of. It helps to know there are other people out there- it would be nice to find a community. I lost my father and grandfather [shortly after the loss of his daughter], I had to handle my grief differently because the expectations were different. When I lost my daughter, my wife connected me to someone she knew, because we had to make decisions but couldn't handle the thought of her laying in a morgue. I was a robot, I was hollow as I was making all these decisions around her funeral… I had to deal with the practical things while I was grieving...If I hadn't had a supportive partner, I probably would have fallen off the planet and hid away from the world. But I had to deal with this, no one wants to hear it because they have their own problems. I have to be happy for everyone else, it's not fair for me to be sad for my kids.

Jared (Case 12.3) shared in a group the fears and flashbacks that he would get regarding his wife's health and well-being, following the terrifying birth of Nikolai. Both Miranda and Nikolai were fighting for their lives as Jared was left with the mantel of making decisions that would impact the lives of both his wife and son as well as their two older children at home. Through further assessment, his experiences would fit in the category of PTSD. Some research has been done on the PTSD experiences of fathers related to their infant's deaths [17, 21, 22]; however, there is little literature on how fathers respond to their partner's possible brush with death following the pregnancy and loss. Like Jared and Martin, many fathers may feel the need to be strong for their partners, and it may fall on them to make medical decisions for the health of both their baby and partner. Some fathers will express tremendous guilt and uncertainty, questioning if they made the right decisions and if deciding differently could have produced a different outcome. The stress of seeing one's partner and child in physical danger fits the criteria for a traumatic experience that can increase the risk of PTSD. Clinicians should explore the psychological distress from this event and screen for PTSD.

Fathers additionally may experience existential and practical crises as they try to explain aspects of the new normal to others. Martin (Case 12.1) shares,

> Do I answer the question 'How many children do you have?' with how many are currently living, then will it seem like I'm not honoring my child who died? If I answer with the number of all of my children, what if there are follow-up questions or people ask to see photos? How do I explain that one child is always missing from photos?

Martin asked himself, "Is it worth it to me to open up about such a painful experience to this person or should I only share the basics so I don't have to expose my pain to another person?"

In previous studies of the experiences of fathers after the loss of their children, three major themes emerged: (a) the need to push forward in order to avoid a breakdown, (b) keeping their child present in everyday life, and (c) finding meaning in their grief experience [23]. It is often assumed that men have difficulty regulating the emotional intensity of their grief and respond to it in a more cognitive manner. Many fathers subscribe to the "keep busy" attitude and can invest time in other areas of their lives. Keeping busy does not deter fathers from processing their loss. In fact, they may find motivation in their surviving children, dedicating attention to them to ease their suffering and help them find meaning in their daily lives. Little research has been done on fathers who have no other children, but they may also respond by investing time in other meaningful areas of their lives. Cathy has shared that her husband, Daniel, seems to grieve in this way as they have no other children and she notices him doing laborious tasks for senior citizens in their town in honor of their son. Alam et al. (2012), who studied the bereavement experiences of mothers' and fathers' after death of a child from cancer, argued that fathers may find a change in their priorities, becoming less satisfied with their employment, for example, and seek out a life that allows them to build a legacy for their child or improve the family home [24].

Families often maintain a connection with their deceased child through memorial rituals such as honoring the infant's birthday with a cake, releasing balloons with a message inside, saying a toast or prayer in their honor, planting a tree, or starting a scholarship fund in the child's name. Fathers also find enjoyment in talking about their child with family, friends, and even strangers.

Fathers may notice that they have an increased sense of empathy and emotional awareness following the loss. Men may strike a balance between the emotional and cognitive aspects of grief. Many fathers find that information-seeking about their infant's condition can be a form of grieving and sense-making following the death of their child.

Almost any bereaved parent would say that nothing can compare to the heartbreak of losing a child. Fathers may also speak about shifting priorities to value the importance of their family's well-being rather than material goods. Addressing Worden's third Task of Mourning is to *Adjust to the environment in which the deceased is missing*, these adjustments occur internally, externally, and spiritually. As providers working with these fathers and families, it's important to acknowledge the changes that have occurred in their lives as well as what things have remained constant, as a way of acknowledging that there is still some stability within their lives.

Maternal Bereavement

> Losing a child is the worst tragedy. I truly believe that nothing can bring the heart, mind, body and soul more pain than this. When he died, a large part of me died too. I will never get that back. Like most grieving parents, I was trying to figure out what to do with myself. Not only had I lost my child, but I felt like I lost my purpose in life. I thought my purpose was to be [his] mommy. –Cathy (Case 12.2)

What can you say to a mother whose infant child has died? What can you do to help? Extensive research has uncovered no generalizable solution. In talking with these mothers in therapy, they will often share: "I don't know what I need." "Nothing can be done" or "All I need is to have my baby back again." As a clinician, it can be heartbreaking to know that you went into a helping profession and still you cannot help. What *do* you say, to a grieving mother?

In the author's experience of working with bereaved mothers, differences have been observed in how bereaved mothers of older children grieve, compared to mothers who have experienced a perinatal loss. No loss is worse than the other, but the mothers who have lost infants speak a lot about the loss of the future. They speak about the hopes and dreams that they had for their children that no longer will be. They describe noticing children who would be about the same age of their deceased child, and wondering if their babies would be doing the same things if they had lived. What would be their favorite toy or food? What would their first word have been? These mothers also describe an arrested sense of time. They often feel that their babies will always be the age that they were at death and that their photographs of the infant are inadequate to capture their lives.

Perinatal loss differs from loss of an older child if the parents had prior knowledge of the impending death. Complications during the birth may be an important factor in their grief, as is their NICU experience. When Miranda shared her birth story, what stood out was how she woke up in the ICU and was told that she and her baby had almost died and that Nikolai had severe brain damage. She met several criteria that would qualify her as having a traumatic birth experience and might have led to PTSD. The harrowing trauma that she experienced prior to the death of her son added another layer to her grief experience.

The research of Wonch Hill et al. explores a woman's sense of her role as mother when she has experienced a poor birth outcome [25]. Women who have lived through a stillbirth or a child's death, rather than a miscarriage, seem to feel more self-blame, with guilt as well as shame. They also report significantly lower self-esteem in comparison to those women who had never experienced these kinds of loss. Riley et al. wrote that a mother's view as her "child's protector" can be shaken when her child has died [26]. This sense of impotence in fulfilling this perceived role can lead to intense guilt and shame, and it is often overlooked by medical providers, leading to psychosomatic symptoms of grief.

Miranda shared some of her reflections after her difficult delivery of Nikolai (Case 12.3):

> After several hours, I remember being excited about how quickly my labor was going. Within a short period later everything suddenly stopped. My cervix began to swell and for 7 hours nothing changed. By the time we decided what the next step was, we acted too late. The next thing I remember was the doctors telling us they couldn't find his heartbeat. They rushed me out of the room and for 8 hours my husband and family were left to wait and hear about news as to what happened and how we were doing. All they were told was that my uterus had ruptured and that my son and I were in critical condition but stable. When I woke up in ICU the next day, I was told I nearly died and the doctors were shocked that I even survived. My son was born with severe brain damage and his condition was questionable.

Miranda not only experienced the devastating loss of the future she anticipated for her son, she also experienced the loss of her ability to have other children after her hysterectomy. In further discussions about this experience, she has shared that she believes she developed PTSD from her birth experience.

After difficult NICU experiences, remembered sights, sounds, and smells can bring unexpected flashbacks. Cathy shared that she had difficulty going into grocery stores shortly after the death of her son, because the sound of the automatic doors at the store reminded her of the sound of the doors in the NICU, when she would visit her son.

Perinatal bereaved mothers who lack other children may also have a different self-image as a mother, because their experiences in early pregnancy have helped them prepare to become a mother, and the loss of their child can challenge this expected role [25]. Women who have other living children may be able to externalize the maternal care that they would have provided their infant, thus fulfilling their motherhood role, but women who do not have other children do not have this outlet.

This author has heard from many mothers, who describe feeling betrayed by their bodies—that their body should have been able to sustain a pregnancy or keep their child safe while inside of them. Miranda spoke candidly about mourning this loss of her womanhood after her uterine rupture. When women experience complications during the pregnancy or delivery, clinicians must be mindful that mothers may not only be grieving for their dead babies but also for their own health.

Mothers may also feel betrayed by their bodies when they are trying to become pregnant again. In Cathy's case (Case 12.2), she experienced three miscarriages following the loss of Lucas. She asked one day: "Why am I now getting pregnant after 14 years of trying?" We discussed how she felt that the pregnancy experience had been tarnished by the many losses; providers would tell her that her body was healthy, yet she felt utter betrayal month after month when her menstrual cycle began and devastation when a miscarriage occurred during her subsequent pregnancies. She spoke of how she and her husband mourned every month that they had tried to become pregnant again, and she felt like a failure as a woman. She felt extreme frustration as she went to fertility doctors, received various treatments, and took medications. None of these interventions worked for her, and she felt slapped in the face when people suggested adoption or surrogacy, giving her another reminder that her body was not "doing what it was supposed to do."

Perinatal losses also carry the weight of physical and psychosomatic pain. Cathy spoke about how she had been "sitting in my grief" for over 7 months after the loss of Lucas. She noticed pains in her lower back and hips, reduced range of motion, and increased fatigue. While some of this she attributed to her body not being the same after giving birth, she also attributed it to grief. She shared that her grief made her much less social: she would stay home, sitting on the couch, just mourning her son. She thought to seek out treatment from her doctor, who recommended a chiropractor and physical therapy, to help her with spinal alignment and exercising her pelvic floor. Some patients may not have the foresight to look into these therapies, so providers should encourage them to get checkups to assess their physical health after pregnancy, since the body may endure trauma during pregnancy.

Like fathers, some women go through an existential crisis following the loss of an infant, especially mothers who do not have other children. Cathy spoke often about her place in the world: "Am I still considered a mother since my baby died?" and "Will I ever be a mother again?" The definition of self can be shattered following such a loss [27], even for those parents who have other children, as they too are trying to make sense of their place in this new world.

Personal growth in the grief process can occur when a mother seeks out instrumental and emotional support when confronted with stressors. Reliance on healthy, consistent social support, in the form of family, friends, or even other bereaved mothers, can provide the grieving parent with care and mutuality, as they search for meaning after their loss. While performing clinical work with bereaved mothers, this author has heard constant feedback that it means the world to bereaved mothers to be around others who understand their experience and be in a space where they could spend time with and parent their absent infant. They find comfort in one another and acknowledge the changes that have occurred in themselves during their grieving processes.

Predictors of Positive Grief Responses

Riley et al. (2007) studied parental grief responses and personal growth following the death of a child [26]. Their research explored optimism in mothers as a dispositional factor that impacts grief reactions. Optimism was characterized as having positive future expectations. Their studies revealed three perspectives: (1) optimism is a protective factor (the more optimistic mothers are, the less they experience intense grief reactions; (2) those who are optimistic remain persistent in their efforts in dealing with adverse events, even when the progress is difficult; in the context of grief, these parents sustained coping efforts as they adapted and changed through their grief process; and (3) optimistic individuals cope by accepting unchangeable life events and are flexible in the goals they have for their lives.

While the sample in this study consisted of bereaved mothers, it is possible that the finding may also apply to the experiences of bereaved fathers as well. The trait of optimism connects to the need to find meaning in the loss of the child and may affect the ability of a parent to accept the reality of her loss. Riley et al. found that bereaved mothers who were action oriented (coping with adversity by taking action and using problem solving skills) had less intense grief reactions [26].

Pregnancy After Loss

> People think being an Angel Mom and having a child after a loss is the best thing but you're always aware that one child is missing from these memories. When you have another child, it's hard to look at pictures because you know that someone else is supposed to be there. -Noelle (Case 12.1)

The effect of an infant loss may also create new challenges for grief management during a subsequent pregnancy. During a pregnancy following the loss of an infant, the pregnant mother can experience many mixed feelings. Noelle was candid in her reflection about her pregnancies following the death of Melody:

> It's probably the most difficult thing you can ever do, especially if it's your 1st child you lose. All of the parenting rules go out of the window when you have your next child. The veil has been shattered and the innocence is lost. Maybe I'm more hyperaware of things and over protective but who wouldn't be, once you lose a child? You don't care what the books say or other mothers say because you just feel like 'I have to do whatever I can and what feels right.' You live by the monthly milestones, not the materialistic things, like baby showers and a layette set. You think 'let me just get to 5 months, 8 months etc… just paying attention to these milestones until you get your baby into your arms.

It is critical to check in with a mother during her pregnancy if she has experienced a prior traumatic birth or loss. As Noelle shared, they may look ahead to the monthly milestones, feeling like they have tunnel vision, trying to make it safely to the next step. Sometimes the mother feels that celebrating the impending birth of their next child will jinx the pregnancy. For mothers who in their first pregnancy had prior knowledge of a severe or lethal fetal diagnosis, these monthly milestones may bring on flashbacks to their last pregnancy and memories, such as doctor's visits at certain milestones where they received a poor prognosis. Clinicians should recognize that it is normal for the mother to feel sad or distressed at times during her pregnancy, as she tries to reconcile her past experiences with her current ones.

The experiences of fathers can't be ignored, as they often experience an increased amount of worry during a pregnancy following a loss. The research suggests that paternal PTSD symptoms may be elevated during a subsequent pregnancy, due to the knowledge fathers have that any pregnancy has a chance of ending in death; however, the symptoms significantly reduce if a healthy child is born [17].

A history of PTSD related to infant loss may impact the behaviors of parents towards any future children they have. Whether it be conscious or not, parents may demonstrate lower levels of attachment with these children, as they may have been preparing themselves for another dead child throughout their gestation. Côté-Arsenault identified *emotional cushioning* as a protective mechanism in pregnancy after perinatal loss in an attempt to reduce their anxiety about another potential loss [28]. This attempt to protect themselves from pain can have long-term consequences on the quality of family life, parenting style, and relationship with future children [17]. Côté-Arsenault and O'Leary (2016) also explore the experiences of fathers in their research [29].

Discussions with a bereaved mom that inadvertently ignores a previous loss may be seen as minimizing their painful experience. One should avoid language that makes it sound like their current pregnancy is replacing the infant who was lost. It helps the clinician to understand the bereaved mother's self-concept by asking her how she chooses to identify herself, the child she is carrying now, and her deceased infant, using their names when they are spoken about. Let parents know that they can parent their deceased and unborn baby simultaneously; they do not have to choose. Some mothers dislike the terms "rainbow baby," "angel baby," or "angel mom" [29].

If the mother is working with a mental health provider, it may be helpful for the provider to refer back to Worden's Tasks of Mourning, Task 3, Adjusting to an environment in which the deceased is missing, and Task 4, Finding an enduring connection with the deceased while emotionally investing into life, when discussing treatment planning with the mother. Additionally, this information can be helpful for other team members to understand the importance of mothers maintain a connection with their baby. A mother can honor her deceased infant and keep a sacred space for them in her life, while also celebrating and creating a new space for the infant about to be born.

> It is in that love that I desire to keep [Lucas'] memory alive and to help other families who have lost a child. I want to take my tragedy and step into a fuller experience of life. I want to say [Lucas'] name and keep his spirit alive. –Cathy (Case 12.2)

The Couple's Experience of Grief

Parents' engagement in grief-related communication with each other is very valuable. Open communication increases marital intimacy and social support, especially in the context of infant loss, where one's partner may be the most significant source of support following the loss. Because it's a shared grief, the other parent may be the only one who truly understands the loss [30]. The use of healthy communication strategies allows parents to have an understanding of each other's needs and allows for their continued mourning to be integrated into their daily lives. Parents symptoms seem to run in tandem to each other [21] allowing them to find balance when they are having a good day or a bad day.

As professionals who work with bereaved mothers and fathers, adopting the mindset that mothers and fathers will always grieve differently because of their gender can cause a biased overall clinical picture. While we can recognize these individual differences due to personality of the circumstances surrounding the death, we must not minimize the experiences of either parent because their grief experiences do not "match" that of the other. It is important for clinicians to respect differences in grieving and also teach families how to respect each other's experiences. Otherwise, we may fall into assumptions that one parent is not "grieving enough" or has moved beyond the death of their infant [31] (see also Chap. 4).

Parenting Grieving Children

Many bereaved parents find it easier to focus on the well-being of their grieving children, rather than their own grief. No matter the age of the children, whether they be in elementary school or high school, how they respond to the loss and as well as how they are grieving should be monitored by parents, family members, teachers, coaches, or any other important adults in their lives so they can provide a supportive atmosphere for the children. Miranda and Jared were very focused on the well-being of their two young boys and sought resources and local support services. They were quick to involve resources at their children's schools and looked for support in other important people in their children's lives. How children mourn a loss is dependent on age, relationship to the deceased, presence during the death, and other factors. Just because a child may be young, it does not mean that their experiences are any less valid or that they are "grieving wrong" if their grief demonstration differs from what is expected. It is important to review how children and adolescents may respond to grief and death from a developmental point of view, so that parents and providers know what to expect. Parenting a child who was born after a child loss has its own set of concerns. Some parents worry that people will think this next child is replacing the child they lost or that the previous loss will eclipse this child's sense of personal identity. If these concerns emerge, parents can reach out to mental health providers and family therapists to discuss their concerns and find a healthy way to integrate the legacy of the infant they lost into the life of their next born child. (See Recommended Resources, Appendix 1, and also Chap. 14, section "Siblings".)

The Role of All Providers

Overview

Providers have an important role in providing context and anticipatory guidance for families. They can ease fear, anxiety, and possible depression. From the first moment when a LLFC is confirmed, the entire interspecialty and interdisciplinary perinatal palliative care team has an obligation to support parents as they try to cope with the diagnosis and make decisions on behalf of the baby. Clinicians can offer compassion and sensitivity to the needs of families and advocate for their patients.

Assess Parental Coping

Providers can first assess the coping disposition of the family and their existing levels of support as they begin to navigate the anticipatory grief period. Clinicians can help families to build their coping strategies in different ways, to mediate their grief. Effective strategies are managing existing stressors, encouraging the use of social support, helping families feel purposeful, and facilitating proactive goal setting [13].

Parenting Through Creating a Birth Plan

In being proactive, the creation of a birth plan helps a family to parent their child in the way they choose. Birth planning can help to reduce anxiety and create a space where the family feels in control of a situation that is out of their control. It also can be very stressful for some parents, making them come face-to-face with the reality of their situation. It may help the parents process their anticipatory grief by facilitating the Tasks of Mourning in advance of death as well as facilitate healthy attachment and grieving [32]. While parents may have limited time with their infant, birth planning helps to maintain their emotional attachment with their child by engaging in meaningful parenting activities [12]. While there is no single template for a birth plan, it is usual to address labor, delivery, and aftercare and may include personalized goals that parents want included in the birth experience (see Chap. 15 for details on birth planning).

Memory-Making

As the family embarks on their grief journey, healthcare providers can facilitate healthy grieving by supporting meaningful parenting experiences in the hospital and after the infant's death that can set the foundation for the mourning process. Memory-making can be facilitated with time spent with the baby, taking photographs with the baby, and creating baby handprints and footprints. Additionally, having their child participate in any religious rites can also be meaningful and provide comfort to parents. Ultimately, the parents' healthy grieving process and having no regrets may be the best possible outcomes.

Follow-Up, Referrals, and Resources

The entire team of providers that work with the infant and family can promote good long-term outcomes. Providers can also facilitate access to aftercare—such as bereavement counseling, support groups, or joining an online community—in order to reduce isolation and complicated grief reactions.

After a perinatal death, follow-up by providers can be an anchor in a sea of confusion. Many times parents do not know where to turn or what decisions need to be made. Following up with families shows that providers care about their lives, giving them access to resources. To serve bereaved parents, clinicians need up-to-date literary and media resources (see Appendix 1), as well as a list of trusted mental health providers and bereavement support services. Not all mental health clinicians work with bereavement, especially infant loss; therefore it is important to identify bereavement specialists on the provider list. Families may follow up with their primary care providers or the team that worked with their child, looking for local resources.

Meeting the Needs of Parents Following Perinatal Loss

When asked "What do you feel was needed following the loss of your infant?" Martin's response was:

....Just the care from the staff after the loss. We had to move out of the room we were in, while dealing with the loss. We were just given a card and told to call this number to get bereavement services. There was a gap between us leaving and getting connected to services. It seemed like once we left the building, the support just wasn't there.

Butler, Hall, Willetts, and Copnell (2015) performed an integrative literature review of parent's experiences with healthcare providers when their child died [33]. The behaviors of healthcare professionals can be mediators for the grief experiences of families. Even if the provider feels helpless to prevent an infant's death, their acknowledgement that they will provide emotional support can help parents feel cared for at a fragile time. Table 12.4 summarizes the study's findings about parents' needs and preferences. It is not an exhaustive list, but it can guide providers as they govern themselves with sensitivity and respect, and communicate appropriately, as they help to shape parent's experiences around their child's death.

Table 12.4 What parents want from their healthcare providers when their child dies [33]

Helpful actions	Unhelpful actions
Staff affect and attitudes	
Parents valued caring and compassionate staff, who were able to remain both professional and "human" to the family members. These staff members were able to display genuine emotional expressions and compassion towards the families	Medical staff who display a cold, non-caring and clinical demeanor. Parents can internalize the demeanor of the staff and be left with the impression that the staff does not care about the family or the child.
Staff who display appropriate empathy and affect, especially when delivering bad news, allow parents to feel bonded with the medical staff	When staff display closed body language (e.g., lack of eye contact), it can leave parents with feelings of suspicion towards the medical staff
	Believing that the staff are in a rush gives the impression that their child is unimportant
	Staff having personal conversations at an unexpected or inappropriate time for the family, especially during or after the death of the child
Follow-up care and ongoing contact with staff members	
Follow-up contact from staff with whom they had a preexisting relationship: Methods of contact can include cards, letters, and phone calls and presence of the staff at their child's funeral	Lack of follow-up care or contact from the hospital staff can leave bereaved families feeling isolated and abandoned
A follow-up bereavement program which contacts and supports bereaved families, especially with the presence of a familiar staff member	

(continued)

Table 12.4 (continued)

Helpful actions	Unhelpful actions
Communication	
Throughout the child's illness and during the immediate bereavement period, parents appreciated the availability of accurate, honest information and explanation of medical procedures	Exclusive use of medical jargon can cause confusion for families and increase distress for parents
Staff using discretion in assessing the appropriate timing for conversations, engaging parents in conversations regarding the "big picture" and maintaining open and honest communication	Giving the impression that staff are unwilling to meet with families unless explicitly requested to do so
Staff displaying patience and understanding that parents may need to hear information multiple times in order to hear what is being said	Giving families contradictory information or withholding information related to prognosis, thus creating false hope
Memento and memory-making activities, e.g., handprints, footprints and photographs, validate the infant's life and create positive memories in a sad time	Giving unexpected news to the families that the child is dying or giving this news at inappropriate times, without thorough previous discussions about the likely outcomes of child's illness and clinical course
Attending to the parents	
Allowing parents to continue to be parents prior to and following their baby's death, enabling them to hold their child, spend time alone, and participate in their child's care	Not allowing parents to be with or hold their child after death
Staff attending to the practical needs of the parents: e.g., providing food, blankets and medical attention, as needed	Not allowing privacy for families to say goodbye to their child
Attempting to soften the harshness of the hospital by allowing families to have privacy and reduced ambient noise in the hospital room	Feeling that the staff are avoiding the room when a child is actively dying can lead to increased anxiety, abandonment, and isolation
Honoring the seriousness of the final days of life and creating "sacred space" within the hospital room for the families. Staff can communicate with the families about how they can be reached during this "sacred time" should family members need anything	
Continuity of care	
Continuity of the staff members who are providing treatment of their child	Multiple changes in care providers can lead to parents' mistrusting staff and having increased anxiety due to unfamiliar people caring for their child
Nursing staff demonstrating familiarity with the child's care and preferences, as well as familiarity with the family	Lack of continuity of information among the medical staff, or having to communicate with too many health professionals, can lead to lack of trust and lack of confidence in the staff
Providing practical support following the death of the child	

Adapted from Butler et al. [33]

Conclusion

When a person experiences the death of a loved one, it may seem that the death is a singular experience that a person goes through. Perinatal loss is a significant loss in one's life, causing a person's life view to change and a continual shockwave that reverberates throughout life. Parents are irrevocably changed after such a loss. As in Noelle's candid reflection, "The veil has been shattered and the innocence is lost." To work with these families, providers must understand that the parents' lives are now divided into before and after: before and after they received a lethal diagnosis; before and after a labor that may have been progressing as expected and suddenly became life threatening; and before and after their infant died. Clinicians must understand and respect variations in normal grieving and identify those with complicated needs to be able to either address or refer to others with more expertise. Excellent anticipatory and bereavement care can provide an anchor of support in a sea of confusion. Most importantly, the lives of the infants who have died can be honored with the reverence they deserve.

Appendix 1 Bereavement Resources for Families and Providers

Bereavement
1. www.bereavedparentsusa.org., National support organization with many resource links [34]
2. https://www.babysbreathcanada.ca/ Baby's breath is Canada's only national foundation focused on SIDS, and more recently also dedicated to reducing all sudden and unexpected infant deaths including stillbirths [35]
3. www.bereavementmag.com, Resource for magazines, (including living with loss magazine—An online magazine), books, cards, gifts, memorials, and music [36].
4. www.compassionatefriends.org Self-help organization for bereaved families [37].
5. https://www.centerforloss.com/ Led by grief counselor and educator Dr. Alan Wolfelt, we are an organization dedicated to helping people who are grieving and those who care for them [38]
6. https://centering.org/ A non-profit organization and retailer providing education and resources for the bereaved and providers [39]
7. http://www.erichad.com/index.html, EriChad describes their work this way: "Grieving the loss of a child is one of life's most difficult experiences. You may think you'll never survive such pain. EriChad can't take away your pain, but we hope to validate it, hold your hand, and help you find life's rainbow." [40]
8. www.griefinc.com, Links to organizations and support groups (founded by Darcie Sims, PhD) [41]
9. http://www.griefnet.org/, On-line grief support provides help to people working through loss and grief issues of many kinds. Has over 50 e-mail grief support groups and two web sites [42]
10. https://grievingdads.com/ Offers support to grieving fathers. Has corresponding book Grieving Dad's: To the brink and back [43]
11. www.journeyofhearts.org/ An online healing place for anyone grieving a loss [44]

12. https://www.newyorklife.com/foundation/bereavement
New York Life's dedicated online resource for bereaved families and those who want to support them [45]
13. http://www.opentohope.com/
Open to Hope is an online community offering inspirational stories of loss, hope and recovery [46]
14. http://www.whatsyourgrief.com/
Promotes grief education, exploration, and expression in both practical and creative ways [47]

Infant loss

1. Beyond tears: Living after Losing a child, revised edition, by Ellen Mitchell. St. Martin's Griffin; revised & enlarged edition (March 3, 2009) [48]
2. Empty cradle, broken heart: Surviving the death of your baby, by Deborah Davis, PhD. Fulcrum Publishing; third edition, (November 1, 2016) [49]
3. Empty arms: Hope and support for those who have suffered a miscarriage, stillbirth, or tubal pregnancy by Pam Vredevelt. Multnomah; second edition (June 30, 2001) [50]
4. The grieving garden: Living with the death of a child, by Suzanne Redfern and Susan K. Gilbert, Hampton Roads Publishing; 1st edition (April 4, 2008) [51]
5. Healing a parent's grieving heart: 100 practical ideas after your child dies (healing a grieving heart series) by Alan Wolfelt. Companion Press; 1st edition (April 1, 2002) [52]
6. Life after the death of my son: What I'm learning, by Dennis L. Apple. Beacon Hill Press of Kansas City (March 10, 2008) [53]

For grieving mothers

1. http://www.firstcandle.org/grieving-families/grief-resources/online-resources/#1
An online resource place providing support for general grief, miscarriage, stillborn loss, loss of an only child, loss of a multiple birth [54]
2. http://handonline.org/
Helping after neonatal death (HAND) is a California non-profit 501(c)(3) corporation, founded in 1981 to help parents, their families and their healthcare providers cope with the loss of a baby before, during, or after birth [55]
3. https://www.mend.org/
A Christian not-for-profit corporation whose purpose is to reach out to those who have lost a child due to miscarriage, stillbirth or early infant death and offer a way to share experiences and information through meetings, the bi-monthly newsletter, and our internet web site [56]
4. http://www.postpartum.net/
The purpose of the organization is to increase awareness among public and professional communities about the emotional changes that women experience during pregnancy and postpartum [57]
5. http://stillstandingmag.com/
Our mission is to help you embrace life for everything that it is after experiencing the loss of a child or infertility. The focus of this magazine can be broken down into three parts: Giving a voice to grief, connecting hearts around the world who have similar life experiences, becoming a resource for friends, family and medical professionals, to know how to support someone enduring child loss and/or infertility [58]

For grieving fathers

1. Grieving dads: To the brink and back by Kelly Farley with David DiCola. Grieving dads LLC (June 8, 2012) [59]
2. Swallowed by a snake: The gift of the masculine side of healing by Thomas R. Golden. G. H. Publishing, L.L.C.; 1 edition (July 1, 2000) [60]
3. The way men heal by Thomas R. Golden. G H publishing, LLC (September 1, 2014) [61].
4. When men grieve: Why men grieve differently and how you can help by Elizabeth Levang. Fairview Press; 1 edition (December 8, 1998) [62]

For grieving children

1. A child remembers by Enid S. Traisman. Centering Corp (March 1, 1994) [63]
2. A terrible thing happened – A story for children who have witnessed violence or trauma by Margaret Holmes. Magination Pr; 1st edition (February 1, 2000) [64]
3. Badger's parting gifts by Susan Varley. HarperCollins; reprint edition (July 16, 1992) [65]
4. Help me say goodbye: Activities for helping kids cope when a special person dies by Janis Silverman. Fairview press; 1st edition (February 23, 1999) [66]
5. Healing the grieving Child's heart: 100 practical ideas for families, friends and caregivers by Alan Wolfelt. Companion Press; 1st edition (April 1, 2001) [67]
6. Helping children cope with the loss of a loved one: A guide for grownups by William C. Kroen. Free Spirit Publishing; 1st edition (January 15, 1996) [68]
7. Helping children grieve: When someone they love dies by Theresa M. Huntley. Augsburg Books; revised edition (September 30, 1991) [69]
8. If Nathan were here by Mary Bahr. Eerdmans books for young readers; 1st edition (march 25, 2000) [70]
9. I miss you by Pat Thomas. B.E.S. Publishing; 1st edition (January 1, 2001) [71]
10. Lifetimes by Bryan Mellonie. Bantam; 1st edition (October 1, 1983) [72]
11. Lost and found: Remembering a sister by Ellen Yeomans. Centering corporation (1999) [73]
12. Reactions: A workbook to help young people who are experiencing trauma and grief. By Alison Salloum (ages 9 through adult). Centering Corp (January 1, 1998) [74]
13. Rudi's pond by Eve Bunting. Clarion Books; reprint edition (October 18, 2004) [75]
14. The fall of Freddie the leaf by Leo Buscaglia. Slack incorporated (June 1, 1982) [76]
15. The invisible string by Patricia Karst. Little, Brown Books for young readers; reprint edition (October 30, 2018) [77]
16. When dinosaurs die by Laurie Kesney Brown and Marc Brown. Little, Brown Books for young readers; reprint edition (April 1, 1998) [78]
17. When someone dies by Sharon Greenlee. Peachtree Publishers (1992) [79]
18. When someone you love dies: A child- caregiver activity book by the National Alliance for grieving children. National Alliance for grieving children; 1st edition (2016) [80]
19. Zora Hurston and the chinaberry tree by William Miller. National Geographic School Pub; 1st edition (December 28, 2000) [81]
20. https://childrengrieve.org/
    National Alliance for grieving children [82]
21. https://www.dougy.org/
    The National Center for grieving children and families [83]
22. www.kidsaid.com
    Safe place for kids to support each other, share artwork, stories, and feelings [84]
23. www.dougy.org/grief-resources/help-for-teens/
    The National Center for grieving children and families [85]
24. https://elunanetwork.org
    The mission of the Eluna foundation is to provide comfort, hope and healing to children and families affected by grief and addiction [86]
25. http://www.sesamestreet.org/sites/default/files/media_folders/Media%20Root/Grief_CaregiverGuide.pdf
    This bilingual kit uses the power of Elmo and the sesame street Muppets to support grieving families. It includes the Muppets, and stories of families coping with the death of a parent; a parent/caregiver guide, and a storybook [87]
26. http://sharedgrief.org/,
    The shared grief project is a multimedia site designed to bring hope to grieving children by sharing the stories of respected athletes and other celebrities who have experienced childhood loss [88]
27. https://centering.org/
    A non-profit organization providing education and resources for the bereaved and providers [39]

References

1. Lang A, Carr T. Bereavement in the face of perinatal loss: a hardiness perspective. In: Becvar D, editor. Handbook of family resilience. New York: Springer; 2013. p. 299–319.
2. Meagher DK, Balk DE. Handbook of thanatology: the essential body of knowledge for the study of death, dying, and bereavement. London, Routledge; 2017. p. 143. p 220.
3. Rando TA. How to go on living when someone you love dies. Lexington: Lexington Books; 1991. p. 11.
4. Worden JW. Grief counseling and grief therapy: a handbook for the mental health practitioner. 5th ed. New York: Springer Publishing Company, LLC; 2018. p. 10. 31–33; 204.
5. Kübler-Ross E. On death and dying. New York: Macmillan; 1969.
6. Stroebe M, Schut H. The dual process model of coping with loss. Paper presented at the International Workgroup on Death, Dying and Bereavement, Oxford, 1995.
7. 4 Phases of Grief. Bowlby and Parkes. 1970. [Internet] Source: https://www.verywellhealth.com/the-four-phases-and-tasks-of-grief-1132550 Accessed 24 Oct 2018.
8. Before the five stages were the FOUR stages of grief [Internet] Source: http://whatsyourgrief.com/bowlby-four-stages-of-grief/. Accessed 24 Oct 2018.
9. Klass D, Silverman PR, Nickman SL, editors. Series in death education, aging, and health care. Continuing bonds: new understandings of grief. Philadelphia: Taylor & Francis; 1996. https://whatsyourgrief.com/continuing-bonds-shifting-the-grief-paradigm/. Accessed 24 Oct 2018
10. Neimeyer RA, Baldwin SA, Gillies J. Continuing bonds and reconstructing meaning: mitigating complications in bereavement. Death Stud. 2006;30(8):715–38.
11. Rando TA. Treatment of complicated mourning. Champaign: Research Press; 1995. p. 43–60.
12. Côté-Arsenault D, Denney-Koelsch E. "Have no regrets:" parents' experiences and developmental tasks in pregnancy with a lethal fetal diagnosis. Soc Sci Med. 2016;154:100–9. https://doi.org/10.1016/j.socscimed.2016.02.033.
13. Rogalla KB. Anticipatory grief, proactive coping, social support, and growth: exploring positive experiences of preparing for loss. OMEGA J Death Dying. 2018;1:30222818761461. https://doi.org/10.1177/0030222818761461.
14. American Psychiatric Association. Diagnostic and statistical manual of mental disorders. 5th ed. Arlington: American Psychiatric Publishing; 2013.
15. Complicated grief overview. [Internet] Source: https://complicatedgrief.columbia.edu/professionals/complicated-grief-professionals/overview. Accessed 24 Oct 2018.
16. Grief vs depression: which is it? [Internet] Source: https://www.verywell.com/grief-and-depression-1067237. Accessed 24 Oct 2018.
17. Christiansen DM. Posttraumatic stress disorder in parents following infant death: a systematic review. Clin Psychol Rev. 2017;51:60–74.
18. Zimmerman GH. Birth trauma: posttraumatic stress disorder after childbirth. Int J Childbirth Educ. 2013;28(3):61–6.
19. Postpartum Support International [Internet] Source: https://www.postpartum.net/
20. PTSD Screening Instruments. [Internet] Source: https://www.ptsd.va.gov/professional/assessment/screens/index.asp. Accessed 21 Nov 2018.
21. Turton P, Badenhorst W, Hughes P, Ward J, Riches S, White S. Psychological impact of stillbirth on fathers in the subsequent pregnancy and puerperium. Br J Psychiatry. 2006;188:165–72. https://doi.org/10.1192/bjp.188.2.165.
22. Christiansen DM, Olff M, Elklit A. Parents bereaved by infant death: sex differences and moderation in PTSD, attachment, coping and social support. Gen Hosp Psychiatry. 2014;36(6):655–61. https://doi.org/10.1016/j.genhosppsych.2014.07.012.
23. Proulx MC, Martinez AM, Carnevale F, Legault A. Fathers' experience after the death of their child (aged 1–17 years). OMEGA J Death Dying. 2016;73(4):308–25. https://doi.org/10.1177/0030222815590715.

24. Alam R, Barrera M, D'Agostino N, Nicholas DB, Schneiderman G. Bereavement experiences of mothers and fathers over time after the death of a child due to cancer. Death Stud. 2012;36(1):1–22. https://doi.org/10.1080/07481187.2011.553312.
25. Wonch Hill P, Cacciatore J, Shreffler KM, Pritchard KM. The loss of self: the effect of miscarriage, stillbirth, and child death on maternal self-esteem. Death Stud. 2017;41(4):226–35. https://doi.org/10.1080/07481187.2016.1261204.
26. Riley LP, LaMontagne LL, Hepworth JT, Murphy BA. Parental grief responses and personals growth following the death of a child. Death Stud. 2007;31(4):277–99. https://doi.org/10.1080/07481180601152591.
27. Côte-Arsenault D, Mahlangu N. The impact of perinatal loss on the subsequent pregnancy and self: Women's experiences. J Obstet Gynecol Neonatal Nurs. 1999;28(3):274–82.
28. Côté-Arsenault D, Donato K. Emotional cushioning in pregnancy after perinatal loss. J Reproductive Infant Psychol. 2011;29(1):81–92. https://doi.org/10.1080/02646838.2010.513115.
29. Côté-Arsenault D, O'Leary J. Understanding the experience of pregnancy subsequent to perinatal loss. In: Black BP, Wright PM, Limbo R, editors. Perinatal and pediatric bereavement in nursing and other health professions. New York: Springer Publishing; 2016. p. 159–81.
30. Kamm S, Vandenberg B. Grief communication, grief reactions and marital satisfaction in bereaved parents. Death Stud. 2001;25(7):569–82.
31. Côté-Arsenault D, Denney-Koelsch E. "Love is a choice:" couple responses to continuing pregnancy with a lethal fetal diagnosis. Illness Crisis Loss. 2018;26(1):5–22.
32. Bennett J, Dutcher J, Snyders M. Embrace. J Perinat Neonatal Nurs. 2011;25(1):72–6. https://doi.org/10.1097/JPN.0b013e318208cb8e.
33. Butler A, Hall H, Willetts G, Copnell B. Parents experiences of healthcare provider actions when their child dies: an integrative review of the literature. J Spec Pediatr Nurs. 2015;20(1):5–20. https://doi.org/10.1111/jspn.12097. Epub 2014 Nov 30
34. Bereaved Parents of the USA. www.bereavedparentsusa.org. Accessed 1 July 2019.
35. Baby's Breath Canada. Baby's breath serves and advocates on behalf of Canadian families who have experienced the tragic loss of an infant. https://www.babysbreathcanada.ca/. Accessed 1 July 2019.
36. Living with loss: hope and healing for the body, mind and spirit. www.bereavementmag.com. Accessed 1 July 2019.
37. The Compassionate Friends: Supporting Family After a Child Dies. www.compassionatefriends.org. Accessed 1 July 2019.
38. Center for Loss & Life Transition. https://www.centerforloss.com/. Accessed 1 July 2019.
39. https://centering.org/. A non-profit organization providing education and resources for the bereaved and providers.
40. Eric Chad Grief Support. Home of loving support for bereaved parents. http://www.erichad.com/index.html. Accessed 1 July 2019.
41. Grief Inc. Lighting the candle of hope. www.griefinc.com. Accessed 1 July 2019.
42. GriefNet.org. Grace happens. http://www.griefnet.org/. Accessed 1 July 2019.
43. Kelly Farley. Grieving dads: to the brink and back. https://grievingdads.com/. Accessed 1 July 2019.
44. Journey of Hearts. An online healing place for anyone grieving a loss. www.journeyofhearts.org. Accessed 1 July 2019.
45. New York Life Bereavement Support. https://www.newyorklife.com/foundation/bereavement. Accessed 1 July 2019.
46. Open to Hope. Helping people find hope after loss. http://www.opentohope.com/ Accessed 1 July 2019.
47. What's Your Grief? http://www.whatsyourgrief.com/. Accessed 1 July 2019.
48. Mitchell E. Beyond tears: living after losing a child, Revised Edition. New York: St. Martin's Griffin, Macmillan; Revised & enlarged edition, March 3, 2009.
49. Davis DL. Empty cradle, broken heart: surviving the death of your baby. Golden: Fulcrum Publishing; 2016.

50. Vredvelt P. Empty arms: Hope and support for those who have suffered a miscarriage, stillbirth, or tubal pregnancy. 2nd ed. Multnomah; 2001.
51. Redfern S, Gilbert SK. The grieving garden: living with the death of a child. Charlottesville: Hampton Roads Publishing; 2008.
52. Wolfelt A. Healing a parent's grieving heart: 100 practical ideas after your child dies. Fort Collins: Companion Press; 2002.
53. Apple DL. Life after the death of my son: what I'm learning. Kansas City: Beacon Hill Press of Kansas City; 2008.
54. First Candle. Saving babies. Supporting families. http://www.firstcandle.org/grieving-families/grief-resources/online-resources/#1. Accessed 1 July 2019.
55. HAND. Helping After Neonatal Death. http://handonline.org/. Accessed 1 July 2019.
56. MEND. Mommies Enduring Neonatal Death. https://www.mend.org/. Accessed 1 July 2019.
57. PSI. Postpartum Support International. http://www.postpartum.net/. Accessed 1 July 2019.
58. Still Standing Magazine for all those who are grieving child loss & infertility. http://stillstandingmag.com/. Accessed 1 July 2019.
59. Farley K, Dicola D. Grieving Dads: to the brink and back. Grieving Dads LLC; 2012. Blog available at www.GrievingDads.com.
60. Golden TR. Swallowed by a snake: the gift of the masculine side of healing. Gaithersburg: G H Publishing, LLC; 1996. 130 pages.
61. Golden TR. The way men heal. Gaithersburg: G H Publishing, LLC; 2014. 58 pages.
62. Levang E. When men grieve: why men grieve differently and how you can help. Minneapolis: Fairview Press, Division of Fairview Health Services; 1998.
63. Traisman ES. A child remembers. Omaha: Compassion Books/Centering Corporation; 1994, Revised 2018. 16 pages.
64. Holmes M. A terrible thing happened – a story for children who have witnessed violence or trauma. 1st ed. Washington: American Psychological Association; 2000. 32 pages.
65. Varley S. Badger's parting gifts. New York: Harper Collins; 1992. 32 pages.
66. Silverman J. Help me say goodbye: activities for helping kids cope when a special person dies. 1st ed. Minneapolis: Fairview Press; 1999. 36 pages.
67. Wolfelt A. Healing the grieving child's heart: 100 practical ideas for families, friends and caregivers. Laguna Hills: Companion Press; 2001. 128 pages.
68. Kroen WC. Helping children cope with the loss of a loved one: a guide for grownups. 1st ed. Minneapolis: Free Spirit Publishing; 1996. 112 pages.
69. Huntley TM. Helping children grieve: when someone they love dies. Revised ed. Minneapolis: Augsburg Books; 2002. 132 pages.
70. Bahr M. If Nathan were here. 1st ed. Grand Rapids: Eerdmans Publishing Company; 2000. 32 pages.
71. Thomas P. I miss you. 1st ed. Hauppage, NY: Barron's Educational Series; 2001. 32 pages
72. Mellonie B. Lifetimes. 1st ed. New York: Bantam; 1983. 40 pages.
73. Yeomans E. Lost and found. Omaha: Centering Corporation; 1999. 32 pages.
74. Salloum A. Reactions: a workbook to help young people who are experiencing trauma and grief. Burnsville: Compassion Books, Inc.; 1998. 49 pages.
75. Bunting E. Rudi's Pond. New York: Houghton Mifflin Harcourt, Clarion Books; 2004. 32 pages.
76. Buscaglia L. The fall of freddie the leaf. Slack Incorporated: Thorofare; 1982. 32 pages.
77. Karst P. The invisible string. Camarillo: Devorss & Co.; 4/30/2001, edition September 1, 2000. 36 pages.
78. Brown LK, Brown M. When dinosaurs die. Reprint ed. New York: Little, Brown and Company, Hatchette Book Group; 1998. 32 pages.
79. Greenlee S. When someone dies. 1st ed. Atlanta: Peachtree Publishing Company; 1992. 40 pages.
80. The National Alliance for Grieving Children. When someone you love dies: a child- caregiver activity book. 1st ed. Lubbock: National Alliance for Grieving Children. 2016.
81. Miller W. Zora Hurston and the chinaberry tree. Reading: Rainbow Book; 2000.
82. National Alliance for Grieving Children. https://childrengrieve.org/. Accessed 1 July 2019.

83. The Dougy Center. The National Center for Grieving Children and Families. www.dougy.org/grief-resources/. Accessed 1 July 2019.
84. www.kidsaid.com. Safe place for kids to support each other, share artwork, stories, and feelings.
85. The Dougy Center. The National Center for Grieving Children and Families. www.dougy.org/grief-resources/help-for-teens/. Accessed 1 July 2019.
86. Eluna (previously Moyer Foundation. https://elunanetwork.org/. Accessed 1 July 2019.
87. When families grieve: a special guide for parents and caregivers. http://www.sesamestreet.org/sites/default/files/media_folders/Media%20Root/Grief_CaregiverGuide.pdf. Accessed 1 July 2019.
88. The Shared Grief Project. http://sharedgrief.org/. Accessed 1 July 2019.

Part III

Models of Perinatal Palliative Care

Structure and Development of Hospital-Based Perinatal Palliative Care Programs

13

Barbara A. Dean, Melanie Chichester, Laurie Hewlett-Miller, Vanita D. Jain, Erin M. Denney-Koelsch, and Michael L. Spear

Introduction

Congenital anomalies are the primary cause of neonatal and infant deaths in the USA and account for approximately 20% of early deaths [1]. Many, though not all, of these anomalies can be identified during pregnancy at the initial 18–20 weeks anatomy ultrasound. Depending on the findings, the prognosis for the child can

B. A. Dean
Neonatal Intensive Care Unit (NICU), Christiana Care Health Services, Newark, DE, USA

M. Chichester
Christiana Care Health Services, Department of Labor & Delivery, Newark, DE, USA

L. Hewlett-Miller
Christiana Care Health Services, Department of Pediatrics, Newark, DE, USA

V. D. Jain
High Risk Unit (PSCU) & Clinic, Division of Maternal Fetal Medicine, Christiana Care Health Services, Newark, DE, USA

Sidney Kimmel SOM, Thomas Jefferson University, Newark, DE, USA

Perinatal Special Care Unit, Clinic & Antenatal Step-Down, Christiana Care Health System, Department of Obstetrics & Gynecology, Division of Maternal Fetal Medicine, Newark, DE, USA

E. M. Denney-Koelsch
University of Rochester Medical Center/Strong Memorial Hospital, Department of Medicine, Division of Palliative Care, Rochester, NY, USA

M. L. Spear (✉)
Pediatric Palliative Care, St Christopher's Hospital for Children, Philadelphia, PA, USA

St Christopher's Hospital for Children, Drexel University College of Medicine, Department of Pediatrics, Philadelphia, PA, USA
e-mail: michael.spear@drexel.edu

E. M. Denney-Koelsch, D. Côté-Arsenault (eds.), *Perinatal Palliative Care*, https://doi.org/10.1007/978-3-030-34751-2_13

range from lethal to serious but treatable, but there is a zone of equivocal findings where postnatal survival and prognosis are very difficult to predict. In all cases when a life-limiting fetal condition (LLFC) is diagnosed, parents are shocked and grieving. Leuthner and Jones described the parents' experiences: "There is a conflict between the expected or anticipated normal sequence of life events and the reality of neonatal death; children are not supposed to precede their parents in death, and pregnancy and childbirth do not evoke thoughts of death" [2].

To care for these grieving and vulnerable families, perinatal palliative care (PPC) programs have arisen out of preexisting pediatric palliative care and perinatal bereavement programs. Before 2007, the literature documented few organized PPC services [2]. Since the American Academy of Pediatrics began to sponsor board certification in Hospice and Palliative Medicine, PPC programs have grown in number and evolved in structure. This chapter will describe the current hospital-based PPC programs, describe their structure and processes, and provide recommendations for building a new program.

Survey on PPC Programs in the USA

Wool, Denney-Koelsch, Côté-Arsenault, and colleagues published the only two articles reviewing PPC programs in the USA [3, 4]. Wool et al. states, "Although recommendations are emerging from research and practice regarding care for parents who choose to continue pregnancy after a life-limiting fetal diagnosis, data are lacking on what actually constitutes high-quality care during pregnancy under these circumstances" [3]. The research team used the framework described by the National Consensus Project (NCP) for Quality Palliative Care [5] to develop a national survey of existing PPC programs. The NCP is organized in eight domains, around which the research team organized their survey:

1. Structure and process. Includes nine subdomains addressing guidelines that focus on holistic care delivered by an interdisciplinary team trained in palliative care and supported in their work.
2. Assessment of pain and symptom management.
3. Psychosocial and psychological implications of end-of-life issues and the need for grief and bereavement services.
4. Assessment of family's social structure.
5. Assessment of the family's spiritual framework and practice.
6. Provision of care with cultural sensitivity.
7. Specific system for end-of-life care.
8. Legal and ethics aspects of care.

The authors created an electronic survey of 48 questions addressing these 8 domains, piloted it with a group of healthcare professionals, and revised it based on their feedback. A total of 136 active PPC programs were recruited through www.perinatalhospice.org [6] and state-by-state internet searches. Qualtrics™ was used to collect the data from 75 programs (55% response rate). The results illustrated for the first time the structural diversity of PPC programs. Some were home-based, and others operated within hospitals, outpatient clinics, and other locations.

What is known about PPC programs in the USA will be described below under each of the eight domains. Many of the components are addressed extensively in other chapters and are marked.

Domain 1: The Structure and Processes of Care

One of the key roles of any palliative care team is to coordinate complex multifaceted care of a seriously ill patient and their family. The PPC team enhances communication between all the appropriate disciplines involved in the care of both parents and fetus. Many people are involved in the care of the family, spread across multiple disciplines, specialties, and sometimes locations. The mother may deliver at one hospital and the palliative services may be at a different children's hospital. Because of the complexity of each family's care, a care coordinator is common and was present in 83% of PPC programs surveyed [4]. The care coordinator role was assumed by providers from a variety of disciplines: physicians, nurse practitioners, nurses, pastoral care representatives, social workers, certified child life specialists, and masters trained persons in psychiatry. This diversity reflects the varied origins of most programs; from our experience, the most interested and passionate person at an institution becomes the main care coordinator.

The overall structure, team members, processes, and philosophy of care for all programs, as well as those that are more advanced, are found in Table 13.1. The varied structures of PPC programs across the country likely result from their development from a nucleus of one or two passionate people. Administrative and clinical responsibilities are often shared among team members, and the shared responsibilities across disciplines are fluid. The survey showed that the most common disciplines in PPC programs were spiritual care, medicine, nursing, social work, hospice providers, and the care coordinator, who could come from several of these disciplines. Less common members were genetic counselors and child life support staff (see Table 13.1). Most but not all (82%) had a team member who could be contacted 24 hours/day, 7 days per week. Having a key person for communication is essential.

Additional detail on Domain 1 is described by Denney-Koelsch et al. [4], in which the authors provide an in-depth analysis of structure and process of PPC programs.

Nearly all programs have weekly or biweekly interdisciplinary team (IDT) meetings to discuss patients and their care plans. Other components include family meetings in which the team assesses parental understanding of diagnosis and prognosis, establishes goals of care for the pregnancy, birth, and ultimate outcome, and provides support throughout these processes. The overall philosophy of care for PPC programs focuses on respect for parent preferences and choices, patient/parent support, respect for the infant, and provision for parent involvement. The reported outcomes that were most important were physical and psychosocial support, parent

Table 13.1 Structure of perinatal palliative care programs [3, 4]

	Team members	Structure and process	Philosophy of care
Essential to all	• Palliative care-trained physician and/or nurse practitioner • Nurse • Social worker • Chaplain • Care coordinator (typically RN or SW) • Administrative support person • Bereavement coordinator	• Interdisciplinary team meetings • Care coordination with patient and family • Care coordination with other specialties • Process for birth planning • Process for documentation and dissemination of birth plan • Development of basic funding and administrative support	• Family-centered care • Interdisciplinary approach • Respect for families' values (e.g., infant and fetal personhood). • Parental involvement in decision-making
More advanced programs	• Genetics counselor • Physicians from other specialties (e.g., maternal-fetal medicine (MFM), neonatology, cardiology, etc.) • Child life specialist • Data manager • Hospice representative • Ethicist	• Increased administrative support • Strengthening connection between home hospice agency and hospital • Data management • Education of other groups (e.g., MFM, neonatology) • Measurement of outcomes ∘ Physical and psychosocial support ∘ Parent satisfaction with decision-making progress ∘ Opportunities to parent the infant ∘ Infant comfort ∘ Positive personal and family growth • Funding for growth ∘ Grants ∘ Grateful donors • Research ∘ Qualitative research on patient experience ∘ Outcome research ∘ Symptom management	• Program growth and sustainability • Improving quality of care

satisfaction with the decision-making process, opportunities to parent the infant, infant comfort, and positive personal and family growth [4].

One of the structural challenges for PPC programs revolves around documentation of a unified care plan. While most programs allowed for documentation in the maternal chart, if the care is being given at a children's hospital, and access to the maternal chart is not possible, an alternative electronic communication system may be needed. This is often an electronic letter to the primary obstetrical or maternal/child provider, but it is often best to ensure that the family has a hard copy, so they can access the care plan in case of emergent delivery.

Funding is a tremendous challenge for all palliative care programs, including perinatal programs. This survey demonstrated that 56% of academic medical centers bill insurance companies for PPC, but only 12% of local hospices and 19% of palliative care organizations do so. Community organizations receive no reimbursement from insurance companies. Philanthropic grants provide support for PPC to 44% of academic medical centers, 24% of regional or community hospitals, 75% of local hospice or palliative care organizations, and 67% of community-based support programs [3].

The remaining domains are covered in greater depth in other chapters (listed below each one).

Domain 2: Physical Aspects of Care

The Wool et al. survey indicated that physical aspects of care were provided by all but one program and included referral to home hospice care, nutritional support, laboratory testing, comfort measures for the infant, and neonatal intensive care [3]. Most physical care is provided to the mother by the obstetrical team and to the infant by the neonatal team. The PPC team may provide direct patient care or make recommendations to the primary team for pain and symptom management. (See also Chaps. 5, 8, and 9.)

Domain 3: Psychological and Psychiatric Services

Nearly all programs (97%) provided a variety of bereavement interventions for grieving families [3]. (See Chap. 12.)

Domain 4: Social Aspects of Care

Most programs included social supports such as support groups for parents, either parent-led or based in a community organization. Social media are being used increasingly for this purpose. Most programs (80%) provided special support for siblings, and child life specialists were often an integral part of this process. They actively engaged the children in both verbal and nonverbal activities to help them process their feelings of loss, anxiety, and stress. (See below, Social Worker, and Chap. 14, section "Child Life".)

Domain 5: Spiritual, Religious, and Existential Aspects of Care

All programs reported addressing spiritual care. Staffing varied, but could include hospital chaplains or pastoral care providers. Some but not all have specific training surrounding perinatal loss; often staff learn these skills on the job. (See Chap. 11).

Domain 6: Cultural Aspects of Care

Culturally sensitive care is of paramount importance. Cultural diversity around loss and grieving is complex. It requires extreme awareness and sensitivity to approach a grieving family in a compassionate manner, respecting their background and beliefs. For example, 69% of programs in the Wool et al. [3] study translated documents appropriately. Interpreter services were used by 99% of services. Providing this support is challenging for smaller programs, but translation of languages can be achieved with an increasing number of methods, including computer-based live video translation. Some programs had "cultural brokers" who were experts in certain cultures and facilitated understanding and communication. (See also Chap. 16.)

Domain 7: Care of the Imminently Dying Patient

Care of the imminently dying patient was provided in 92% of programs. This care included comforting the baby, supporting the family, and helping them make memories, as described in other chapters. (See Chaps. 8 and 9, section "Special Considerations During End-of-Life Care" and "Symptom management".)

Domain 8: Ethical and Legal Aspects of Care

The percentage of perinatal programs that had written policies and protocols is 55%. Others used textbooks, journal articles, and organizational algorithms and process maps. The majority of programs (95%) had ethics boards to provide consultation. (See Chap. 3.)

PCC Program Development in Canada

Stenekes et al. conducted a descriptive qualitative investigation of three large Canadian tertiary referral centers to determine the depth and scope of palliative care in this country [7]. Providers from multiple disciplines were interviewed: physicians, nurses, respiratory therapists, midwives, social workers, chaplains, ultrasonographers, and other health care providers. The disciplinary breadth of this sample suggests that the authors took an inclusive approach to palliative care. Focus groups and individual interviews were conducted, and analysis revealed three main themes, all involving communication: (1) connecting through proximity, (2) protected time and dedicated space, and (3) flexibility and formality. *Connecting through proximity* was challenging when team members worked in different facilities, e.g., a children's hospital separate from an obstetrics hospital with separate billing systems and electronic records. Respondents reported that establishing clear lines of electronic communication, or providing written documentation of all encounters, was important. Often the parents themselves carried the information from one caretaker to another, if the electronic medical records of each institution were not linked. *Protected time and dedicated space* were standards to enable clear palliative care communication, including dedicated meeting times and private space for discussions within the team and between team and family. *Flexibility and formality* were also considered a hallmark of effective communication. Every family situation has its own nuances, and the team needed to be able to adapt to each situation.

The Canadian study identified three phases of program development across all institutions: emerging, developing, and integrated [7]. Many programs began as a "grass roots" voluntary process. To develop sustainability, funds were needed for personnel time and space, which required administrative approval and support. In many hospitals, extramural funding was needed to supplement patient revenue. Efforts were needed to explain to hospital administrators how palliative care programs can save money. A fully integrated program had the following characteristics: an interdisciplinary team approach, a formal collaboration between specialties for decision-making, regular staff training, bereavement planning and follow-up care provision, and administrative support (see Table 13.1). Overall, Canadian programs are struggling with similar growing pains as those in the USA.

Building a Perinatal Palliative Care Program

Programs can grow in several ways. Kobler et al. advocate for program growth out of bereavement programs, which have been established much longer than PPC programs [8], and the principles and organizational system of perinatal bereavement programs provide an appropriate foundation because they already have standard processes and infrastructure that can be adapted for PPC. These include (1) access on any hospital unit at any time of day, (2) staff education, (3) relationship-based care, (4) family-centered philosophy, (5) tailored interventions, (6) follow-up, (7) consistency with legal and institution guidelines and policies, and (8) assessment of quality. In making the transition, it is important to ensure adequate staffing to accommodate increased patient volume, and newly organized PPC teams would benefit from additional training from a nationally recognized bereavement training program and/or training in palliative care specific skills such as symptom management. Kobler et al. stress the need for an overall coordinator, as well as a key group of individuals qualified to guide and support decision-making around the desired plan for the pregnancy, about labor and delivery, and plans after birth.

As an alternative, PPC programs can also be developed out of existing pediatric palliative care programs, which have well-established processes for communication surrounding very sick patients, supporting families through difficult journeys, and addressing symptom concerns. An increasing body of literature describes detailed processes that PPC programs can offer as the family traverses the multiple specialties they encounter during this complex time of decision-making in the midst of hope and grief [9–12].

It is paramount for the PPC team to include a key person or persons with sufficient time dedicated to coordinating care of the family during their journey. This can be the physician, a nurse or nurse practitioner, or social worker. Since palliative care revenue is often insufficient to sustain a salary, programs may require grants and other sources of income (e.g., hospital support). Some key steps to formation of a PPC Program are outlined in Table 13.2, based on the authors' and editors' experience.

Table 13.2 Key steps to formation and growth of a perinatal palliative care program

Steps		Comments/considerations
Brand new programs		
Step 1	Identify your care coordinator	A nurse, social worker, physician: whoever is the most passionate, and organized, and has time
Step 2	Meet with key stakeholders (from MFM, neonatology, genetics counseling, etc.)	Gauge interest and understanding of role of palliative care
		Assess readiness to begin collaboration
Step 3	Establish your structure and processes	Who will be the key members of the IDT
		Which patients will be seen?
		All congenital anomalies or only likely lethal anomalies?
		Premature babies or other post-birth diagnoses?
		Where will you see patients (hospital, clinic, home)?
		Referral process
		IDT meeting schedule
		Care coordination process
		Documentation and dissemination process
		Initial parent feedback
		Team professional growth
		Self-care of team members
Step 4	Plan funding	Can you do it initially on minimal funding within existing job descriptions?
		Billing to insurance (usually MD or NP required to bill)
		Institutional funding
		Grants/philanthropy
Established and growing programs		
Step 5	Quality outcomes and data management	What will you measure and how?
		Who will track data and analyze?
		QA/QI training for team?
		Reevaluate your structure and process if needed
Step 6	Managing growth	Additional hiring?
		Training process for new team members?
		Expansion to hospitals/clinics?
		Requesting additional funds from institution vs philanthropy

IDT interdisciplinary team, *QA/QI* quality assessment, quality improvement

A Program Example: PPC Program Structure and Processes at Christiana Care Health System

Program Initiation

In the remainder of this chapter, we will give examples of how programs are structured and function at Christiana Care Health system, the largest hospital system in Delaware and the only tertiary care hospital for the state. The hospital has a delivery service of 6000 births/year with a 72-bed, level 3 NICU. The PPC team is known as IMPACT, or Infant Maternal Pediatric Advanced Care Team. The team is led by a neonatologist who underwent an intense training process at The Harvard Palliative Care Education and Practice Program and is Board certified in Hospice and Palliative Care. Members also include a second neonatologist and two pediatric residents, RNs from labor and delivery and the NICU, chaplain, and social worker. The PPC team currently averages 24 consults each year. The patients are a mixed group ranging from patients referred from an outside facility who has been diagnosed with a serious fetal anomaly to patients being seen for the first time when they have received a questionable anatomy ultrasound. Infants born at less than 25 weeks are automatically given a palliative care consult. Case 13.1 describes the case that spurred formation of the program at Christiana.

Case 13.1 Muhammed

Muhammed was born in 2008. His diagnosis of Trisomy 18 had been previously confirmed by an amniocentesis. His condition was complicated with cardiac abnormalities— ventricular septal defect, patent ductus arteriosus, and dysplastic valves. Despite extensive discussion of the life-limiting nature of his condition, his parents remained hopeful, picturing their son someday playing baseball, and requested full resuscitation. He was intubated at birth. A PDA ligation and pulmonary artery banding were performed on day of life 6. He was placed on medication for congestive heart failure. He developed a pleural effusion on day of life 21 and required a chest tube. He was unable to be extubated because of long apneic periods. His parents continued to want full support. His congestive heart failure worsened and he developed pneumonia. On day of life 36, he died after a prolonged period of aggressive resuscitation.

At the time of Muhammed's birth, PPC was not available at the institution. No debriefing was offered to the staff. Few staff members had knowledge about palliative care as part of practice. They were distressed after Muhammed's death, wondering how this family might have been better supported and how Muhammed's life might have had more quality and less suffering.

PPC awareness was becoming a topic of interest and discussion during this time and after attending a lecture at a national conference, a core group of interested physicians, neonatal nurse practitioners, and NICU nurses met to discuss forming a program. First, they conducted an extensive literature search and attended national training programs. Next, information was shared with physicians and nursing staff in journal clubs, lectures, and case presentations. Debriefings were offered to staff after each death that occurred in the NICU [13]. Finally in 2012, a regional conference was held, bringing in expert speakers to enhance the staff's understanding of PPC.

After the conference, the palliative care team started to receive antenatal consults on families faced with life-limiting fetal diagnoses. Initially neonatologists felt that they did not need help in supporting families of NICU infants, but because medical teams frequently change in the NICU of a teaching hospital, it was soon realized that a palliative care team could offer better support and consistency to families with critically ill infants or those with a short life expectancy. As consults, both antenatal and neonatal, increased in frequency, team members were added, including a chaplain, social worker, and a labor and delivery nurse. Grant and gift money was used for supplies and continuing education. Although some protected time is available, staff positions in PPC are not yet available.

Role of the Neonatologist

The role of the attending neonatologist varies somewhat depending on the structure at each institution. Prenatally, the neonatologist's input is invaluable regarding implications of the baby's condition for neonatal care immediately after birth and beyond, the care options for delivery room and NICU care, and prognostication. (See also Chap. 7.) After birth, the neonatologist is typically the primary attending physician for the baby's care, with the other specialists, including palliative care, providing consultative service. The neonatologist makes all the moment-to-moment decisions about the baby's care and orchestrates the multiple consultants. Ideally the neonatologist and palliative care physician work in tandem to provide comprehensive care to the patient and the family. Often, the neonatologist's work load is considerable: rounding on large numbers of patients, performing medical procedures, teaching rounds, etc. These can prevent the kind of in-depth conversations that may need to occur with the parents. By working in tandem with the palliative care team, the patient and family can receive multiple physicians' expertise and focus on the key issues involved. The palliative care team always complements the primary team and never tries to replace them in the process.

Role of the Palliative-Care-Trained Physician

The role of the palliative physician is multifaceted; working closely with the primary medical team is required. In the NICU, multiple physicians often care for each infant and family, as they rotate through the unit. Patients who survive beyond the NICU will likely have a different group of physicians. The palliative care physicians may serve as a more constant source of support for each family. In some institutions, they attend the delivery of each of their patients, to provide that continuity, from the prenatal through the postnatal period. After birth, they provide the same source of support and continuity throughout the course of the child's life. Parents have reported that this added layer of physician support is invaluable to the process of understanding, acceptance, and loss. In addition, palliative care physicians often are the most highly trained experts in complex symptom management, especially at the end of life. They play a key role in advising the team about the best approaches to balancing complex medical care with attention to comfort and symptom control. They are highly trained in complex pain and agitation management, including last-resort options such as palliative sedation for intractable symptoms.

While much of this role could be provided by any advanced practice provider (nurse practitioner or physician's assistant), some situations may be easier when a physician is advocating for the patient or family with the physicians from other teams. This is particularly true in situations when there is disagreement (within the team or between team and family) or ethical dilemmas arise about the best course of action. Negotiation and coming to an agreement can sometimes be easier between physicians.

Another role of the palliative care physician can be direct education of other physicians and team members about the essential, basic palliative care skills all providers should know. Providing inservices on pain management or presenting grand rounds to the MFM team can allow palliative care specialists to "spread the word" about the importance of palliative care, dispelling common fears and myths about it. (For further discussion, see Chaps. 8, 9, and 10).

Role of Maternal-Fetal Medicine Physician

The first ultrasound is often the transition from what could be a normal to a more complicated pregnancy. A pregnant mother's first interaction and "visualization" of her child occurs typically in the first trimester with the measurement of the crown-rump length and fetal heart rate by her obstetrician. Although ultrasound imaging is improving, and earlier diagnosis of lethal and congenital anomalies are made in the first trimester, the current standard of care typically involves an anatomy ultrasound for all pregnancies at 18–20 weeks [14]. This ultrasound is a life-changing turning point for pregnant mothers who are carrying a fetus with a serious anomaly.

After a LLFC is found, the American College of Obstetricians and Gynecologists recommends a thorough discussion with the family of all the findings and possible risks, benefits, or alternatives to various options, which can range from termination of the pregnancy to fetal intervention to continuation of the pregnancy and consideration of perinatal palliative care [15]. The physician who interprets the ultrasound and/or the patient's obstetrician is often faced with sharing this new knowledge with the patient. This is an important interaction wherein the physician should try to establish communications with the parents, share valuable knowledge, and help the parents understand the diagnosis [16]. It is usually after multiple conversations with her obstetrical providers that the mother will meet the PPC team. This section will review the intersection of the MFM specialist with the PPC team. Extensive discussion of obstetrical management can be found in Chap. 5.

Communication between the parents and the MFM physician can be crucial in shaping how the parents perceive their options. Information regarding the fetal anomalies should be given in a supportive manner with empathy and respect for the baby and the family. Once the anomalies have been identified, the family must consider their options and may be considered a candidate for referral to a PPC program.

Currently, most referrals to the IMPACT program at Christiana are for fetuses with a life-limiting diagnosis involving genetic aneuploidy or severe birth defects. However, another group of patients are those who face an extremely premature birth (<23 weeks gestation) whether due to maternal complications warranting delivery or fetal testing that suggests significant problems. The parents need to hear the full spectrum of possibilities. Failure to address all possibilities with any parent can lead to frustration, confusion, anger, and even moral angst or guilt. As noted by Carter, a mother anticipating an extremely preterm delivery also requires support that respectfully provides information and assesses her hopes, values, and perception that she is making the right choice for her child or family in keeping with her cultural and spiritual values and appreciation of societal norms [17]. At present, at Christiana Care, this subgroup of women is not referred to the PPC, but we hope the program will soon expand to include them. Some institutions include extreme prematurity in their PPC programs, while others leave this group to the pediatric palliative care team.

As noted by Wool and colleagues, PPC programs vary across the country in how they are set up and how they function [3]. At Christiana Care, MFM plays a crucial part in all eight Domains of care as outlined earlier in *Development and Structure of PPC Programs.* During antenatal care, the physical care of the mother and fetus is provided entirely by the primary obstetrician in consultation with MFM or by the MFM provider after transfer of care (Domain 2, Assessment of pain and symptom management). Prenatal care involves scheduled routine prenatal visits, more frequent visits if requested by the families, and frequent ultrasounds. MFM typically also coordinates referrals for the various pediatric subspecialists, genetic counseling, and then any other indicated imaging (fetal MRI, fetal echocardiogram). The MFM also provides counseling and information regarding diagnostic testing via amniocentesis or, most recently, cell-free fetal DNA. Other programs leave this role to the genetics counselor (see also Chap. 6).

As soon as possible after completion of the evaluation and prior to completion of the pregnancy, the obstetric provider should initiate the PPC referral. All records, imaging studies, diagnostic testing, prenatal lab work, and consultation reports are forwarded to the neonatal and palliative care team for review. Often, a meeting or phone call between the MFM and neonatologist is scheduled to fully review the scope of the anomalies and to communicate the family's desires and any concerns of the MFM specialist. In addition, all fetal anomalies are reviewed monthly at the 1–4 hour fetal therapy meeting attended by MFM physicians from the entire state of Delaware, as well as the pediatric subspecialists. Cases are reviewed along with birth plans, pregnancy-related goals, and post-natal outcomes, if available. In addition to this meeting, the neonatal palliative care team meets quarterly, along with a member of the MFM division, to review cases, address potential issues of management and concern, and identify solutions.

Somewhere in the third trimester, the patient's finalized birth plans are circulated and formalized among the divisions. The birth plan typically has two parts, the MFM and the neonatal components. The MFM section typically addresses such things as when the mother will be admitted for delivery, mode of delivery, what monitoring (if any) will be performed, and who will be in attendance [18]. The parents may also specify their desires for anesthesia and this is documented in the chart. Anesthesia preferences should be carefully discussed with the mother and documented, because some options will limit the mother's consciousness during a time when bonding with the infant will be important and their time together may be brief [18]. It is essential for the MFM department to have a single coordinator who handles the referrals and compiles the chart for any provider who may care for the mother. This record-keeping ensures that timing and mode of delivery are appropriately communicated to the in-house generalist obstetrical team, should the patient come in unanticipated prior to her scheduled delivery date. All providers need to be aware of patients who are receiving PPC, to keep the PPC team informed about any changes to the patient status or care plan [19].

For some mothers, transfer of care from her local obstetrician to the Christiana High-Risk Clinic (staffed by MFM) is arranged to facilitate her delivery in the care of the PPC team. This decision relates to Domain 2, but also Domain 4 (Assessment of family's social structure). Maternal and family values will determine which birth setting will be most acceptable to the parents [7], based not only on medical needs, but on the mothers' concerns for her family (e.g., proximity to her other children). At times, the severity of the fetal or maternal complications requires prolonged inpatient hospitalization that can also have significant social impacts.

At Christiana Care, the MFM group assists with memory-making (Domain 7: Care of the Dying Patient) by recording of the heart beat for "heart beat bears" or 3D pictures or other video imaging of the fetus as desired by the family. During all visits during antepartum care, MFM providers work to address and include cultural aspects of care (Domain 6). The hospital provides both telephone language lines and in-person translators to assist in the cultural aspects of care. Although interpretation alone may not be enough, it is an essential strategy to clarify the patient's and family values. At these follow-up appointments, MFM may also address options for grief counseling, psychiatric counseling, chaplain/faith-based services, and social work (Domains 3, 4, 5).

As noted by Wool and colleagues, the majority of PPC programs do not have formal palliative care training for all care providers [3]. At Christiana, although most MFM providers see and counsel these patients, apart from fellowship training and years of experience attending "un-routine" deliveries (https://www.smfm.org/members/what-is-a-mfm) [20], no formal training in palliative care has been undertaken by any of the divisions' members. It is important that providers delivering news of a life-limiting diagnosis should learn how to discuss with families their concerns about infant pain control and whether intervention/therapy for the fetus may increase suffering and provide progress status/updates to the family [18]. Domain 7 counseling is most often completed by the neonatologist or PPC physician. Though the MFM provider may initiate conversations based on an anomaly discovered by ultrasound, final determination of the neonatal plan of care is appropriately left with the neonatal providers.

Lastly, often the MFM may face barriers that fall under Domain 8 (Ethical and Legal). Although the MFM division has intimate knowledge and understanding of the PPC options, referral into the program is often resisted by primary care providers and mother's themselves. Such barriers to palliative care referral often include equating palliative care with care of the "dying," not knowing when to consult the palliative care team, perception that the parents "aren't ready yet," perception that termination of pregnancy is a better option for the mother's health, not wanting to reduce parental hope, self-confidence that the primary obstetrician can provide complete care, and/or cultural, language, or religious obstacles [19].

In setting up the palliative care team, the MFM palliative care champion has focused on education of other MFMs to enable them to value the potential benefits of referral for PPC. They share published protocols about indications for PPC consultation that emphasizes the benefits of PPC, including parental understanding of the fetus's trajectory and outcomes and knowing all reasonable care options; clinician's understanding of the family's narrative and their perspectives on desired information, as well as parent's hopes and acceptable outcomes; and lastly, informing parents about the potential risks, harms, and pain related to procedures that could be performed on their child [19]. Education is provided to palliative care team through grand rounds, an annual PPC conference, and department business meetings.

The Role of the Social Worker

The role of the social worker in PPC involves a combination of understanding and supporting the parents, the members of the palliative care team, and the nursing staff. In some programs, the care coordination of the entire PPC team is done by a social worker. At Christiana, once the fetus or infant has been identified as having a LLFC, it is explained to the parents in detail by the MFM physician. If the family decides to continue the pregnancy, they are referred to the palliative care team for an outpatient consult. It is ideal for the social worker (or an RN in some programs) to establish a relationship with the parents at this consult or a subsequent prenatal consult, to develop trust and begin the process of assessment [21]. The assessment and screening process allow perinatal social workers to discover the issues that need to be addressed and strengths within each family. Perinatal social work assessments highlight the areas of need to be addressed and strengths within each family (Domains 3–6).

If timing prevents meeting the parents prenatally, the relationship can be established in the NICU. At Christiana, once a baby is identified as needing an IMPACT consult, the team is notified, is given a summary of the Birth Plan and Goals, reviews the chart, and meets with parents [22]. NICU mental health professionals strive to meet with all parents/primary caregivers within 1–3 days of admission to establish a working relationship, normalize emotional distress, and evaluate risk factors for all forms of emotional distress.

Although the nursing and medical staff provides most direct patient care and spends a great deal of time with families in the NICU, the social worker is a key team member at Christiana who usually gets to know the family at a deeper psychosocial level than other members [21]. Assessments by perinatal social workers help conceptualize interactions between race-ethnicity, culture, patient health and well-being, and the larger family system. Issues that need to be addressed and strengths within each family can be used to enhance communication between all disciplines involved in the care of the parents and the newborn.

The goal of the social worker is to act as a liaison between the parents, the care team, and IMPACT members to coordinate the palliative care delivery plan, maximize infant care and family satisfaction, and confirm that their needs are being met. This care coordination role is often fulfilled by nurses in other programs across the country. There are important topics to investigate with parents at the initial visit, while other questions may be better received when the relationship is further established. In addition to demographics, it is important to understand each family's structure, including relationship with father of the baby, number of siblings and their ages, previous losses, primary support system at home and in the community, mental health history, religious preference, and current ability to cope with their difficult situation. The social worker should be a good listener and encourage expression of concerns and feelings, ask parents to explain the current care plan and expectations for their infant, and be certain that the family is oriented to the NICU and its resources. The social worker should also ask if they have questions, concerns, or things they would like done differently.

Prior to the emergence of PPC in the year 2000, Catlin and Carter recognized that palliative and bereavement care were often provided in a fragmented approach, with many disciplines operating in their own "silos," each offering advice without knowing what has been said to overwhelmed families [17]. The social worker can play a key role in bridging these gaps. In addition to enhancing communication, the perinatal social worker takes a proactive role as problem solver, as well as provider of insurance information and community resources, and assists with funeral services and discharge planning if appropriate. Families are offered bereavement services and psychosocial support options for the entire family, both during the hospitalization and after. A key component of mentoring parents in the NICU is to recognize, address, and normalize their distress as a common and expected response to their situation. Educating parents about self-care during this difficult journey is important as well and may include not only psychosocial and psychological support but also proper nutrition, exercise, rest, and open communication with their personal support system.

Social workers are particularly well suited to support emotional self-care for staff, as well. The IMPACT team offers critical incident stress debriefings that provide emotional support. At Christiana, these confidential meetings are led by a physician, social worker, or chaplain in a private room. The purpose is to offer a forum for mutual support to staff, and no one is obligated to participate [23]. Caring for children with life-threatening conditions can have a profound effect on health care professionals. Without the ability to manage one's grief response after the death of a patient, health care professionals may experience physical, emotional, cognitive, behavior, and/or spiritual distress, which can affect their professional practice and personal health. If a staff member is not comfortable in a group setting, they can meet individually with any IMPACT team member, chaplain, or trained peer supporters in our Care for the Caregiver Program. (See also below: Caring for the Care Team.)

The Roles of the Nurse

Nurses fulfill multiple roles as part of the perinatal palliative care (PPC) team; however it is unlikely that any one nurse would fulfill all of the roles described below. They work in a variety of overlapping settings and responsibilities and can be the fiber that twines all team members into an even stronger rope. Once a woman or couple has learned the devastating news of a LLFC during an office visit or ultrasound appointment, the office nurse may be the first person they seek out to try to comprehend what they have just been told. Whether an office nurse, nurse practitioner, or clinical nurse specialist, the nurse provides emotional support and clarification of information. She may assist with scheduling a follow-up visit, more in-depth testing, or a specialty consult. The office nurse may be a companion, gatekeeper, and advocate for parents through a maze of decisions over the next few days, weeks, or months, arranging specialized prenatal visits, neonatology consults, detailed ultrasounds, childbirth classes, and family birth planning [10, 24]. The nurse's role as emotional supporter, educator, and grief counselor begins when the bad news is given. Ideally, she remains a consistent person to promote care from office, to hospital, and afterwards to home or in the community [2, 11].

One of the fundamental roles of the nurse is to clarify information for the family. After the parents have been told about a diagnosis, or an unexpected outcome, they often need to have the information repeated or translated into simpler terms. The nurse can then feed information back to the PPC team to better inform them about the parents' comprehension [12, 25]. The nurse can establish a trusting relationship that will continue throughout perinatal care. Following the "bad news visit," the nurse may simply act as medical translator, to enhance the family's ability to make decisions [26, 27]. She offers written information to the family, as well as key websites or books. At each prenatal visit, the nurse maintains trust, provides support, answers questions, assesses grief, maintains hope, and empowers development of a birth plan for labor, birth, welcome, treatments or limitations, the dying process, and memorial items [28, 29]. Ideally the same nurse is present at all care team meetings for consistency in care and information, as these families report higher satisfaction when supported compassionately through this life-altering experience [30]. Whether or not team members change over this period, communication between caregivers is essential. For many families this means assisting them in making meaningful memories, such as taking ultrasound pictures or a video during which only "normal" things are discussed, such as fetal movement or a facial profile. The effectiveness of the nurse in improved patient satisfaction is well-supported in the literature [31, 32].

Parents of a fetus with a LLFC are not likely to feel comfortable participating in traditional childbirth education alongside joyfully expectant couples [10]. These parents still need information about pregnancy milestones, preparing for labor and birth, pain management options, labor support, postpartum/recovery, and parenting, as well as anxiety, stress, grief, postpartum depression, and hope. The nurse can contact a childbirth educator or other nurse willing to meet with the parents one-on-one.

As mentioned, there are times when the nurse as part of the PPC team can help the family create a birth plan. A PPC birth plan needs to be both comprehensive and flexible, because circumstances, diagnosis, and perspectives may change up until the time of delivery. Communication of the birth plan to other providers is essential [7, 29], including admitting, labor and delivery, NICU, postpartum, and consulting providers. Components of a PPC birth plan include "normal" labor concerns, timing of delivery, evaluation of condition and trial of resuscitation, memories hoped for if time permits, and transition to comfort care and saying goodbye [9]. The nurse (or other member of the PPC team) sits with the parents and walks through labor and delivery plans with them, exploring both their dreams and fears.

During the birth planning process, families may wish to discuss organ, tissue, and cord blood or breast milk donation as a means to help others and create a legacy for their infant. This can be thought of by some parents as a way to honor their infant; knowing that their baby made a difference may soften the grief process [33]. The nurse caring for the infant should be knowledgeable and explore the options available with the family, informing them of how much time they are likely to have with the infant and by helping them make choices that are best for them. She can assist them with referrals to the appropriate agencies and arrange meetings with key people, as needed. Accurate instructions about any donations should be spelled out in the birth plan so that the obstetric team caring for the patient has all the information needed to facilitate the family's wishes. Communication and dissemination of the plan is critical.

When the parents arrive in labor and delivery (L&D), the labor nurse will be their companion up through the immediate postpartum/recovery period [34]. With good birth plan dissemination prior to arrival, all labor staff can be aware of the family's special needs or requests and thereby ensure a warm welcome and supportive care. A lactation nurse may also provide assistance. The nurse may also collaborate with the chaplain or family spiritual leader for a formal ceremony of naming and blessing, in accordance with the family's cultural and religious beliefs [2, 9]. L&D, NICU, or PPC nurses can take footprints and pictures, and parents deeply appreciate the opportunity to create the sacred bond of family [9]. An environment of teamwork and collaboration between labor, postpartum, and NICU nurses provides support and encourages the family and friends to work and be together [35].

Case 13.2 Rose

A 21-year-old primigravida patient, Meg, presented to the PPC team during her 36th week of pregnancy. The infant had been diagnosed early with anencephaly, trisomy 13, and associated anomalies. She had been given options for intervention and instead decided to choose comfort care only.

The first meeting was focused on relationship building and assessment of the parents' knowledge, feelings, and expectations. While her fiancé was unable to attend this meeting, he attended a subsequent meeting. The infant was named Rose, after Meg's favorite color. They had explored the internet and were familiar with the baby's anticipated differences. The physician and NICU nurse members of the team met with her to discuss their relationship with the unborn baby, plans and expectations for delivery, and ways to make memories after their daughter's birth. Meg was given numerous books to help prepare for the birth and the grief to follow.

After the initial meeting, a birth plan was sent to all disciplines that might be caring for Meg and the plan was also placed in designated areas where staff knows to find them. An open line of communication with this patient was available to address her concerns as she got closer to her day of delivery.

Meg learned through an online support group that a planned cesarean delivery would afford the best chance of a live birth, giving her the opportunity to meet her daughter alive. After discussion with her obstetrician, a date and time for delivery was set. A nurse from labor and delivery contacted the anesthesia department to discuss pain medication options and to make them aware of the sensitivity of this delivery. They requested that the patient's arms be freed as soon as possible after a cesarean section in order to hold the baby, not knowing how long the baby would survive.

The primary palliative care nurse helped the family locate a Now I Lay Me Down to Sleep photographer who would be present to take photographs. Knowing rose was the mother's favorite color, she gathered rose scrapbooking supplies, rose-colored ink, ribbon, a pink bunny, an ornament, and a silk rose. She found volunteers to make a hat that would tie under her chin.

On the day of delivery, many labor and delivery (L&D) nurses volunteered to care for this family. The L&D admitting nurse welcomed and greeted Meg with compassion, already knowing her story. Many of the L&D staff wore something of rose color to honor baby Rose.

Rose lived less than 2 hours after her birth, but during that time she was surrounded by love and caring by her family and so many others. One L&D nurse made a "Welcome Rose" sign for the infant warmer bed in the operating room and played the happy birthday song on the computer. Her bassinet was decorated in rose-colored blankets and her mother, a hair stylist, was able to carry out an important wish by trimming what little hair that she had on the back of her neck. She and her fiancé bathed and dressed Rose and shared her with other family members. Many photographs were taken and prints and impressions of her hands and feet were made. The PPC nurse was present throughout the morning to guide the family in carrying out their birth plan.

Meg and Rose were then moved to the antenatal floor and remained together for 36 hours. The chaplain and a bereavement/grief counselor from the palliative care team met the family. Questions about cremation, burial, and funeral planning were addressed. On the day of discharge, the family left with a memory box, teddy bear, a pink bunny, many photographs, and encouragement to attend a monthly support group.

Although the grief of losing a child is known only to those who experience it, when families are served with love, compassion, and excellent care, the grief process can be less intense. The PPC team left that day feeling they had provided high-quality palliative care in action-planning, communicating, teamwork, and creating positive memories for not only the family, but for the health care team as well.

The time parents have with their infant may be very brief, less than an hour, or several days, even weeks. Hence flexibility on the part of the nurse is key. The parents may have been told their infant would only survive a few minutes, but then the baby could still be alive after several hours. When this happens, the nurse needs to continue providing companionship for the family, reassuring them, and contacting the pediatric or neonatal team so they can reevaluate the infant and help the parents be comfortable with the situation. Conversely, if the parents plan for a full trial of care and evaluation at birth, and prospects for infant survival are poor, the labor nurse and the NICU nurses together will need to support the parents as they transition from possible curative care to comfort care. Collegial knowledge-sharing across departments is an essential part of optimal family-centered care for these families [36]. Regardless of the details of the plan, it needs to be agreeable to the parents, the obstetric team, and the neonatal team, and flexible enough to accommodate changes in diagnosis and prognosis. Dissemination of the plan is a critical part of the birth plan, between the time and location when the mother presents for delivery can be unpredictable [37].

Changes in neonatal care have resulted in infants surviving longer in the neonatal intensive care unit (NICU) over the last two decades [38]. Parents will often choose a trial of support for their infant born at the threshold of viability. Sometimes the antenatal diagnosis is ambiguous, or the family does not accept the life-limiting diagnosis. In these cases, the infant will be admitted to the NICU for additional diagnostic testing. These families, holding on to hope, may insist on aggressive intensive care for their infant. In these uncertain cases, palliative care and intensive care team need to collaborate proactively [39]. Treatment in the NICU may give families "a gift of time" with their infant [40]. In these circumstances, an experienced NICU nurse is a vital member of the palliative care team. As she establishes a trusting relationship with the family, she will encourage the parents to engage in their infant's care and create precious memories while facilitating bonding and parenting. The NICU nurse can provide added support to the family by listening to their worries and needs, clarifying information, and determining what hopes they might have for their baby. She may also assist the palliative care team in celebrating milestones and holidays with crafts utilizing pictures or footprints.

Communication between the physician provider and the family is of upmost importance but may be brief due to workload restrictions. Families not wanting to take too much of the physician's time will talk to the nurse about their concerns and fears [41]. When parents comprehend the complexities of the diagnosis, their anxiety associated with the unknown may decrease. Taking time to listen to their story is meaningful; there is a direct relationship between how much the family speaks during an encounter and their satisfaction with the meeting [42]. Regardless of the setting, the nurse works to promote parenting opportunities. As parents learn to assist with basic care, such as changing the diaper or providing gentle or calming touch or bathing, the nurse can assist with taking photographs which will aid them later in remembering these special moments. Encouraging them to talk and read to the infant and engage in early skin-to-skin holding will foster the bonding process and memory-making.

Many goals and principles of palliative care, including pain control, are universally applicable in the NICU [39]. Pain and symptom management depends on the nurse's frequent assessment. Clustering care can decrease stress and promote sleep. The nurse can act as the gatekeeper to promote clustered care by other providers. Non-pharmacologic approaches such as swaddling, sucking on a pacifier, or providing drops of breast milk or sucrose might provide comfort, especially during painful procedures. Pain scales are used to assess the degree of pain and the nurse acts as advocate for the infant when the non-pharmacologic approaches are not enough (see also Chaps. 8 and 9). At any point in the family's care, any nurse may reach out to one with specialty PPC training for suggestions, a different perspective or assistance in implementing a novel approach to care.

As the infant's condition worsens or becomes futile, or diagnostic testing validates a life-limiting condition, goals of care will need to be revisited [43]. The nurse may request a family meeting or encourage the parents to initiate the request. This meeting should include the neonatologist, specialists, PPC team members, the parents, and any outside support persons that they desire. If the family chooses a compassionate extubation, plans will be made as to when and what wishes might be carried out before their final goodbye. The nurse can help the family explore whether to bring a special outfit for the baby and invite others to be present. Visiting rules can be flexible under these circumstances. Parents may wish to let their infant taste chocolate or go outside and feel the sunshine or go home to die. "Fulfilling wishes at the close of life is deeply meaningful to families but also profoundly moving and gratifying for staff members." [39] Parents may desire to do skin-to-skin holding before or during a compassionate extubation. Prior to removing the life support, families' need a clear understanding of what will happen when the endotracheal tube is removed, what physical changes they can expect as death approaches, and what will happen after death [41]. During the last moments of the dying process, not only does the nurse monitor the infant's comfort, administer medications, and check heart rate but also continues to support the parents, anticipating and meeting their needs. The nurse also supports grandparents, friends, and in the absence of a child life specialist, the siblings if present. At the end-of-life, she assists in taking final photographs (if desired) making footprints and handprints and molds and collects items for the memory box. She ensures that their cultural and spiritual wishes are carried out. She discusses milk suppression or donation and gives appropriate literature on this topic, as well as possible referrals for ongoing support in the weeks, months, and years to come.

Case 13.3 Asher

Casey, a 41-year-old primigravida woman, and, her soon-to-be husband, Ron, were excited to be pregnant when they were told early in pregnancy that the baby had trisomy 21. Although not what they had planned, they were eager to meet their son Asher and make him part of their family. At 25–4/7 weeks gestation, they were devastated to learn that Casey had contracted intrauterine parvovirus. Within the next month, ultrasounds showed fetal ascites, pleural and pericardial effusion, intrauterine growth restriction, and oligohydramnios. At each visit to MFM, the perinatologist disclosed more and more devastating news, but made no offer of a neonatalology or PPC consult. At 28 weeks gestation, Casey was admitted for hypertension. At this point, neonatology was consulted to explain usual care of an ill, 28-week gestation infant. The parents were not offered the option of comfort care. Two weeks later baby was delivered by C-section for poor Doppler flows and severe maternal hypertension. Asher was gravely ill, and at 6 hours of life, a neonatologist met with the parents to discuss goals of care. Asher's nurse was not part of this discussion, nor was a social worker, other family members, or a chaplain invited. The parents chose to continue aggressive care at that time.

Asher's first day and a half of life was complicated by high frequency ventilation, nitric oxide, umbilical line placement, four chest tubes, a brief need for chest compressions, an abdominal paracentesis, vasopressors, fluid boluses, and frequent blood product transfusions. The next evening, at 36 hours of life, Ron and Casey asked the neonatologist about Asher's chance of survival and were told it was less than 2%. They returned to their son's bedside and shared their concern about his quality of life with his nurse, who had previously received palliative care education. They worried that Asher was suffering. The nurse called the neonatal nurse practitioner who was a member of the novice PPC team, requesting a health care team meeting to include the primary care nurse, neonatologist, and neonatal fellow to discuss goals of care. With the team, the parents decided to redirect the focus to less aggressive and more palliative care, which would allow them to hold their son. The respiratory therapist suggested changing the ventilation mode to conventional and chest tubes were clamped. The charge nurse contacted a Now I Lay Me Down to Sleep photographer to photograph their parenting moments as they bathed, dressed, and held Asher. Family members also visited and took turns holding him. After the extended family left, Casey expressed that she was still not ready to take out his breathing tube. The nurse offered the option of kangaroo care. The chest tubes remained clamped and the morphine and vasopressor drips continued. The parents were given reclining chairs and Asher was placed skin-to-skin on Casey's chest. Lights were dimmed and monitor alarms were turned off. Asher was able to feel his mother's heart beat for approximately 5 hours until his own heart beat for the last time. They were given a "gift of time" as they bonded with him in his last moments. They have since expressed that their grief process was easier knowing that he left this earth in a peaceful manner.

At the time of Asher's birth, the PPC team at this institution was in its early stages. Offering palliative care, or even discussing the option, was not a routine part of interdisciplinary rounds. During team building, many learning opportunities were offered to staff. Asher's nurse's understanding of palliative care was a reflection of this training. Referrals from MFM were sporadic, and many of the neonatologists had not yet embraced the concept or need for a PCC team. Neonatal nurse practitioners, while better versed in PPC, may not have felt recommendations for PPC would be heard. Had there been an interdisciplinary palliative team meeting with Casey and Ron when Casey was first admitted, relationship building between the family and the health care team could have prepared them for what was to come. There would have been discussions about Asher's diagnosis along with their hopes and fears. They would have been encouraged to read, play music, and talk with him and to journal these experiences. They would have received reading material to prepare for worst-case scenarios. A birth plan could have been developed so that their wishes might be carried out at the time of birth. A NICU tour to prepare them for his stay there would have been offered. Frequent discussions after Asher's birth would have helped the parents understand how he was responding to treatment. Although the end of Asher's life was peaceful, a palliative care team could have helped support this family earlier during this difficult time.

At the time of maternal discharge, the L&D nurse remains responsible for standard education, as for any mother who has just delivered a baby, including normal postpartum bleeding, pain management, and reasons to call their provider. In rare cases, infants may survive long enough to go home for the remainder of their life, or parents may strongly desire to have time at home as a family. Either the L&D or the NICU nurse can engage a social worker to coordinate home health care, transport, and hospice care, so the family can continue their journey in the sanctity of their own space.

Regardless of the final setting for an infant's death, one topic that may have been discussed was funeral planning. Some parents, holding on to hope, may resist early discussion of this topic and feel that to pre-plan the funeral would be giving up or admitting that their child will die. After the infant's death, however, the nurse is typically the team member who sits down with the parents to inquire about their thoughts for caring for their infant's body. The options of cremation or burial are discussed, as well as a funeral or memorial service, if desired. If parents hesitate to plan a funeral or burial due to concerns about prohibitive costs, the PPC nurse coordinator can enlist the resources of the social worker and/or the chaplain to aid with burial and memorial service planning [2, 44]. She can help by providing information on the variety of options available and on organizations that offer funds to assist families who find this expense to be a burden.

And finally, one facet of the nurse's role in high-quality PPC that might not be immediately evident is palliative care research. Nurses, as frontline clinicians, are in a key position to ask questions about practice and have long been actively involved in research. They can ask questions, design protocols, and gather data to validate and improve perinatal end-of-life care [45]. Much of PPC planning revolves around the uncertainty of the diagnosis and outcomes; participating in ongoing research may result in evidence to help the PPC team support families through this experience. The clinical research nurse, nurse educator, care coordinator, or nurse clinician all can be driven by a wish to make a difference and enhance family outcomes through evidence-based practice. A nurse contributes to the health care team as a key stakeholder in compassionate family-centered care [46] and is a natural team member to track research data and assist with quality improvement activities.

Caring for the Care Team

Health care providers who care for families as they lose an infant are at risk for stress and compassion fatigue and can face ethical dilemmas [47, 48]. The PPC members who care for these families experience grief, need to process the loss, recover from and integrate the experience, and maintain their mental and emotional integrity. This is best accomplished through preparation and education, peer support and compassion, and self-care [49, 50]. Many health care workers do not receive sufficient (or any) end-of life education [48]. Integral care for the caregivers means ensuring ongoing education, use of debriefing, enlisting the chaplain, or reminding colleagues to take personal time to find how they can best honor the memory of an infant's death and remain emotionally and spiritually whole [51]. (See also Chap. 15.)

Conclusion

A team approach is of paramount importance in all kinds of palliative care, and PPC is no exception. While all of the domains of PPC that we have discussed—family assessment, pain management, psychological support, spirituallty, bereavement services, culturally concordant end-of-life care, and ethical discussion—can be carried out by more than one or overlapping disciplines, the infant and family derive optimal support and compassionate relationship-based care from the diverse perspectives and skills that a well-oiled team brings together through shared responsibility.

New and growing interdisciplinary PPC programs are gradually developing high-quality standards of care, enhanced by functional structures and processes, ongoing team education and communication, and effective support of team resilience. They have developed a culture of care that enables them to embrace an infant's family to develop respectful, holistic, and flexible goals of care. Ultimately, the goal of PPC programs is to affirm the life and value of the infant who will be loved and cherished as a part of a family, regardless of birth outcome or length of life, and provide families with the best care so they can grieve moving forward.

References

1. Osterman MJK, Kochanek KD, MacDorman MF, et al. Annual summary of vital statistics: 2012–2013. Pediatrics. 2015;135:1115–25.
2. Leuthner S, Jones E. Fetal concerns program: a model for perinatal palliative care. MCN Am J Matern Child Nurs. 2007;32:272–8.
3. Wool C, Côté-Arsenault D, Black B, Denney-Koelsch E, Kim S, Kavanaugh K. Provision of services in perinatal palliative care: a multicenter survey in the United States. J Palliat Med. 2016;19(3):279–85. https://doi.org/10.1089/jpm.2015.0266.
4. Denney-Koelsch E, Black B, Côté-Arsenault D, Wool C, Kim S, Kavanaugh K. A survey of perinatal palliative programs in the United States: structure, processes, and outcomes. J Palliat Med. 2016;19(10):1080–6.
5. National Consensus Project (NCP) for quality palliative care. https://www.nationalcoalitionhpc.org/ncp/. Accessed 1 June 2019.
6. Perinatal Hospice & Palliative Care. https://www.perinatalhospice.org/. Accessed 1 June 2019.
7. Stenekes S, Ens C, Harlos M, Chochinov H, Mytopher K. A descriptive study evaluating perinatal healthcare providers' perspectives of palliative programming in 3 Canadian institutions. J Perinat Neonat Nursing. 2014;28:280–9.
8. Kobler K, Limbo R. Making a case: creating a perinatal palliative care service using a perinatal bereavement program model. J Perinat Neonat Nursing. 2011;25(1):32–41. https://doi.org/10.1097/JPN.0b013e3181fb592e.
9. Wool C. Clinician confidence and comfort in providing perinatal palliative care. J Obstetr Gynecolog Neonat Nursing. 2013;42(1):48–58. https://doi.org/10.1111/j.1552-6909.2012.01432.x.
10. Wool C. Clinician perspectives of barriers in perinatal palliative care. MCN Am J Matern Child Nurs. 2015;40(1):44–50. https://doi.org/10.1097/NMC.0000000000000093.
11. Platt M. Continuous care across teams: principle of nursing practice G. Nurs Stand. 2011;25(34):31–3.
12. Montgomery KE, Sawin KJ. Communication during palliative care and end of life: perceptions of experienced pediatric oncology nurses. Cancer Nurs. 2017;40(2):E47–57. https://doi.org/10.1097/NCC.0000000000000363.
13. Dean B, McDonald K. Nursing perspectives: building an interprofessional perinatal palliative care. NeoReviews. 2014;15(10) https://doi.org/10.1542/neo.15-10-e422.
14. Wax J, Minkoff H, Johnson A, Coleman B, Levine D, Helfgott A, O'Keeffe D, et al. Consensus report on the detailed fetal anatomic ultrasound examination. J Ultrasound Med. 2014;33:189–95.
15. The American College of Obstetricians & Gynecologists. Committee Opinion 501. Maternal-Fetal Intervention and Fetal Care Centers. ACOG; 2011 (reaffirmed 2017).
16. Denney-Koelsch E, Côté-Arsenault D, Lemcke-Berno E. Parents experiences with ultrasound during pregnancy with a lethal fetal diagnosis. Global Qual Nurs Res. 2015;2:1–8.
17. Carter BS. More than medication: perinatal palliative care. Acta Paediatr. 2016;105:1255–6.

18. Quinn M, Gephart S. Evidence for implementation strategies to provide perinatal palliative care in the neonatal intensive care unit. Adv Neo Care. 2016;16:430–9.
19. Carter BS. Advance care planning: outpatient antenatal palliative care consultation. Arch Dis Child Fetal Neonatal Ed. 2017;102:F3–4.
20. Society for Maternal-Fetal Medicine. https://www.smfm.org/members/what-is-a-mfm.
21. Cross JaNeen. Perinatal social work practice in health care settings. Practice perspectives. National Association of Social Workers. Spring Issue; 2017.
22. Hall SL, Phillips R, Hynan MT. Transforming NICU care to provide comprehensive family support. Newborn Infant Nursing Rev. 2016;16(2):69–73.
23. Keene EA, Hutton N, Hall B, Rushton C. Bereavement debriefing sessions: an intervention to support health care professional in managing their grief after the death of a patient. Pediatr Nurs. 2010;36(4):185–9. quiz 190
24. Tosello B, Dany L, Bétrémieux P, Le Coz P, Auquier P, Gire C, Einaudi MA. Barriers in referring neonatal patients to perinatal palliative care: a French multicenter study. PLoS One. 2015;10(5):e0126861. https://doi.org/10.1371/journal.pone.0126861.
25. Gordon S, Aydam J, Hamm K, Rocha M, Northcut A, Roberson B, Shook M. Improving communication and coordination of complex perinatal patients. MCN Am J Matern Child Nurs. 2015;40(3):167–73. https://doi.org/10.1097/NMC.0000000000000128.
26. Peiritsch H. Bundle payment program initiative: roles of a nurse navigator and home health professionals. Home Healthcare Now. 2017;35(6):335–8.
27. Cole J, Moldenhauer J, Jones T, Shaughnessy H, Zarrin H, Coursey A, Munson D. A proposed model for perinatal care. J Obstet Gynecol Neonatal Nurs. 2017;46(6):904–11. https://doi.org/10.1016/j.jogn.2017.01.014.
28. English NK, Hessler KL. Prenatal birth planning for families of the imperiled newborn. J Obstet Gynecol Neonatal Nurs. 2013;42(3):390–9. https://doi.org/10.1111/1552-6909.12031.
29. Sumner L, Kavanaugh K, Moro T. Extending palliative care into pregnancy and the immediate newborn period: state of the practice of perinatal palliative care. J Perinat Neonatal Nurs. 2006;20(1):113–6.
30. Wool C, Repke JT, Woods AB. Parent reported outcomes of quality care and satisfaction in the context of a life-limiting fetal diagnosis. J Matern Fetal Neonatal Med. 2017;30(8):894–9. https://doi.org/10.1080/14767058.2016.1195362.
31. Munson D, Leuthner SR. Palliative care for the family carrying a fetus with a life-limiting diagnosis. Pediatr Clin N Am. 2007;54(5):787–98, xii
32. Tho PC, Ang E. The effectiveness of patient navigation programs for adult cancer patients undergoing treatment: a systematic review [review]. JBI Database System Rev Implement Rep. 2016;14(2):295–321. https://doi.org/10.11124/jbisrir-2016-2324.
33. Akard TF, Duffy M, Hord A, Randall A, Sanders A, Adelstein K, et al. Bereaved mothers' and fathers' perceptions of a legacy intervention for parents of infants in the NICU. J Perinat Neonatal Nursing. 2018;11(1):21–8. https://doi.org/10.3233/NPM-181732.
34. Price S, Noseworthy J, Thornton J. Women's experience with social presence during childbirth. MCN Am J Matern Child Nurs. 2007;32(3):184–91. https://doi.org/10.1097/01.NMC.0000269569.94561.7c.
35. Gold KJ, Dalton VK, Schwenk TL. Hospital care for parents after perinatal death. Obstet Gynecol. 2007;109(5):1156–66.
36. Williams C. Can you help me? Knowledge sharing within the nursing profession. Nursing Women's Health. 2013;17(2):139–42. https://doi.org/10.1111/1751-486X.12022.
37. Breeze AC, Lees C, Kumar C, Missfelder-Lobos H. Palliative care for prenatally diagnosed lethal fetal abnormality. Arch Dis Childhood Fetal Neonat Edition. 2007;92(1):F56–8.
38. Marc-Aurele KL, English NK. Primary palliative care in neonatal intensive care. Sem Perinatol. 2017;41(2):95–100.
39. Carter BS, Brown JB, Brown S, Meyer EC. Four wishes for Aubrey. J Perinatol. 2012;32(1):10–4. https://doi.org/10.1038/jp.2011.171.

40. Kidszun A, Linebarger J, Walter JK, et al. What if the prenatal diagnosis of a lethal anomaly turns out to be wrong? Pediatrics. 2016;137(5):e20154514. https://doi.org/10.1542/peds.2015-4514.
41. Kenner C. The role of neonatal nurses in palliative care. Newborn Infant Nursing Rev. 2016;16:74–7.
42. Williams C, Munson D, Zupancic J, Kirpalani H. Supporting bereaved parents: practical steps in providing compassionate perinatal and neonatal end-of-life care- a North America perspective. Sem Fetal Neonatal Med. 2008;13:335–40.
43. Samsel C, Lechner BE. End-of-life care in a regional level IV neonatal intensive care unit after implementation of a palliative care initiative. J Perinatol. 2015;35:223–8.
44. Ilse S. Empty arms, coping with miscarriage, stillbirth and infant death. 43rd printing. Maple Plain: Wintergreen Press; 2016.
45. Bakitas MA. On the road less traveled: journey of an oncology palliative care researcher. Oncol Nursing Forum. 2017;44(1):87–95.
46. Gray TF. How Can I Change My patients' treatment decision making by becoming a nurse scientist? Clin J Oncol N ursing. 2017;21(2):263.
47. Zhang W, Lane BS. Promoting neonatal staff nurses' comfort and involvement in end of life and bereavement care, Nurs Res Pract. 2013:365329. , 5 pages. https://doi.org/10.1155/2013/365329.
48. Robertson MJ, Aldridge A, Curley AE. Provision of bereavement care in neonatal units in the United Kingdom. Pediatr Crit Care Med. 2011;12:e111–5.
49. Petrella K, Tepner L, Chichester M. When a friend's baby dies: empowering nurses to balance professional and personal care. J Obstet Gynecol Neonatal Nurs. 2013;42(1):S108. https://doi.org/10.1111/1552-6909.12212.
50. Jonas-Simpson C, Pilkington FB, Macdonald C, Mcmahon E. Nurses' experiences of grieving when there is a perinatal death. Sage Open; 2013. Retrieved August 30, 2015 from http://sgo.sagepub.com/content/3/2/2158244013486116.
51. Riotte C, Kukora S, Keefer P, Firn J. Identifying the types of support needed by interprofessional teams providing pediatric end-of-life care: a thematic analysis. J Palliat Med. 2018;21(4):422–7. https://doi.org/10.1089/jpm.2017.0331.

Community-Based Perinatal Palliative Care

14

Alyssa W. Gupton, Lauren M. Zwetsch, and David N. Korones

What Is Community-Based Perinatal Palliative Care?

There is no single standard definition of community-based perinatal palliative care (PPC). Kaye et al. write that community-based *pediatric* palliative care is:

> …pediatric palliative care that is provided outside of the hospital setting with the goal of offering pediatric palliative care resources and services in private residences, community-based clinics or settings, long-term care facilities, and local respite or hospice facilities. Community-based pediatric palliative care may be managed through formal pediatric palliative care programs, home health or hospice agencies, or other community-based clinicians, with support provided in person, by telephone or by electronic correspondence; when linked with hospital-based PPC services, Community-Based Pediatric Palliative Care programs provide continuity of care for patients who journey between inpatient and outpatient settings, optimizing quality of life across the care continuum [1].

Community-based *perinatal* palliative care is an extension of this definition to include women with fetuses with life-limiting diagnoses and their families. Those unborn infants may have a variety of chromosomal abnormalities or congenital defects that are likely to result in a complex chronic condition from which the child may or may not recover. Community-based PPC, like pediatric palliative care, allows PPC teams to "meet these families where they are at" both literally and figuratively, whether that might be in their homes, at high-risk obstetric visits, on bed rest in the hospital, or after the infant is born, in the NICU, at a cardiac PICU, at a subspecialist clinic visit, or in the home. Like any aspect of palliative care, PPC is

A. W. Gupton (✉) · L. M. Zwetsch
Lifetime Care Home Health Care and Hospice, CompassionNet, Rochester, NY, USA
e-mail: alyssa.gupton@rochesterregional.org

D. N. Korones
Lifetime Care Home Health Care and Hospice, CompassionNet, Rochester, NY, USA

Department of Pediatrics, University of Rochester Medical Center, Rochester, NY, USA

E. M. Denney-Koelsch, D. Côté-Arsenault (eds.), *Perinatal Palliative Care*,
https://doi.org/10.1007/978-3-030-34751-2_14

interdisciplinary, bringing to the fore not just the palliative care pediatrician, nurse, and nurse practitioner, but a skilled pediatric social worker, child-life specialist, chaplain, and more. Also like any community-based palliative care program, perinatal programs come in different shapes and sizes – affiliates of hospitals or part of larger community-based palliative care programs [2].

Essential Elements of Community-Based Perinatal Palliative Care

The key elements of a community-based PPC program do not differ in substance from those of any community-based palliative care effort, but there are a few important distinctions. Key elements include developing a relationship with a maternal fetal medicine program, a neonatology group and the local hospital that houses them, integrating the perinatal program into a pediatric palliative care program, and assuring that there is broad interdisciplinary representation within the perinatal program.

Developing a Working Relationship with Maternal-Fetal-Medicine and Neonatology Groups

Perhaps the most daunting aspect of developing such a program is the need for a strong working relationship with the local hospital that is home to a maternal-fetal medicine (MFM, sometimes called perinatology) program and a neonatal intensive care unit (NICU). The approach to care by palliative care specialists (less medicine-focused, spending a lot of time at the bedside with parents, grandparents, siblings) is very different from the high-intensity, brisk-paced world of the perinatologist and neonatologist, and the things that attracted clinicians to one versus the other may be very different. But common bonds exist: the desire to provide the best possible care for a family and child, the desire to communicate clearly with a family, and the importance of including them in medical decision-making. Through these common bonds, the creation of effective working relationships is critically important. This can be fostered through a willingness of palliative care teams to attend hospital-based medical meetings, meet busy clinicians at the hospital, open invitations to hospital-based teams to attend meetings in the community, and respect for the relationship between the obstetrician or neonatologist and patient. The palliative care team's intent is not to take over all conversations regarding goals of care but to collaborate with the hospital-based team and to advocate for families and help them process information and treatment options to make decisions consistent with their values. A hospital-based champion in the obstetrics and/or neonatology world can be quite effective in opening doors. Just as it is crucial to forge relationships with the perinatologists and neonatologists, so too, it is important to coordinate care with hospital-based pediatric palliative care teams so that palliative care services are reiterated and reinforced; thus parents are not confused by conflicting communication.

Perinatal Palliative Care as a Part of a Pediatric Palliative Care Program

While there may be some larger centers that have independent and free-standing community-based PPC programs, most community programs would be more likely to embed PPC as part of their pediatric palliative care services. The volume of children with complex chronic conditions requiring community-based PPC services is not large, so it is a very practical consideration to extend the perinatal palliative care into an existing interdisciplinary pediatric palliative care team. While the latter requires additional experience and training, it is not so different as to require creation of an entirely new team. For example, the authors' community-based pediatric team had years of hands-on clinical experience in community-based palliative and end-of-life care before initiating the perinatal program. When the idea of expansion of the team to include PPC was born, several team members championed the effort, underwent training, developed the program, and then trained other team members.

Interdisciplinary Perinatal Palliative Care

Finally, one additional key element is the need for the team to be interdisciplinary, as is the case for any palliative care team. How interdisciplinary a perinatal team is depends, in part, on the resources available to support team members and the availability of highly specialized pediatric palliative care experts in smaller communities. The ideal team should include the following, all with specialty training in pediatric and perinatal palliative care: a pediatrician, a pediatric nurse practitioner (and/or RN), a pediatric social worker, a pediatric chaplain, and a child life specialist (Fig. 14.1). The latter is particularly important because a major stressor for many families is what and how to tell their young children about their soon-to-be born ill sibling. Child life specialists work with these children, and through therapeutic medical play and diagnostic teaching, learn what they are thinking and help them absorb the impending change in their lives. This is particularly well-suited to a home-based program since interaction with these siblings in their own home is more practical and a safe place for them.

Unique Benefits of Community-Based Perinatal Palliative Care Teams

There is no question that a hospital-based PPC team is an essential component of good perinatal care. Such teams "live" under the same roof as perinatologists and neonatologists and therefore can develop good working relationships. In addition, the hospital-based palliative care team is well-poised to respond to unexpected events, such as an expectant mother hospitalized or the birth of a baby in distress or a baby's turn for the worse. But a community-based team is well-poised to offer continuity, providing family-centered care in a safe place (home) to support parents, siblings, and extended family, effectively complementing the work of a hospital-based team.

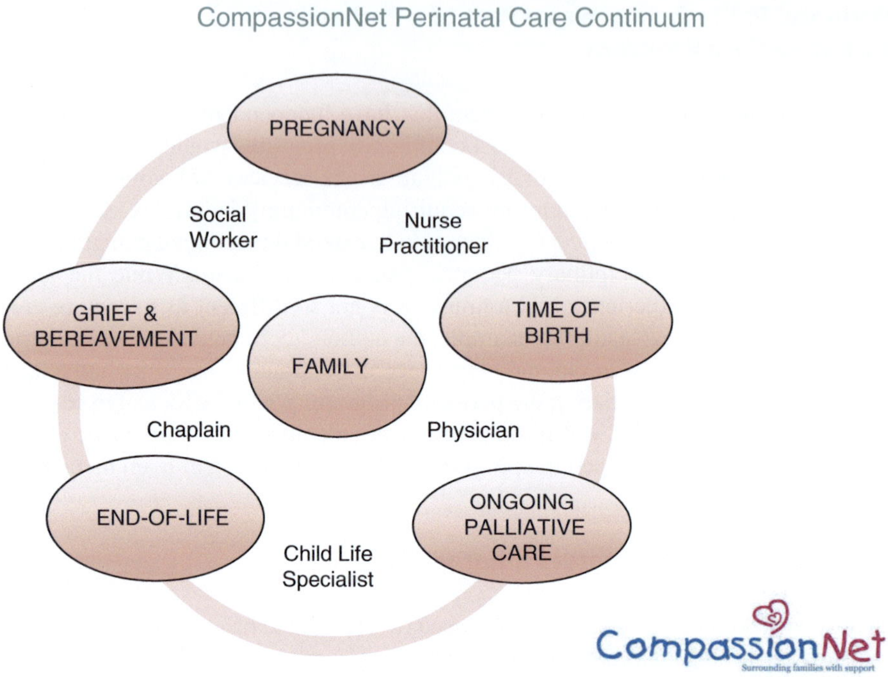

Fig. 14.1 Key members, role and the care continuum of an interdisciplinary community-based perinatal palliative care program. *Nurse practitioner/RN* – provides support and guidance regarding medical diagnoses, birth planning, goals of care, end-of-life care, and bereavement. *Social worker* – provides emotional support and guidance to the family regarding anticipatory grief, goals of care, and bereavement (support extending for up to 3 years after the death) and provides referrals for community psychosocial, logistical, and financial support throughout care continuum. *Child life specialist* – provides support and guidance to parents regarding developmentally appropriate communication with children and works directly with siblings throughout care continuum providing developmentally appropriate interventions (medical and therapeutic play, diagnostic teaching, memory-making, bereavement) to promote effective coping and understanding. *Chaplain* – provides spiritual support for immediate and extended family, including siblings, across the care continuum. *Physician* – provides consultation to family and team, reviews goals of care, addresses complex symptom management, facilitates perinatal MOLST, and supports family as liaison to hospital-based subspecialty teams

Continuity

A community-based PPC team is accustomed to travelling. It is a palliative care "team on wheels." Two or three team members (or more, depending on the need) coordinate to go to a family's home and help the family process difficult news they have heard about their unborn baby. Sometimes a home visit following a medical visit can be extremely helpful. It gives the family time to digest what they have heard and the team can help them formulate questions to ask at the next visit. The team will follow up with regular home visits, the frequency dependent on the severity of the problem and the needs of the parents. A perinatal team can also meet a family at an obstetric visit and, if the obstetrician is in agreement, even accompany and support the family at selected visits. Such a team can visit the mother if she is hospitalized for complications of pregnancy or for delivery. In short, a community-based team is mobile and has the flexibility to literally "meet a family where they are at" (i.e., meet with the family in their preferred location; home, clinic, hospital, or even local coffee shop) at the time that best meets their needs. Over the course of several months, a close working relationship is often developed and families quickly learn that their community-based team is an important source of support. While hospital-based teams can also provide some continuity, they often do not have the breadth of staff or the flexibility of scheduling to meet families at obstetric visits, especially if those visits occur outside the hospital.

Siblings

One of the biggest stressors for parents whose unborn child has a significant medical problem is their concern for that child's older siblings and the potential impact on their emotional well-being. Should they be informed about what is happening? If so, how much information should they receive? And from whom? Oftentimes the siblings are overlooked because the focus is understandably on the ill child or fetus. However, the needs of siblings at this difficult time are significant. Having a sick or terminally ill baby sibling, coupled with an absent mother or father who spends much of his/her time at the hospital, is profound and can have a lifelong impact [3].

Expectant parents often need guidance on what to tell their children and when. There is general consensus that siblings, even young siblings, cope better in the short and long term when they are more fully informed about what is happening with their ill baby sibling [3–5]. It is a challenge guiding parents to understand and accept this because it is our instinct as parents to protect our children from bad things. It requires time and patience on the part of the PPC team to explain to parents that, despite their well-intended efforts to protect their children from the sad reality of their very ill sibling, this approach will likely not serve the children well over time. In fact, there is potential for more harm by withholding information than by sharing it [6]. Palliative care teams, home- or hospital-based, should be a resource to guide families in this regard. However, it is more of a challenge for a hospital-based team, particularly working directly with the older siblings, since prenatal visits do not typically include siblings and even if so, the physical space and logistics of spending time with a young child at a doctor's office is a challenge.

Community-based PPC teams are uniquely suited to attend to the needs of siblings. Since these teams visit families in the home, siblings are far more likely to be present and to feel safe in their home environment. In addition, with frequent home visits, these teams can develop a relationship with the child, just as they do with the parents. They can learn from the parents, and often directly from the siblings, the types of questions the siblings have, what their personalities are like, and how to best explore their feelings about their soon-to-be-born sibling. It is an important opportunity to acknowledge parents as "the experts" on their child and an opportunity to impress upon them the importance of informing the children in some way that their unborn sibling is going to be sick and life is going to be different.

The Child Life Specialist

While most members of a palliative care team have the expertise to guide parents on the importance of including siblings and how to talk to them, it is the certified child life specialist (CCLS) who has the unique skillset to work directly with children of all ages, explore what they know, and explore their hopes and fears. CCLSs are specially trained health-care professionals who focus on developmental, emotional, and psychosocial needs of children and adolescents facing the life-altering impact of illness, injury, and/or death. Through developmentally appropriate interventions, CCLSs collaborate within the interdisciplinary team to promote effective coping through play, preparation, education, and self-expression activities in the hospital, home, and other community settings. Becoming a child life specialist requires rigorous training, hands-on experience through internships, and passing a certification exam. CCLSs are a vital part of the health-care team in virtually all children's hospitals. Their expertise extends beyond the child-patient; they can advise parents as well, and also explore the needs, hopes, and fears of siblings of ill children. For younger children in particular, as many expectant mothers and their families have concerns, the CCLS can be particularly effective. Through therapeutic and medical play, they can learn what young children are thinking, and based on their "play" sessions, they can offer parents and health-care teams their advice on how to support the sibling whose expectant or new baby brother or sister is seriously ill. For those infants who are discharged from the hospital and die at home, the CCLS often takes the lead in memory-making, saving locks of hair, making hand prints or footprints, making sure photos are taken, and including the siblings in all these rituals.

The CCLS can be a safe person for the child to talk with about his/her worries or ask questions they might be too afraid or worried to ask their parents. She/he can offer guidance to parents about a child's developmental understanding and help parents to find the words to share or explain difficult news. As children get to know and form a therapeutic connection with the CCLS, he/she becomes an important source of support for children during the pregnancy, the subsequent hospitalization of the mother and baby, and for those infants who do not survive, at the time of death and into bereavement. Such support, while focused on the siblings, is a huge support for distressed parents as well.

Not all community-based PPC teams may have the resources to support a child life specialist as a part of their perinatal program. Therefore other members of the team may need to consider the needs of the siblings, identifying appropriate and available resources to best address their needs.

A Safe Place

The opportunity to meet with a family in distress in their own home is a privilege. The willingness of a team to travel and meet the family at their home is tacit acknowledgement of their distress and the importance of meeting them on their own turf. That said, there are challenges unique to the home setting such as creating an intimate space when in a big living room with all the seats and couches far apart from each other and being able to focus on hard discussions amidst noisy and busy households with young siblings clamoring for attention, babies crying, and doorbells and phones ringing, for example. But home is home, a place without the constraints of a timed appointment, a place where a family can feel more relaxed and free to talk about what they have been told and how scared they are about what lies ahead.

Different Approaches of Perinatal Palliative Care Programs

There is hardly a one-size-fits-all approach for PPC programs. They are put together on the basis of resources and expertise available, volume of families served, who might be a local champion and where that champion works, and local services already available within the community. It is difficult to get a firm sense of all the community-based PPC in the USA, where they are housed, and what is the makeup of their teams. In a recently published study of PPC programs, of 75 programs surveyed, programs were housed in "academic centers, regional or community hospitals, local hospice or palliative care organizations or community-based support systems" [7]. While most of the programs offered services in the hospital (87%), 49% also offered services in the home, suggesting that community-based services are available to many families, regardless of where the program is actually based. In this same study, makeup of PPC teams was also reviewed; the vast majority of programs included a chaplain, physician, nurse, and social worker, and most had a care coordinator. At least some programs also included a geneticist, ethicist, or child life specialist. It is not known whether community-based teams differed from hospital-based teams in terms of team makeup.

Barriers to Developing and Sustaining a Community-Based Perinatal Palliative Care Program

The barriers to developing a community-based program are considerable and similar to the barriers to developing and sustaining any pediatric palliative care program. These barriers include financial resources to develop and sustain a program, the challenges of a community-based group working with a tertiary care center, and inherent biases and misunderstanding on the part of the medical community about what a palliative care team does.

Financial Barriers

PPC programs around the USA are interdisciplinary and include variable combinations of physicians, care-coordinator (often a nurse or social worker), nurse and/or nurse practitioner, social worker, child life specialist, chaplain, geneticist, ethicist, and bereavement specialist. Clearly the cost of maintaining an interdisciplinary staff is considerable, especially for medium-sized communities or smaller towns in rural areas. In many places, the volume of affected families is not high enough to sustain a large interdisciplinary staff like this, particularly when services of many staff (important though those services are) are not reimbursable by third-party payers. In the previously noted survey of 75 PPC programs in the USA, reimbursement sources included insurance companies, local hospice organizations, and philanthropic support; the source of financial support varied depending upon where the program was housed (e.g., an academic center vs in the community) [2]. Program cost-savings may be realized by incorporating PPC programs into pediatric programs and training a subgroup of practitioners with particular skills in the perinatal aspects of palliative care. Exploring potential opportunities to partner with local insurance companies or alternate funding sources, such as is the case with CompassionNet's model, may be helpful and provide viable options. The development and details of CompassionNet's model of care will be fully described and illustrated later in this chapter.

Community-Based PPC and Tertiary Care Centers: Two Different Worlds

Collaboration of hospital-based palliative care teams with medical subspecialty teams is challenging enough, but the challenge is even greater when the palliative care team does not even work within the hospital and/or may be part of a different health-care system. Perinatologists, neonatologists, and even hospital-based pediatric palliative care teams work in a very different environment than the community-based team, and respect for their perspective is paramount for forging a good working relationship. Once a working relationship is established, there needs to be mutually agreed upon triggers for palliative care referrals. Some programs may choose to focus on supporting families with fetuses with lethal or very poor prognoses (e.g., anencephaly, Potter syndrome, or Trisomy 13 or 18), while others might want to "cast the net wider" offering support to families whose infants face more chronic conditions with less certain prognoses but are still potentially life-threatening (such as hypoplastic left heart or other complex congenital anomalies). In either case a next step is a systematic trigger to remind busy hospital-based practitioners when a palliative care referral is warranted for a woman with a high-risk pregnancy. This can be done through automatic triggers in an electronic medical record or a nurse or care manager who works with a perinatology group.

"De-Stigmatizing" Palliative Care

Although palliative care is far more mainstream than it was only a decade ago, it still carries a stigma within the medical and lay communities. This barrier is not unique to PPC, although obstetricians, who deal largely with a young and healthy patient population, may be less likely to encounter palliative care scenarios with their patients. It is incumbent upon the team to teach the obstetric team what PPC is, reminding them that its scope is far broader than hospice or end-of-life care. It can be helpful to suggest ways they might bring up the possibility of a palliative care referral to their patients. If they are not armed with the right words or do not understand what palliative care is, they are likely to be less comfortable bringing it up to their families. Phrases that resonate with families include "an extra layer of support" or "helping to make sure your voices are heard" and "making sure everyone is on the same page regarding the care of your baby."

CompassionNet: A Community-Based Perinatal Palliative Care Model

We share our own experience with our community-based PPC program as an example of what such a program can look like. We recognize that programs may differ widely based on the needs of a community and the expertise available in the community. Our program, CompassionNet, is a community-based pediatric and PPC program that provides support to families across Upstate New York caring for a child with a potentially life-threatening illness and families anticipating the birth of a child with a serious medical condition. CompassionNet was born in 2001 through a partnership between Lifetime Care Home Health Care and Hospice, Inc., and Excellus BlueCross BlueShield, Inc., with a shared goal of improving care for children with potentially life-limiting disease and their families. CompassionNet strives to meet families where they are, both literally and figuratively. Care is provided primarily within the family's home, but can also happen in the hospital or a doctor's office.

CompassionNet's team includes social workers, nurse practitioners, child life specialists, physicians, registered nurses, a chaplain, and volunteers. Every CompassionNet family has a supportive care social worker or specialist who provides emotional support and practical case management support, helping connect families with financial, therapeutic, and community resources. The CompassionNet medical team specializes in palliative care coordination and consultation as well as pain and symptom management. Child life specialists help the children and their siblings understand and cope with their diagnosis, treatment, and emotions. Some children are discharged from CompassionNet when their condition improves, while others remain on the program as they continue to receive treatment. If a child's condition worsens, the team provides compassionate end-of-life and bereavement care to the family.

CompassionNet began as a pediatric palliative care program, serving families caring for a child from birth through 21 years of age, and did not initially include a perinatal component. But as the CompassionNet team cared for an ever-increasing number of families with newborn infants who faced serious illnesses and bore witness to how so many of these families were ill-prepared for what lay ahead, it seemed only natural to extend this same model of care to families who learned during their pregnancy of their baby's serious medical condition.

How CompassionNet's Perinatal Program Started

We quickly learned that family stress and suffering begins at the time of diagnosis of a serious, potentially life-limiting condition, even when that diagnosis is made prenatally. The CompassionNet perinatal program was designed to provide support beginning with the diagnosis. While in some ways it is an extension of CompassionNet's pediatric palliative care program, in many ways, it is very different.

We began the development of our community-based PPC by researching and contacting PPC programs around the country to learn what was being done elsewhere. We also knew that we needed to forge a bond with the local tertiary care center, where so many ill infants were born. CompassionNet was already a well-established, multidisciplinary, community-based pediatric palliative care program but we seldom, if ever, crossed paths with the high-risk obstetrics group. Our team was fortunate to already have close ties with our pediatric palliative care colleagues at the University of Rochester Medical Center, the major academic center in our community. Through those ties, CompassionNet was invited to participate in the planning and development of a multidisciplinary perinatal clinic, soon thereafter named the Perinatal Supportive Care Clinic (PSCC). The clinic was comprised of representatives from high-risk obstetrics, neonatology and associated support staff, and the hospital-based pediatric palliative care team. The offer was extended to our own staff to attend, and as a consequence, relationships with the hospital-based subspecialist teams were established. Assisting in developing and then attending the PSCC gave us the opportunity to learn more about the unique medical and psychosocial concerns of mothers and families, as well the unique medical challenges faced by the obstetric and neonatology staff. It also gave us the opportunity to teach the staff and families about our program and ultimately led to more referrals to our program. This direct and personal relationship with the perinatology staff resulted in mutual trust and respect for our complementary roles in caring for families in distress.

Eligibility Criteria

As the perinatal program grew, we recognized the need to further develop and define our eligibility criteria. A baby with a fetal condition very likely to be lethal (like Trisomy 18, anencephaly) would be an obvious candidate, but we were undecided with less certain prognoses such as hypoplastic left heart, holoprosencaphaly, or gastroschisis. Should we restrict our support to families with infants with diagnoses very likely to be lethal? Or should we "cast the net wider" and include babies whose conditions place them at significant risk to die, yet may not be definitely lethal, consistent with our approach to medical eligibility for our pediatric palliative care population? We opted for the broader approach but recognize that this might vary from one program to the next. For example, a program that is just starting and might not have broad interdisciplinary support might want to focus the program on infants with diagnoses most likely to be lethal; the numbers of patients are fewer and the staff can focus their energies on the most needy parents and sickest of infants. Regarding timing of eligibility, we decided to enroll families at any point during the pregnancy when they learned of a potential life-threatening diagnosis. The rationale for this approach is that grief and a sense of loss begin at the time of diagnosis and that is a starting point from when the support is needed.

Education

Once the population was identified and the eligibility criteria established, staff training began. Initially, CompassionNet sent a social work case manager, an RN, and pediatric nurse practitioner to a two-day intensive educational conference, Resolve Through Sharing (RTS) [8]. RTS, a premier perinatal bereavement educational organization, offers conferences to train professionals caring for those anticipating perinatal or neonatal loss. This training was very beneficial to our perinatal program in its infancy. We learned that even though we were very experienced in pediatric palliative care, we had much to learn about perinatal palliative care and loss. We also learned that there are few, if any, programs like CompassionNet that offer community-based PPC. Those who attended the initial training went on to develop an education day for other team members who would be working with our perinatal patients. Eventually, several other interdisciplinary team members attended the RTS training, and ultimately, an RN and PNP attended an RTS Train the Trainer conference to continue to share the expertise with newer staff.

How the CompassionNet Program Works: Phases of Involvement

Prenatal Involvement: Referrals and Initial Visits

Families are most often referred to CompassionNet's perinatal palliative care program by the high-risk maternal-fetal medicine group (often through their genetics counselors) or in cases of congenital cardiac anomalies diagnosed in utero, by the pediatric cardiology group. (See Appendix A for referral form.) Upon referral and eligibility determination, each family is assigned a supportive care social worker and pediatric nurse practitioner, who promptly reach out to the family by phone to introduce the program and coordinate an initial visit. Visits are most frequently conducted in the family's home, though sometimes the team will meet with a family at an office or other location based on wishes and needs of family. Sometimes additional interdisciplinary team members (chaplain, child life specialist, or physician) will join in the initial visit, but the team strives to be mindful that meeting so many people at once can be overwhelming to a family, especially in the intimacy of the home environment coupled with the emotional impact of their baby's diagnosis. Thus visits typically include only two or three team members. Establishing and maintaining a trusting relationship is at the core of all care provided and is thus the primary focus of the initial visit and early subsequent visits. The amount and frequency of prenatal visits vary with the family and is dependent on a number of factors, most significantly how far along in the pregnancy the mother is, the gravity of the diagnosis, and the particular needs of the family.

Case 14.1 Part 1

Dorothy was referred to CompassionNet when she was 26 weeks pregnant, shortly after a fetal ultrasound revealed that her son Adam had hypoplastic left heart syndrome (HLHS). Treatment for this complex defect typically entails three open-heart surgeries before a child turns 5, and the need for a heart transplant as a teenager. There are risks for many serious long-term complications and a guarded prognosis. The team went out to meet with Dorothy, her husband, and Dorothy's sons, ages 7 and 13 for an initial visit.

The Visits

Meeting with families in their home, on their own turf (or in any location of their choosing), empowers parents to feel more in control in a circumstance where so much is outside of their control. This is particularly important during those first visits when the subject matter to be discussed is difficult, and the team and family are just starting to build a relationship. The home visit also fosters unique opportunities for the care team to get to know the family more intimately or in more depth than possible in a hospital or outpatient environment. Rather than hearing about a family's environment, the team has the opportunity to experience it firsthand. Instead of the family describing their baby's nursery from a fluorescent-lit, sterile exam room, they can show the team. Similarly, the team can see or experience examples of a family's cultural and/or religious norms or traditions, within the home, sometimes even beyond seeing and hearing, such as through smelling dinner cooking. In addition, the visits provide an opportunity to meet and support siblings in the home.

The focus of the first home visit is on building rapport, getting to know the family, and gathering important information about their understanding of their baby's medical condition and prognosis and includes exploring questions, fears, and worries they may have. It is also an opportunity for the team to obtain a medical and psychosocial history without the time constraints of an office visit, in a more comfortable setting that helps facilitate open conversation. It is essential to explore their prior pregnancy history and any loss history to help assess current and future needs and coping.

Case 14.1 Part 2

During the first home visit, Dorothy explained that she felt a "lack of support for her, her baby, and her family from the hospital staff," and she was glad to be connected with a program that could support the family through her pregnancy. Dorothy was not close with her own family, and James' family lived out-of-state. CompassionNet was able to help them arrange for a doula, along with massage therapy for the parents and a music therapist to work with Dorothy's sons. At our third visit, Dorothy and James shared that they had not been offered any options other than termination or aggressive surgical interventions after Adam was born. As we talked, it became clear that the parents did not want Adam to undergo multiple surgeries and a possible heart transplant. This did not feel like a good "quality of life" to them. The parents explained that their holistic approach to life was more compatible with comfort care with minimal interventions.

It is important for any team (community- or hospital-based) to understand that not everything can get accomplished in a single visit. For example, it was not until the third visit that Adam's parents brought up the fact that they were pondering comfort care. It takes time to gain trust and make certain that the efforts made to care for the baby are in line with a family's values and beliefs. Ideally over time, the community-based team can broach these hard issues with the family and eventually put together a birth plan so that everyone is on the same page regarding care for the baby and family throughout labor and delivery and once he or she is born (See "Birth Plan," Appendix B). In addition, as needed, the team can explore how to support the parents' older children, bringing in the child life specialist, as discussed previously.

CompassionNet, 2010–2018

To give the reader a sense of the specifics of a palliative care program, we provide some data on the children and families we have served. Other community-based programs may have a different approach, and developing programs might choose different eligibility criteria depending on the available staff and needs of the community. From the perinatal program's inception in 2010 through April 2018, the CompassionNet program has enrolled 125 families with 137 infants (Table 14.1).

Of the 126 infants who delivered, 63 survived and 63 have died, 11 of whom died prior to delivery. An additional 11 had not yet been born at the time of data compilation. Details of the infants enrolled and their outcomes are listed in Table 2. Of the 137 infants, only 21 had what are traditionally regarded as "lethal diagnoses": Trisomy 18 (13), Trisomy 13 (3), renal agenesis (2), fetal skeletal dysplasia (2), and anencephaly (1). A summary of children's diagnoses are enumerated in Table 14.2.

Table 14.1 Outcomes of infants enrolled prenatally in the CompassionNet Program, 2010–April 2018

Pregnancies	125
Infants	137
Alive	63
Enrolled in CompNet	33
Discharged from program	30
Died	63
Prior to birth	11
First day of life	19
First month of life	19
First year of life	12
After 1 year	2
Not yet delivered	11

Table 14.2 Diagnoses[a] of infants enrolled in CompassionNet, 2010–April 2018

	Total[b]	Alive	Died	In utero
Cardiac anomaly	50	27	20	3
Respiratory	1	1		
Neurologic disorders	11	6	4	1
Renal anomalies	7	2	5	
Congenital anomalies	39	9	26	4
Malignancies	1	1		
Newborn complications	28	17	8	3

[a]Diagnosis based on ICD9 codes for 10 complex chronic conditions
[b]Includes 11 living in utero infants

Involvement at Labor, Delivery, and Birth

The role of the CompassionNet team at the time of labor, delivery, and birth is variable, depending on the family's needs, the resources in the family's community, the training of nurses in L&D, and the palliative care staff available in a given hospital. Typically, we do not "take call" for our perinatal deliveries. However, there have been instances when there is a planned C-section and anticipated fetal demise, in which we are asked by the family to be present at the birth and death. The involvement of a community-based team in a hospital-based birth and death is something that must be carefully negotiated between members of community-based and inpatient palliative care teams and obstetric staff. Our goal, when present at birth, is to be a familiar face at a difficult time, an advocate, an added support to the family, and to assist with photography and memory-making as indicated. Many major teaching hospitals with level IV NICUs, and often smaller community hospitals, have staff with expertise in perinatal and neonatal loss and have child life specialists available to help with sibling support. Often these institutions have RTS trained staff. It is helpful to become familiar with the local resources and training of the staff at the hospital where the mother delivers to assess if there are needs and openness for additional support. We often support families through advocacy to ensure their expressed cultural and spiritual needs are addressed, sometimes serving as a liaison between family and staff as desired. The PPC team works together with hospital staff to assist with memory-making activities and legacy building with siblings.

Case 14.1 Part 3

When Adam's parents learned about the lifelong effects and multisystem complications of a child with a hypoplastic left heart, it confirmed for them that this was not the life they wanted for their son, and they decided to pursue comfort care. The team consulted with the hospital-based subspecialty teams to confirm the diagnosis and prognosis and to be certain that a comfort-oriented approach to care was a reasonable one. The team then worked with the family over the course of several home visits to develop a birth plan consistent with their values and goals of care, which was shared and further discussed with their maternal-fetal-medicine team. Through these difficult conversations, Dorothy and James decided they did not want medical interventions, intubation, or resuscitation. They wanted to bring Adam home and perhaps have a home funeral. The social worker was able to provide information and guidance about a home funeral. In addition, Dorothy's two sons started meeting with the child life specialist and music therapist who helped them understand and cope with Adam's diagnosis and prognosis.

Role of the Community Team after Birth

The role of the community-based PPC team after the birth of the baby is also highly variable depending on the condition and prognosis of the baby and the local hospital resources. If the baby lives and needs an extended stay in the NICU, the role is that of support and advocacy. If the baby dies shortly after birth, the team can assist with memory-making, sibling support, funeral planning and assistance, and bereavement. If the family chooses to take the baby home and it is anticipated that the baby will die at home, the community-based palliative care team is available to provide end-of-life care or work with the local community health agency and/or hospice to coordinate care for the baby and family.

Case 14.1 Part 4

Dorothy went into labor and delivered a beautiful, healthy-appearing baby boy via *C-section. The neonatologist met with the parents shortly after delivery and told them that an echocardiogram confirmed that Adam had HLHS. Upon hearing this, the parents declined any medical interventions and confirmed their wish that Adam not be resuscitated in the event of a cardiac or pulmonary arrest. Adam roomed in with his parents on the labor and delivery unit and began to breast feed.*

When Adam was 3 days old, his parents decided to take him home. This would have been difficult without the CompassionNet team which was not only available for medical and psychosocial support at home but also had an established and trusting relationship with the entire family. Adam did well at home that first day, but the next day he rapidly declined. The parents were very worried about Adam's breathing and called the on-call CompassionNet pediatric nurse practitioner (PNP) at 4:30 a.m., who came over and guided the family on how and when to give the prescribed medications. Dorothy was also encouraged to give Adam her breast milk through a syringe. Later that afternoon, Adam declined further and appeared to be actively dying. At the parents' request, the entire CompassionNet team was present to support Adam and the family. The CompassionNet PNP guided the parents on when to give oral fentanyl and lorazepam for Adam's respiratory distress. His parents and brothers all took turns holding and loving him. The social worker arranged for a photographer to come, and the child life specialist helped the boys with memory-making. Early in the evening, Adam died peacefully in his mother's arms surrounded by his loving family and their trusted palliative care team.

At CompassionNet, we are fortunate to be affiliated with Lifetime Care Home Health Care and Hospice, and specifically in the Rochester, NY area, our team is able to partner with Lifetime's pediatric palliative care nursing team. When the death of a baby is anticipated, and the family chooses to have the baby die at home, our CompassionNet team is able to partner with the pediatric palliative care nursing team to provide 24 hour on-call nursing and medical support.

When a baby dies at home, the interdisciplinary team is usually able to be present at the time of death if the family wishes (and most do). At time of death we assist with tending to the care of the body and provide emotional support to the family, often helping parents inform the siblings of the baby's death and encouraging and guiding sibling participation in rituals and memory-making when possible. We also help the family with funeral planning, offer and guide memory-making activities and, as with a hospital death, arrange for a photographer when desired.

Case 14.1 Part 5

Dorothy and James washed Adam and kept him swaddled in a blanket and cooled with ice packs. They kept Adam home with them for a few days with the support of an understanding funeral director, whom the CompassionNet team contacted. They chose to have a home wake and rode with Adam in their arms directly to the cemetery. Following a moving graveside service, Adam's father laid him in the grave wrapped in a shroud. For the past three years, Adam's family has received bereavement support from the CompassionNet team. In addition to ongoing home visits, the team has provided access to other services including massage therapy, acupuncture, child life, and music therapy supporting meaningful outlets to help the family cope in their grief. Ultimately, the family shared that they are comfortable with the care they were able to provide to their son and how grateful they remain for the photographs and memory keepsakes the CompassionNet team facilitated for their family and the continued support provided.

Role of the Community Team in Bereavement

- *"I look forward to your visits. It's the only time I can count on the chance to talk about my baby, about how much I still sometimes long to hold her in my arms and rock her, about the details of her tiny feet that I'm scared will slip away as the months and years pass, or just about how I wonder what she might look like or sound like now."*
- *"I like when you come see me because then I can talk freely, without worrying about my friends or family thinking I'm crazy, or broken, or that I just need to move on already."*
- *"I look forward to your visits because when you bring up my daughter, say her name, and talk with us about our memories, she doesn't feel quite as far away."*

Each sentiment above, shared by a different mother or father receiving bereavement support from CompassionNet after their baby died, illustrates a need frequently faced in perinatal loss and addressed through a community-based model. While each person's grief is unique, there are specific elements recognized as recurrent themes in perinatal loss and distinct ways in which community-based PPC is uniquely poised to address these needs. (More on bereavement theories and care can be found in Chap. 12). Included among these themes are the propensity for disenfranchised grief, i.e., grief that is not acknowledged or understood by others; the related need for validation of the loss; and the threat to attachment and related need to foster continued bonds with the baby [9]. These themes significantly contribute to the complexity and intensity of the perinatal grief experience. It is well recognized among bereavement professionals and within the literature that men and women tend to grieve differently, and that specifically with perinatal loss, such differences might be further amplified. We acknowledge and validate this in our work with families. Not only do there tend to be gender differences within grief reactions and needs, but in perinatal loss, we also find differences due to the physical nature and bonding opportunities of having carried the baby versus being the parent who did not carry the baby, also a factor for same-sex couples [10]. A community-based model is particularly well-suited to assess and respond to the unique individual needs of each parent, as visits can be arranged at a time when both parents can be present or the team can even meet separately with each parent based on their needs and wishes, to respond to and address support.

Two primary aspects of community-based PPC, illustrated through CompassionNet's model of care, demonstrate unique opportunities to address these needs from a community-based model: (1) care provided across all phases of the care continuum – pregnancy, birth, death, and ongoing bereavement – by a consistent interdisciplinary team and (2) family-centered care provided in the home and community versus a clinical or hospital-based setting.

The PPC continuum integrates bereavement care and grief support throughout the family's experience. This is essential as the family's grief, complex and multifaceted, truly begins at the time they learn of their baby's condition, encompassing both concrete and symbolic losses: loss of a healthy pregnancy; loss of joy and positive emotions of pregnancy; loss of role or identity of being a parent/or sibling; loss of future hopes and dreams; and loss of social circle (e.g., other expecting couples) [11]. The juxtaposition of anticipating a loss at a time expected to be filled with such joy, hope, and excitement further intensifies the profound and complex anticipatory grief experienced.

Case 14.2 Part 1

Ellie was diagnosed prenatally with Trisomy 18, a large omphalocele, congenital cardiac anomaly, and intracranial abnormalities at her 18 weeks ultrasound. Shortly after learning of her complex, life-limiting medical condition, Ellie's parents were referred to CompassionNet's PPC program for support as they continued their pregnancy. The CompassionNet social worker (SW) and pediatric nurse practitioner (PNP) first met Ellie's family, including her 5- and 2-year-old sisters, at their home when Ellie was 21 weeks gestation. A married couple, Ellie's parents were practicing Catholics, who found much strength and meaning in their faith. Their primary support system, in addition to their strong faith and support within their marital relationship, included Ellie's maternal aunt and great aunt, and Ellie's paternal grandparents. Ellie's mother and father also each had social support through friends and colleagues at work.

CompassionNet's community-based model of care spans all phases of perinatal palliative care and enables a family to continue with the same consistent care team throughout all phases, including ongoing bereavement support, which is available for up to 3 years following the death of their baby. This consistency fosters opportunities to build and maintain trusting relationships with the care team.

For many families, the time during their pregnancy is the only time they have with their baby alive. Families often identify and express a sense of comfort with members of the team, because they are among the few people who "knew them when," or "knew their baby" during the pregnancy, when their baby was alive, and who appreciate how special that time is. Capitulo explains grief for parents in perinatal loss as being "particularly susceptible to being disenfranchised, as only parents may have known the baby, felt it move, or seen it through ultrasound" [12, p. 390]. This can only add to the already complex impact of their grief.

For parents who learn of their baby's life-limiting condition during pregnancy, the time of the pregnancy itself may be their only opportunity to parent their baby [13]. Often their earliest acts of parenting involve making life and death decisions for their child, an intense and devastating introduction to parenthood. Yet for some parents, the opportunity to make decisions that will bring their baby comfort or protect them from pain is where they find meaning.

Case 14.2 Part 2

From the very first visit with CompassionNet, Ellie's parents openly expressed their shared wishes for a live birth, acknowledging the devastating reality that her life would likely be brief. Upon further discussion regarding goals of care, they also articulated their wish to hold and spend time with Ellie, and if possible, to bring her home. As a community-based team, CompassionNet's PNP and SW were well-equipped to assist Ellie's parents in exploring options and resources to realize these goals. From this point forward, joint home visits from the PNP and SW continued on a biweekly basis from 21 weeks gestation until delivery at 37 weeks. Community-based child life support was introduced and offered, as parents sought guidance about how to most appropriately communicate with their young daughters about their baby sister and her medical conditions. The child life specialist met the girls in the home beginning at 31 weeks and continued to see them on a regular basis. The PNP and SW also introduced the concept of the birth plan at the enrollment visit, and based on continued discussions regarding the family's wishes and goals of care for baby, the CompassionNet physician joined the SW and PNP at a visit to discuss formally placing limits on aggressive care at birth.

Anticipatory bereavement care provided by a community-based PPC team centers around supporting families to parent through goals of care and decision-making consistent with their wishes and values, equipping them with information about options and choices available, exercising control where they are able, and helping to minimize regret moving forward [14]. Care provided by a consistent team across all phases enables the family to count on seamless support through their grief, both anticipatory and after their baby dies. Helping to foster attachment becomes a key component to validating the meaning of the baby's life and is central to the bereavement care provided. Opportunities can be found during pregnancy and after to assist with fulfilling this very important need (See Chap. 12).

Meeting families early on in their care continuum – when bereavement starts – helps validate their complex grief and allows time to develop trust. This proves especially helpful in supporting siblings, who may struggle with the abstract nature of pregnancy based on their developmental understanding. A community-based team can work with parents to help children bond with their baby sibling through talking to the baby in their mom's belly, touching her belly, and seeing ultrasound pictures or video.

Case 14.2 Part 3

Ellie was born at 37 weeks and died shortly after her birth. Because her parents were able to discuss goals of care with one another and the care team in the weeks and months prior to her birth, they were able as a couple to focus on meeting Ellie and keeping her comfortable. With the support of the CompassionNet team, their faith, and their supportive marital relationship, they were able to spend over 24 hours in the hospital with Ellie. They held her, made and captured memories through photography, and spent time as a whole family as they introduced their young daughters to their baby sister. The trust and rapport CompassionNet's child life specialist developed with Ellie's sisters during the pregnancy led to the parents' request that the child life specialist come to the hospital. Partnering with her hospital-based counterpart, the child life specialist provided support when the siblings came up to meet their baby sister and encouraged opportunities to actively participate in her care, and be big sisters to Ellie. This also helped build their memories and validate their big sister role.

Through ongoing bereavement visits in the home with families, community-based palliative care providers seek opportunities to encourage parents and siblings to maintain bonds and memories with their baby, often discussing and looking at photos and mementos together in the home. Families frequently share that they look forward to these visits because they know it is a time they can talk about their baby without worrying about how it might impact friends or family. Some families have shared that their CompassionNet providers are the only people who bring up their baby or ask questions and encourage them to remember.

As siblings grow developmentally, experts recognize they understand their loss in new ways, and thus re-grieve based on their new understanding. CompassionNet's model, offering community-based bereavement support for 3 years after the loss, enables siblings to continue or intermittently access bereavement support as needed without starting all over with a new provider and with a history of trust and rapport to build upon.

Case 14.2 Part 4

Ellie's family engaged in bereavement support through continued home visits with their CompassionNet team. Ellie's sisters continued to benefit from the support of the child life specialist in expressing their feelings in their grief and fostering continued bonds with their baby sister. Ellie's parents expressed healing and comfort in opportunities to talk about Ellie and their grief with their CompassionNet SW and PNP, which deepened their continued bond with Ellie and validated her life and their loss.

Conclusion

In conclusion, community-based perinatal palliative care programs provide invaluable support to mothers, fathers, unborn children, sick infants, and their siblings. The unique contribution of home-based teams is their ability to provide such support within the safety of the home, to guide parents on how to help young siblings through this difficult time, be a constant presence throughout the pregnancy and beyond, and in the case of infant loss, provide expert bereavement care to the parents and siblings. Such teams function best when they partner with hospital-based perinatal, neonatal, and palliative care teams so that the care of these families is seamless from home to hospital and back home.

Appendix 14.1 CompassionNet Perinatal Referral Form

Perinatal Referral for All-Inclusive Care Program
Please fax referral to (585) 475-8801or toll free 1-800-290-0410
For assistance, call Referral Coordinator at (585) 475-8835.
If you have not heard from us within 2 business days, please contact to confirm.

CompassionNet
Surrounding families with support

Mother's Name: ______ Home Phone: ______
Address: ______ Cell Phone: ______
______ Work Phone: ______
Mother's Insurance: ______ Policy #: ______ (Required) DOB ______
Father's Name: ______ Home Phone: ______
Address: ______ Cell Phone: ______
______ Work Phone: ______
Father's Insurance: ______ Policy #: ______ (Required) DOB ______
Siblings (and ages if known): ______

Pregnancy and Baby Information

Baby's Name (if known): ______ Gender (circle): M F
Maternal Age: ______ Current Gestation: ______ EDC: ___/___/___ G___ P___ ___ ___

Diagnoses	ICD10 Code		Diagnoses	ICD10 Code

Please check which of the following criteria are met by the baby's current medical condition:

	Condition for which treatment options are available but may fail
	Progressive condition in which treatment is exclusively palliative after diagnosis
	The baby's prognosis is guarded but not clearly defined

Please provide pertinent medical history justifying medical eligibility (i.e. U/S, genetics, testing):
______
______
______

Immediate Needs: ______
Has family been made aware of this referral to CompassionNet: YES NO
Has family had a palliative care consult: YES NO

PLEASE NOTE: Eligibility determinations will be made as soon as possible. Additional information may be requested by CompassionNet medical staff.

Team member to contact for additional medical eligibility information: ______
Phone: ______ Email: ______
Team member to notify regarding eligibility determination: ______
Phone: ______ Email: ______
Please **Print** name of **Perinatologist/Obstretrician:** ______ (If different than referring physician)
Phone: ______ Email: ______

Please **Print** name of **Referring** Physician **(REQUIRED):** ______
Referring Physician Signature **(REQUIRED):** ______ Date: ______
For use by Compassion Net Staff: Ins. Eligible: Yes No Medically Eligible: Yes No Confirmed by: ______
Date Notified of Eligibility ______ by ______
V12-18 SW/SCS & PNP./RN: ______ C ______

Appendix 14.2 CompassionNet Birth Plan

CompassionNet
Surrounding families with support

Birth Plan

About this birth plan: *If you are reading this birth plan, you have likely been told that your baby has a serious medical condition. This can be a very difficult time for families, and we want you to know that your CompassionNet team is here for you.*

This birth plan allows you to indicate your preferences as you continue on your pregnancy journey. Although some decisions may be out of your hands, it can be helpful to express your wishes regarding the choices that you can make. Before you begin, it is important to know that some sections ask you to consider difficult scenarios (page 5 in particular). Please keep in mind that not all parts of this birth plan apply to every family, and you are not required to complete every section. We encourage you to spend some time working through this birth plan with your care team. Once you are finished, please share this document with your obstetrician and the rest of your team. It is also a good idea to bring a copy with you when you go to the hospital to deliver.

About you:

Today's date: ____________ Due date: ____________

Parent's name: ____________ Phone: ____________

Parent's name: ____________ Phone: ____________

Baby's name: ____________ Sex: M F

2nd Baby's name (if twins): ____________ Sex: M F

Diagnosis: ____________ Date informed: ________

Your care team:

OB/GYN: ____________ Phone: ____________

Pediatrician (if known): ____________ Phone: ____________

Specialist: ____________ Phone: ____________

Your CompassionNet team:

Supportive care social worker / specialist: ____________ Phone: ____________

Pediatric nurse practitioner / nurse: ____________ Phone: ____________

Child life specialist: ____________ Phone: ____________

CompassionNet
Surrounding families with support

Prenatal appointments:	**Completed**	**Would like**
Tour of the labor and delivery unit	☐	☐
Tour of the neonatal intensive care unit (NICU) (Specialized unit for babies who need medical support)	☐	☐
Meeting with a neonatologist (Pediatrician who cares for sick and premature infants in the hospital) Name: ________________ Phone: ____________	☐	☐
Meeting with a pediatric palliative care physician (Pediatrician who focuses on the relief of pain, stress, and other symptoms of serious illness. Palliative care can be offered at any stage of an illness and can be provided along with treatment meant to cure.) Name: ________________ Phone: ____________	☐	☐
MOLST (Form that highlights decisions regarding life sustaining treatment)	☐	☐

Prenatal testing:	**Completed**	**Would like**
Ultrasound (sonogram)	☐	☐
Genetic testing / counseling	☐	☐
Amniocentesis	☐	☐
Other (please specify): ____________	☐	☐

Delivery plans:

☐ We have discussed delivery options with an obstetrician

☐ Vaginal birth

☐ C-section (__repeat or __for baby's health)

☐ The NICU team plans to be present at the delivery

Support person we would like present during labor and delivery:

Name: ________________ Phone: ____________

Support person

Name: ________________ Phone: ____________

During labor, we would like:

☐ Our baby's heart rate checked from time to time

☐ Continuous monitoring of our baby's heart rate

☐ IV pain management and/or an epidural

CompassionNet

After delivery, we would like to:

- ☐ Hold our baby as soon as possible
- ☐ Hold our baby skin-to-skin
- ☐ Bathe our baby
- ☐ Use our own blankets and clothing
- ☐ Have pictures taken with our camera / phone
- ☐ Have our baby stay with us for as long as possible
- ☐ Delay any non-urgent medical procedures (weighing baby, testing, etc.) to give us more time with our baby

Support person we would like to accompany our baby to the NICU if necessary and be informed of all testing and care:

Name: ______________________________ Phone: _______________

Support person we would like to remain with the mother if our baby is taken to the NICU:

Name: ______________________________ Phone: _______________

Feeding:

- ☐ If our baby is able, we would like to breast feed
- ☐ If our baby is able, we would like to bottle feed
- ☐ Formula preference if our baby is unable to have breast milk: ____________
- ☐ If our baby cannot suck, we would like feeding via dropper or tube

Spiritual support:

- ☐ We would like spiritual care support:
  - ☐ During pregnancy
  - ☐ At time of birth
  - ☐ After our baby is born
- ☐ We are interested in meeting with a chaplain
- ☐ We have our own spiritual support person

  Name: ______________________________ Phone: _______________
- ☐ Religious / cultural rituals that we would like to do shortly after birth: ______

  ____

CompassionNet
Surrounding families with support

Sibling support:

Sibling Name: ______________________ Gender: M F Age: _____

Sibling Name: ______________________ Gender: M F Age: _____

Sibling Name: ______________________ Gender: M F Age: _____

Sibling Name: ______________________ Gender: M F Age: _____

- ☐ We have told our children that: ______________________

  ____

- ☐ We would like to talk to someone about how to explain our baby's diagnosis to our children
- ☐ We would like our children to receive support from a child life specialist (Professional who helps children and teens understand medical conditions and treatment using supportive conversation, activities, and play)
- ☐ A child life specialist is already involved with our children

  Name: ______________________ Phone: ______________
- ☐ We have a family member / friend who will care for our children during labor & delivery

  Name: ______________________ Phone: ______________
- ☐ We would like our children brought to labor & delivery shortly after our baby's birth

If the hospital can provide the following, we would like:

- ☐ Pictures
- ☐ Footprints / handprints
- ☐ Lock of hair
- ☐ Crib card
- ☐ Clothing / hats / blankets
- ☐ Ring
- ☐ Stuffed animal
- ☐ Baptismal / blessing certificate
- ☐ ID Bracelet

If there is anything else that you would like to share with us to help us better care for you and your family, please note here: ______________________

____

____

CompassionNet
Surrounding families with support

If our baby is born still or dies soon after delivery, we would like to:

- ☐ Have our baby be swaddled and handed to us as soon as possible
- ☐ Hold our baby skin-to-skin
- ☐ Bathe and dress our baby ourselves
- ☐ Have our baby be bathed and dressed by a: nurse / friend or family member: _______
- ☐ Use our own blankets and clothing
- ☐ Have pictures taken with our camera / phone
- ☐ Spend time alone with our baby
- ☐ Stay with our baby for as long as possible
- ☐ Bring our children / family in as soon as possible after the delivery
- ☐ Include our children in memory-making activities

  Alternative plan for our children: ____
- ☐ Engage in the following religious / cultural rituals: ______________________________
- ☐ Learn more about the possibility of organ donation
- ☐ Have an autopsy performed
- ☐ Talk with someone about how to make funeral arrangements
- ☐ Use this funeral home (if known): _________________________ Phone: ___________

For the remainder of our stay in the hospital, we would like to:

- ☐ Remain on the labor & delivery unit if possible
- ☐ Move to the postpartum floor as soon as medically safe
- ☐ Move to a floor that does not have newborn babies

If the hospital can provide the following, we would like:

- ☐ Footprints / handprints
- ☐ Moses basket
- ☐ Monitor strip
- ☐ Memory box
- ☐ Sealed bags for clothing and other items to preserve our baby's scent

  Professional photographs of our baby and family

  Photographer (If known): _________________________ Phone: __________________

If there is anything else you would like to share with us to help us better care for you and your family, please note here: ____

____

References

1. Kaye EC, Rubenstein J, Levine D, Baker JN, Dabbs D, Friebert SE. Pediatric palliative care in the community. CA Cancer J Clin. 2015;65(4):316–33. https://doi.org/10.3322/caac.21280. Epub 2015 May 7
2. Wool C, Côté-Arsenault D, Perry Black B, Denney-Koelsch E, Kim S, Kavanaugh K. Provision of services in perinatal palliative care: a multicenter survey in the United States. J Palliat Med. 2016;19(3):279–85. https://doi.org/10.1089/jpm.2015.0266. Epub 2015 Dec 14
3. Fanos JH, Little GA, Edwards WH. Candles in the snow: ritual and memory for siblings of infants who died in the intensive care nursery. J Pediatr. 2009;154(6):849–53. https://doi.org/10.1016/j.jpeds.2008.11.053. Epub 2009 Apr 1.
4. Gaab EM, Owens GR, MacLeod RD. Siblings caring for and about pediatric palliative care patients. J Palliat Med. 2014;17(1):62–7. https://doi.org/10.1089/jpm.2013.0117. Epub 2013 Dec 6
5. Lovgren M, Sveen J, Nyberg T, Wallin AE, Prigerson HG, Steineck G, Kreicbergs U. Care at the end of life influences grief: a nationwide long-term follow-up among young adults who lost a brother or sister to childhood cancer. J Palliat Med. 2018;21(2):156–62. https://doi.org/10.1089/jpm.2017.0029. Epub 2017 Sep 26
6. Spinetta JJ, Jankovic M, Eden T, Green D, Martins AG, Wandzura C, et al. Guidelines of assistance to siblings of children with cancer: report of the SIOP working committee on psychosocial issues in pediatric oncology. Med Pediatr Oncol. 1999;33(4):395–8.
7. Denney-Koelsch E, Black B, Côté-Arsenault D, Wool C, Kim S, Kavanaugh KA. Survey of perinatal palliative care programs in the US: structure, process, and outcomes. J Palliat Med. 2016;19(10):1080–6. Epub 2016 Aug 25
8. Resolve Through Sharing. www.rts@gundersonhealth.org. Accessed 28 Mar 19.
9. Gupton AW. Addressing the unique and profound psychosocial impact of perinatal loss: implications for expansion of social work leadership in multidisciplinary learning and care [unpublished manuscript]. NYU Silver School of Social Work, Zelda Foster Leadership Fellowship in Palliative and End-of-Life Care; January 20, 2017.
10. Côté-Arsenault D, Denney-Koelsch E. "Love is a choice:" couple responses to continuing pregnancy with a lethal fetal diagnosis. Illness Crisis Loss. 2017;26(4):293–315.
11. Côté-Arsenault D, Denney-Koelsch E. "My baby is a person:" family experiences with life-threatening fetal diagnosis. J Palliat Med. 2011;14(12):1302–8. https://doi.org/10.1089/jpm.2011.0165. Epub 2011 Nov 11
12. Capitulo KL. Evidence for healing interventions with perinatal bereavement. MCN Am J Matern Child Nurs. 2005;30(6):389–96.
13. Côté-Arsenault D, Krowchuk H, Denney-Koelsch E, Jenkins Hall W. "We want what's best for our baby": prenatal parenting of babies with lethal conditions. J Prenat Perinat Psychol Health. 2015;29(3):157–76.
14. Côté-Arsenault D, Denney-Koelsch E. "Have no regrets:" parents' experiences and developmental tasks in pregnancy with a lethal fetal diagnosis. Soc Sci Med. 2016;154:100–9. https://doi.org/10.1016/j.socscimed.2016.02.033. Epub 2016 Feb 26

Interdisciplinary Perinatal Palliative Care Coordination, Birth Planning, and Support of the Team

15

Emilie Lamberg Jones and Steven R. Leuthner

Context for Care

For many, pregnancy is a joyful time of preparation. Although almost half of all pregnancies in the United States are unintended [1], by mid-pregnancy couples are making preparations to become parents and transitioning from *being pregnant* to *having a baby*. By the time of an anatomy ultrasound around 19–20 weeks, women may look forward to the opportunity to "see the baby," learn gender, and expect to be reassured that "everything is ok." Normal test results can decrease anxiety, resolve ambivalence, and enhance bonding between the mother [2] and her partner. The process of bonding includes preparing siblings to become big brothers or sisters, choosing the baby's name, decorating a nursery, and planning welcoming rituals such as baby showers. These developmental tasks of pregnancy facilitate the acceptance and identification of parenthood [3].

The terms "parents" and "baby" are used throughout this chapter as many women and their partners consider themselves parents of a child who has died, regardless of the gestational age or circumstances. However, it must be acknowledged that some individuals will grieve their loss as the loss of a pregnancy rather than the loss of child and that some women will not share this loss with a partner. We use the terms "parents" and "child" for simplicity. Relationship-based care practices will allow the care provider to individualize care and terminology, as appropriate.
Anecdotes from family and provider interactions interspersed throughout this chapter offer examples to illustrate concepts and show how suggestions for care can be applied in clinical practice. Pseudonyms have been used.

E. L. Jones (✉) · S. R. Leuthner
Children's Wisconsin, Fetal Concerns Center, Milwaukee, WI, USA
e-mail: elambergjones@chw.org

E. M. Denney-Koelsch, D. Côté-Arsenault (eds.), *Perinatal Palliative Care*,
https://doi.org/10.1007/978-3-030-34751-2_15

Contrast this joyful process to the shock of discovering that the baby may have a life-limiting fetal condition (LLFC). "The identification of abnormalities transforms the pregnancy experience," [3, 4] making expectant families face a real or potential fetal concern. They must cope with grief over the loss of a "normal" pregnancy and the stigma of being identified as "at increased risk" [5]. Parents describe experiencing a multitude of losses: loss of their healthy baby, of the normal pregnancy experience, and of the future parenting of their child [6]. Ultrasounds no longer carry with them reassurance but become diagnostic procedures to find out "what is wrong." Joyful preparation is replaced with anxious meetings with maternal fetal medicine and pediatric specialists. Instead of deciding about the baby's name and what color to paint the nursery, parents must decide about continuation of the pregnancy, relocation of care for greater access to specialized neonatal care, possible fetal interventions, and potential end-of-life planning [7, 8]. The opportunity for partners to begin to bond with the unborn baby and learn to parent together is often replaced with a sense of separation and ultimately a feeling of loss of control. Parkes described this loss as "the loss of the assumptive world"; parents lose what they assumed they would have [7, 9]. These concepts and parent experiences are discussed further in Chap. 2 and Chap. 4.

Birth Planning Is a Process, Not a Document

The development and implementation of a comprehensive pregnancy, birth, and neonatal plan (often called a "birth plan" for simplicity) offers opportunities for parents to regain some of what they have lost. This decision-making process helps them to fulfill their roles as a parent [6, 10], develop parenting competence, and regain some control over their baby's future. Birth planning is a process, not just a written document, through which parents can develop trusting relationships with a perinatal palliative care (PPC) interdisciplinary team (IDT) as they work to set goals and plan for achieving them. Interdisciplinary PPC teams are described, including team members, roles, and basic structure, in Chap. 13, Table 13.1.

An IDT led by a dedicated PPC care coordinator provides necessary tools and guidance to parents as they face the challenge of parenting a child who may have a very short life. This chapter will focus on the IDT's role in developing a birth plan that honors the parent's goals and values as well as the care coordinator's work to disseminate the comprehensive plan to the broader interspecialty and interdisciplinary team.

The Process of Birth Planning as Parenting

The goal of perinatal palliative care (PPC) planning is to facilitate a process by which parents define and cultivate a relationship with their baby. This relationship may have begun at the emotional level prior to conception and will continue for the rest of their lives. Thus, PPC planning is about how and to what extent to embrace the pregnancy, birth, time with baby, and integration of the baby into a family story.

One fetal center states, “The perinatal palliative care consultation is focused on navigating medical choices and validating good parenting, which derives directly from the broad view that perinatal palliative care acknowledges the very idea of parenthood” [11]. At the Fetal Concerns Center at Children’s Wisconsin, which was developed in 2000 by this chapter’s authors, we have found that aspects of PPC may help any family facing a difficult fetal diagnosis, even when the baby is expected to survive [5, 12].

Families should begin to receive PPC services as soon as possible after a concern for a LLFC is identified, given the importance and extent of specialized care needed. Care planning helps families to embrace relationship-making opportunities, parenting opportunities, and decision-making throughout their pregnancy. When the outcome for a baby is concerning but uncertain, PPC services are just as necessary, and perhaps more valuable, than when an outcome can be predicted with more certainty. PPC consultation can be beneficial whenever a baby has complicated and concerning prenatal findings; uncertainty should open the door to PPC services rather than become a barrier to these concepts [8, 13, 14]. Meeting parents soon after diagnosis also allows the IDT to develop a relationship with them [15], help them clarify their values, and define their goals. The parents and care providers may revisit these goals as new information emerges and as they have time to think through their decisions [16].

Goals of Care Coordination and Planning

The goals of developing a palliative care birth plan are to empower the family to define what they have lost, to gain control of what they can control, and to help them define themselves as good parents. (See examples in Table 15.1.) The PPC IDT works with a family to develop a care plan for the remainder of the pregnancy, birth, and care of the baby.

Table 15.1 Goals of interdisciplinary perinatal palliative care planning

Goal	Considerations and examples
Name what has been lost by the fetal diagnosis	PPC team’s role is to help the parents define their relationship to the fetus/baby and parenting role in the context of the pregnancy and their life experiences
	Example: Does the woman define this as a pregnancy loss or the loss of a baby with an identity? A woman for whom this was an undesired pregnancy may define the loss differently from a woman for whom the pregnancy is the result of many years of infertility treatments
	Knowing the meaning of the loss, providers can then tailor their interventions. As one family explained, “they did not focus on the impossibility of curing the trisomy, but rather on the meaning of the child’s life and the healing of the family” [17]
Restore control and empower decision-making	With their role defined, parents become a member of the team: “...the family gets a consistent message indicating that they are the architects of this plan to the degree they wish” [18]
	Example: PPC team speaking to parents, “This is your opportunity to make plans for your birth and your baby and to think about how you’d like that time to be”

(continued)

Table 15.1 (continued)

Goal	Considerations and examples
Assess goals of care	The PPC team must learn the parents' goals for the pregnancy, birth, and neonatal period. These will vary from family to family. Examples of parent goals may include:
	"I don't ever want her to leave the arms of her family"
	"I need the neonatal team to be at the birth, assess him and try to resuscitate so that I know I gave him a chance"
	"We want him to be born alive so the first words he hears are his dad calling him to prayer"
	"We just hope that she is comfortable"
Provide a framework from which a goal-aligned care plan can develop	The care team can facilitate reasonable interventions to support the family's goals, keeping in mind that the obstetric and neonatal plans should be congruent
	Example: If the goal is to minimize the need for a surgical delivery and to allow for a natural death, the family may choose to omit antenatal or intrapartum fetal monitoring
Provide opportunities to parent	Parents want to be competent, good parents. PPC team can facilitate parenting through:
	Enabling decision-making so that parents feel "reassured that they have carried out their rights and responsibilities" [10]
	Encouraging memory-making during the pregnancy: Including maternity photos, capturing time spent doing activities like traveling or reading books to the baby
	Baby/birth showers
	Time with family and baby's siblings
	Baptism and other rituals before or after birth
	Bathing/dressing the baby
	Feeding the baby, skin-to-skin positioning for mom and other family members
	Legacy creation through memory-making
	Plans for funeral, celebration of life, and respectful disposition
Treat parents and their baby with care and respect	Team members communicate that providing palliative care does not mean "doing nothing" or "not providing care." Instead it includes concrete plans for what care WILL be provided:
	Pain and symptom management, possible attempts at life-sustaining care, if desired
	Facilitation of memory-making
	Respectful disposition
Provide anticipatory guidance	Give families concrete examples of what might happen, what to expect in the delivery room and NICU and how they can be managed so there are no surprises. One parent said: "I truly didn't know where to start or even that there was such a person as a palliative care neonatologist or that I could meet with a lactation consultant. You anticipated my needs before I could even verbalize them"
Provide documentation of a written plan for care	A written plan for pregnancy and birth and for the immediate care of the family helps communicate to others all the parents' hopes and goals as well as logistical issues, so they can focus on compassionate care: "It was a heart-breaking experience, but it really helped to have had great people to talk with us ahead of time. We felt like we were treated with a lot more understanding and compassion even though we arrived unexpectedly in the middle of night"

Members of Interdisciplinary Care Team

Leuthner described the team as a key component of an effective program that provides compassionate, nonjudgmental care through a consistent team for the

Table 15.2 Network of caregivers for fetus/infant

Parents
Parents' identified support network
The perinatal palliative care coordinator
Perinatal palliative care interdisciplinary team
Neonatology providers
Maternal fetal medicine providers
Obstetrics/family practice providers
Sonographer
Social worker
Lactation consultant
Child life specialist
Spiritual care provider (community and/or hospital based)
Childbirth educator
Labor and delivery staff
Photographer
Psychologist/psychiatrist
Hospice team
Pediatric specialists such as cardiology, surgery, and others based on diagnosis
Doulas
Lay support and parent advocates
Funeral directors
Perinatal pathologist
Language interpreters

family and infant [5]. Members of the care team vary depending on the size and structure of the program, availability of resources, and individual family needs, desires, and goals. In addition to the members of the PPC specialist team (Chap. 13, Table 13.1), many other specialists and team members interact with the parents (listed in Table 15.2). At a minimum, the team must include the pregnant woman and her support system, her obstetrical provider, and a pediatric provider. Obstetrical providers – the primary obstetrician along with a maternal fetal medicine specialist (MFM) if needed – are critical to address fetal and maternal health concerns and support delivery planning. Pediatric providers, who might include the primary care pediatrician, neonatologist, and other pediatric medical, surgical, and palliative subspecialists, are critical for explaining the diagnosis, prognosis, and natural history of the condition and to provide symptom management.

Role of the Care Coordinator

In many PPC programs, a case management process is led by the care coordinator, who arranges consultations based on the individual fetal diagnosis and family needs and goals [5, 11]. For example, a family with older children may benefit from meeting with a child-life specialist. A mother who hopes to donate her breast milk may meet a lactation consultant prenatally. A family whose faith is critical to their decision-making and setting of goals should be encouraged to include their own church leader or a hospital chaplain on their team.

The care coordinator facilitates communication with the family and all members of the care team to provide consistent care [12]. Research findings suggest that "care lacked continuity and coordination" if the care team did not consult with each other [6]. Without adequate internal communication to develop a cohesive plan, each specialty provides different, often contradictory, guidance to families [18, 19]. "The care coordination through PPC can mitigate the potentially negative impact of the fragmented care system by providing holistic care, sharing not only information specific to the needs of the infant but a plan for how their care is organized" [16, 18].

> "*This experience has really opened my eyes to realize how important it is to have people like you (the care coordinator) who help patients navigate through a healthcare system that is so complicated when the patient is focused on her emotions, the diagnosis, and still soaking in all the information. You really humanized the experience for us and have blessed us in so many ways.*" (quote from the mother of Rodrigo, who was delivered at 22 weeks following a diagnosis of Trisomy 13)

Despite the wide range of PPC programs, services, sites of care, and differing missions in the United States, most share the common goal of providing a single point of contact for each family [16, 20]. This contact person may provide administrative support by scheduling appointments and consultations or offer direct patient care and facilitate the birth planning process. The care coordinator may be a nurse, social worker, genetic counselor, chaplain, midwife, doula, palliative care physician, or trained lay provider, among others. No matter the care coordinators' background or training, they are a single point of contact, an advocate and communicator, and a holder of hope.

Single Point of Contact

Parents often describe not knowing where to start, especially soon after learning that the baby has a LLFC. At a time when patients may be exhausted physically, mentally, and emotionally, they are expected to quickly learn a great deal of medical information and then quickly make significant decisions, often involving ethical and moral considerations. The care coordinator can suggest members of the care team with whom to meet and arrange consults, serving as a point of contact not only for the family but also for the entire team, so that care is seamless.

Advocate and Communicator

The care coordinator knows the family's story, shares that story with the other members of the team, and advocates for efforts to meet the family's goals. He or she communicates the plan to all care providers and is readily accessible so that the plan can be followed. The presence of the care coordinator during prenatal visits and at the delivery is often welcomed. As a "familiar face," they advocate that the care provided be consistent with the determined goals, e.g., the extent of resuscitation efforts, initiation of comfort measures, or inclusion of religious rituals or memory-making activities [5, 11, 21].

"Holder of Hope"

Hope for a miracle often exists simultaneously with hope for comfort. Hopes can shift and change [6], and the care coordinator can support and guide families as they reevaluate and revise their goals. For example, a parent might share: "At first I just hoped that the doctors were wrong and that he would be born healthy. Now I just hope that we might get a little bit of time with him and that he doesn't suffer." Families experiencing a pregnancy with an LLFC tell us that they want several things from their primary health care providers: provision of accurate, comprehensive information in a balanced manner; respect for their decisions; treatment of their unborn child as an individual; and the maintenance of some degree of hope [22]. They do not want to feel pressured into any decisions but want to be provided support. The PPC IDT should provide balanced and personalized counseling, integrating appropriate hope about the uncertainty of the child's birth, life span, or about the value of the short time parents might have with their child [22].

Relationship-Based Care

Relationship-based care is essential to the roles of the care coordinator. There may be months or only a few hours in which to establish a relationship with parents and help guide them through a complex array of information and decisions. Developing a PPC plan is not as simple or straightforward as following a checklist; one must consider how to begin the conversation and how to enter into a relationship with a family. High-quality, individualized, compassionate PPC is based on the principle that relationship, in itself, is an intervention [15].

Establishing a relationship between provider and patient/family serves many of the goals in Table 15.1. The provider must deeply understand the meaning of the loss for the family and their goals and fears in order to individualize value-aligned care. The care provider guides the family through learning opportunities that will allow them to feel competent in the care of and decision-making for their child. This helps them to regain some control, facilitates parenting, and ultimately makes possible the creation of a birth plan.

By this means, the relationship established between family and care provider becomes an intervention of its own. The care coordinator becomes part of the baby's story and the compassionate relationship acts as an anchor for the family in an otherwise swirling sea of emotions and decision-making. One family said this in a letter to their care coordinator:

> *I can't express how thankful we are to have you in our lives. You made this experience so memorable with Rodrigo. You made me feel like a mother birthing her son. Even after Rodrigo came and went, you checked in and provided support that is continuing to help my husband and myself through this. We are so thankful and can't express it. We've been blessed with you and your team.*

Establishing the Relationship

In this section, we will review the steps and considerations in establishing relationship-based care with a PPC family. These steps can be done by anyone on the PPC IDT, but typically the PPC care coordinator fulfills this role. Table 15.3 lists the basic steps that are described in more detail.

Time and Place

In an ideal situation, referral to PPC should occur early on, so the care team has weeks or months to establish a relationship and work on care planning over time. However, medical and legal circumstances may necessitate that this work be done very rapidly, over the course of hours or days. The time around initial diagnosis and decision-making is often most distressing, morally challenging, and exhausting for prospective parents. Parents must learn "a new language" of medical terminology and then use this knowledge to make life-changing decisions for themselves, their baby, and their entire family. They must do this work at a time when they may be

Table 15.3 Steps to establishing relationship-based perinatal palliative care

Steps	Examples of wording
1. Establish best time and place	"I know that you just had your ultrasound and received some concerning news. Would you like to take a break and talk later or do you have questions that you are ready to discuss?" and/or "What are the things you are most concerned about today?"
2. Introduction and acknowledgment	"Congratulations on your pregnancy. I'm sure this may be a bittersweet time for you"
3. Extent of relationship	"I'm here to answer questions and offer information and guidance as needed. How can I be most helpful?"
4. Share their story	"Tell me a bit about how things have gone so far"
	"Help me understand what this pregnancy means to you"
5. Clarifying the family understanding	"What have you been told about your baby's condition and how she may do after she is born?"
6. Meeting the family where they are	"I know these are difficult things to discuss and I'm so sorry that you are going through this. Please let me know what would be helpful to know today and what you'd prefer to talk about another time"
7. Setting goals	"Knowing what we now know, what are your hopes for Madeline's birth?"
8. Exploring fears	"What things worry you the most about as you think about meeting Madeline?"
9. Providing anticipatory guidance	"It may be helpful to talk about what to expect and what sorts of things may happen as she is dying"
10. Shared decision-making	"Do you feel like you and the doctors (or you and your partner) are 'on the same page' about how to take care of Madeline?"
11. Documenting the plan	"I'm going to document your plan for Madeline's birth in your electronic medical record so that it's available to everyone who may take care of you, day or night"

physically and mentally exhausted and they are certainly emotionally upset after hearing that their desired baby may have a very short life. Decisions may need to be made very quickly if there are legal constraints around a choice of termination or when an impending birth is imminent. Skillful counseling, provided through relationship-based care and guided participation, can assist families in achieving a sense of peace and purpose in their decisions, minimizing the suffering of both babies and their parents.

Consultation may take place in a hospital or clinic/outpatient setting, or it may be community-based in churches, homes, or other settings. At times, care planning may take place with the assistance of technology, using video calls for conversations or emails to share edited care plans [21].

Introduction and Acknowledgement of Their Experience

To begin, introduce yourself, your role, and how you hope to be helpful. Offer both congratulations for the pregnancy and condolences that they are having to face such difficult conversations about a baby who they had hoped would be healthy. One dad provided this feedback after the neonatologist introduced himself: "You were the first person at the hospital who said, 'Congratulations.'"

Acknowledge that they are in a difficult situation with challenges and that these are difficult conversations and difficult questions to ask. Assure the family you are there to support them and that you can approach different issues as they are ready or as care necessitates.

Clarify the Extent of Relationship with Care Team

One of the first and ongoing assessments to make is the extent of a relationship which the family needs or wants from the care providers [23]. Some families will welcome their care team into their lives as "part of their family's story," while other families may feel confident and competent to rely less heavily on the care team's presence. Some families may not want to talk about the baby's diagnosis and prognosis at all. The use of relationship-based care will allow the providers to tailor their involvement over time as appropriate, building a foundation of trust and comfort on which many difficult conversations can take place.

Sharing Their Story and Clarifying Understanding

Asking the family to share their story of the pregnancy is useful in several ways: it clarifies how the family interprets the diagnosis, defines how they think about their loss and their role as a parent, and helps to identify the family needs for an individualized care plan that supports their goals [12]. The use of open-ended questions, such as, "Tell me a little about what's happened so far and how I may be of help to you today" can elicit cues about how the patient and partner define themselves and their pregnancy [10]. Do they refer to a baby by pronouns or given names, or use language such as "fetus" or "pregnancy?" After hearing the diagnosis of a LLFC, some individuals will embrace the role of parent while others may attempt to distance themselves; hence, different families will appreciate different interventions [24, 25].

Having listened to the parents' story, the provider may have the opportunity to clarify medical diagnostic or prognostic misunderstandings, legal concerns, and options and decisions that are before them. Families often struggle to understand exactly what is going on and what to expect. It is critical to reassure the family that there is no one "right way" to proceed and let them know that you will offer all available options and be present for them. Offering choices nurtures trust and gives the parent some sense of control [10]. Staying responsive to families' changing needs and desires also helps to create a trusting relationship; an option that at first sounds foreign to them may later feel familiar [10].

Meeting the Family Where They Are

Part of the care coordinator's role is to trust that the family will cope as they need to, want to, and are able to. Use of a relationship-based care approach supports parents' belief in their own ability to get through each circumstance. Some families embrace relationships with their babies, while others will withdraw emotionally to protect themselves from pain. Care providers need to meet them "where they are," without judgment but with awareness and acceptance. Many families desire a relationship with their baby. Sharing with them the concepts of perinatal bereavement can be a blessing, giving them options for bonding and memory-making. However, bonding and memory-making may also challenge a patient's attempts, desire, and/or need to protect themselves. No matter how a couple decides to proceed with their pregnancy, parents need an experienced, knowledgeable, compassionate care provider to offer a safe space where they can do what is meaningful to them [10, 25].

Setting Goals and Exploring Fears

The core of PPC planning is helping and supporting families as they identify their goals and alleviating their fears. While many parents can verbalize and articulate their goals soon after diagnosis, these goals may well change many times over time. Pregnancy is a dynamic process for both maternal and fetal health that often brings new information, a clearer prognosis, and more or fewer options, all of which might modify the family's goals. Goals might also change after birth, when the baby's condition and needs are better known [26]. Several authors have used the term "regoaling" to described this process [3, 27] (see also Chap. 4, Table 4.1). A useful question can be, "Knowing everything that you now know, what are you hoping for?" Parents may respond in various ways, such as:

- "We just hope to have some time with him, you know, while he's still alive."
- "We don't want her to leave our side."
- "I need the doctors to be there in the delivery room and give her a chance. If, after she's born, they still say that she can't make it well, then, I'll know that I gave her every chance."

As Côté-Arsenault and Denney-Koelsch describe the process, "palliative care approaches in other settings use empathic counseling, sometimes over several visits, to reframe a family's expectations from hope for the loved one's long-term survival to hope for a meaningful life and peaceful death with dignity" [6].

Acknowledging fears is just as important as identifying goals in the parents' experience with an LLFC. It is crucial for the care coordinator to explore fears; parents may find it difficult to admit to concerns they have been, until now, too frightened to articulate. Families are reassured to hear that their concerns, questions, and fears are normal. For example, families may ask,

- "Will he suffer?"
- "I'm not sure I can hold him right away."
- "What if this happens in the middle of the night with doctors I've never met?
- "Will you be there?"
- "How am I going to be able to leave the hospital without my baby?"
- "What is going to happen to her body?"
- "I'm scared of making the wrong decision."

At times, parents won't be able to verbalize their hopes and goals nor their fears. In these cases, the care coordinator might offer to provide an overview of options. For example:

- "Let's start with what you may expect the day your baby is born. I can mention some things other families have done. There is no right or wrong. See what fits for you."
- "Be open to the possibility that what doesn't seem right today might be right later on."
- "I cannot guess what may be too painful to discuss so please let me know if you'd like to postpone some discussions for later. Know that I am available to talk about these things when you are ready."

A LLFC may carry with it feelings of shock, disbelief, and inability to process unfamiliar, technical information. Ideally, these are not one-time conversations, but introductions to topics that can be explored as the pregnancy progresses and the family is ready to enter into decision-making. When timing or clinical needs demand more hurried discussions, the use of guided participation allows the provider to identify the most immediate needs and time-sensitive decisions which need to be made, guiding the family gently as they cope with the process of decision-making [23, 28].

To help parents envision themselves and their babies in an unfamiliar situation, accurate, detailed descriptions of concrete examples for care, whether comfort or curative, can be comforting. Families appreciate hearing what they can do, not only about what cannot be done. Many families find it helpful to hear other parents' stories of what they chose for their babies. Suggestions of books, support groups, and web-based resources on perinatal hospice may be welcomed [21]. Some may appreciate a guided tour of the birth center and/or neonatal intensive care unit.

Shared Decision-Making

A study of prospective parents' perspectives on antenatal decision-making found that most participants "desire a shared role in decision-making alongside their providers" [29]. Nonetheless, many parents verbalize the emotional burden of feeling that they will be responsible for ultimate decisions made and fear that, later, they will feel responsible for their child's death. Care providers must balance providing options with offering guidance and even recommendations, depending on the parents' goals and their medical expertise and experience.

While the pregnant woman is often the focus of many of these discussions, it is important to include the woman's partner and other sources of close support. Family members and friends may hold back their emotions in an attempt to protect the mother and have been described as the "forgotten mourners" [30]. They appreciate acknowledgement of their unique loss. It is also important to recognize that there may be disagreement between parents and other family members regarding goals. For example, parents may say:

- "I'm not sure I want to see her after she's born but my husband does."
- "My grandmother says that all of you doctors are wrong and my baby is going to be fine."

The care coordinator must identify who the woman defines as her family and work to bring each individual into the conversation. This can allow for more open discussions and enable more individualized care.

The care plan may also include information about practices the family does not want, even when they are part of more routine perinatal bereavement practices. For example, a family may decide that they do not want to see or hold their baby after birth and do not want photographs or other memory-making rituals. In this case, after careful assessment of the families' needs and goals, the care coordinator can communicate their wishes to birth center staff, while recognizing that individuals may (or may not) change their minds at the time of delivery. "Whether parents want to be with their baby or not, parents need an experienced, knowledgeable, compassionate bereavement care provider to offer a safe and sacred space where they can do what is emotionally and spiritually meaningful to them" [28].

Individualized Care

It is important to recognize that palliative care birth planning is a philosophy of care, not a prescribed process used only in specific circumstances. Birth planning is not restricted to cases where there is a confirmed life-limiting diagnosis nor to families who decide to continue a pregnancy to an expected due date. Care planning can be used at any gestational age and with any mode of delivery. For example, it can help a family choose aggressive, life-sustaining treatments, or only a comfort-oriented approach to care. A common scenario in which parents often choose a comfort approach is when they are expecting a baby who has anencephaly. The parents may choose to continue the pregnancy as long as possible and plan that their newborn will receive care that will keep him or her comfortable and keep the family together in the same place as they allow for a natural death. A fully comfort-oriented approach is one with which most are familiar, but family choices vary depending on their goals. Sometimes PPC is provided when fetal interventions have been offered to a pregnant woman whose fetus is at high risk of in utero or neonatal death. While the family may consent to the treatment with the hope and goal of cure, they can benefit from resources and relationships to support them if the fetal intervention is not successful. The medical and ethical complexities of these cases are discussed at length in Chap. 3 (see also section "Individualized Care Plan Scenarios", Chap. 4). The clinical scenarios below illustrate variations in care choices made by parents with the same diagnosis.

Clinical Scenarios

In each of these examples, there is a prenatal diagnosis of Trisomy 18 with associated bladder outlet obstruction, anhydramnios, and a high likelihood for pulmonary hypoplasia. In each case, care planning is tailored to help parents clarify their hopes and goals for their child and consider interventions that correspond to those goals.

Case 15.1

Family 1 expresses that their primary goal is to keep their son comfortable and to avoid any separation. While they are hopeful that they will be able to meet him alive, they have declined a cesarean section delivery for fetal distress and thus have declined continuous fetal monitoring during labor. His mom hopes he will be able to breastfeed or at least be comforted as he is skin-to-skin with her. They choose to have only medical intervention which will bring him comfort, and thus their neonatal plan is to "allow for a natural death." They plan to joyfully celebrate their son's birthday. Their care plan specifies that their birthing room will be a place for celebration, complete with balloons, a birthday cake, and many family members present for the party.

Case 15.2

Family 2 shares many of the goals of Family 1, but it is of vital importance that their son be born alive so that he can be baptized immediately after birth. The mother has chosen to undergo twice-weekly antenatal testing and continuous fetal monitoring during labor in order to minimize the risk of stillbirth. Despite being 22 years old and in her first pregnancy, she consents to a cesarean section if necessary, with full understanding of the surgical risks and potential risk for complications in future pregnancies. Her care plan includes documentation of her monitoring plan so that her labor and delivery providers are aware of her goals, as well as the confirmation of availability of physicians who are willing to perform a surgical delivery in this situation. The care plan also includes the name and cell phone number of their priest who will be present at the time of birth.

Case 15.3

Family 3 requests that they and their baby "be treated like a normal pregnancy" and request all medical interventions that are available to assist their son in living as long as possible. In addition to antenatal testing and fetal monitoring during labor, their care plan indicates that the neonatal intensive care team should be present at the delivery with a plan for full resuscitation efforts. They have discussed the risks and benefits of artificial ventilation and nutrition and would like these interventions to be taken, if required.

Case 15.4

Family 4 did not have confirmatory genetic testing. Their prenatal screening tests indicated that their baby is at increased risk for Trisomy 18, and, while the structural anomalies apparent on ultrasound appear to correspond with that diagnosis, they feel that they "can't be sure" until after delivery. Their care plan includes a plan for limited resuscitation measures at birth if needed (transitional bag/mask ventilation but not escalation to CPR or heroic measures that may be potentially painful). They plan for an initial assessment and evaluation in the NICU. They are open to transitional artificial feeding measures but "don't want him to be hooked up to tubes for the rest of his life."

Case 15.5

Family 5 was devastated at the news that their baby was diagnosed with Trisomy 18, especially as this was the first time they were able to continue a pregnancy past the first trimester. They conceived this baby with assisted fertility treatment after three miscarriages. Despite their baby's prognosis, they have embraced their role as parents and are prepared to continue the pregnancy with a plan for meeting their baby near her due date and then enjoying "whatever time we get with her." Sadly, their baby developed hydrops at 21 weeks and the mother developed mirror syndrome, a life-threatening maternal condition in which the pregnant woman "mirrors" the symptoms of the baby and develops edema and high blood pressure. The couple was counseled that early delivery was now medically indicated to prevent further maternal complications. The couple was shocked to hear that a delivery at 21 weeks was defined as an "abortion," an option they never considered for their pregnancy. Their care coordinator assured them that their delivery and baby would be treated with respect and they would have all of the same options for memory-making and spending time with their daughter that they would have had if she had been delivered nearer to her due date. They delivered their daughter 2 days later, were able to hold her while she lived for "32 wonderful minutes" and found comfort in the mementoes they received at the hospital.

While a comfort-oriented approach is commonly chosen in the case of LLFC, PPC is also offered to parents who consider that the best-interest decision for their child is to begin treatment and allow evaluation after birth for a condition that is critical. The parents may wish to set limitations on curative care, as more information is gathered [2]. The grief reactions of Family 5 are like those of parents with any other perinatal loss. Relationship-based care allows the care provider to integrate established bereavement practices into the care of families who consider ending a desired pregnancy after a life-limiting fetal diagnosis [31]. It is important to recognize that letting parents determine for themselves when and how to deliver a baby following a significant maternal or fetal diagnosis acknowledges the parent's ability to make decisions about what is best for themselves and their baby. This decision-making can help to restore some sense of control and parental authority. Therefore, individualized PPC may include the choice to terminate a much-wanted pregnancy and deliver a much-loved baby early [31].

These case examples exemplify that there is no "one right way" for a family to care for their child nor one "correct" set of goals to have. Instead, the goal of PPC planning for the family is to determine what is "right" for them and will bring them the most comfort and peace.

Development of a Written Palliative Care Birth Plan

Once the care team has established a relationship with a family and their goals have been clarified, they begin to work together on developing a written care plan. Documentation of the plan should be done as soon as possible in the pregnancy, with the understanding that it is a "living" document that is likely to evolve as parents revise their goals or the baby's condition changes [8]. Having a blank template of your organization's care plan available during consultation is useful, but the goal of initial care-planning meetings is not to "fill out the form," but rather, to use each section as a means to introduce ideas, and provide anticipatory guidance. Then families need time to consider what feels most comfortable for them.

Written care plans, much like checklists, are important tools to promote and guide care, guide conversations, and confirm that all elements of the plan are in place, but they do not replace individualized care planning [21]. Care providers must engage parents in conversations about their options, emphasizing each parent's right to make decisions, accommodating a variety of grief reactions, and taking into account the uniqueness of each parent, family, and circumstance. Cultivating a caring relationship with parents is what makes individualized care possible and effective [20].

A key component of care is creating a written document that is readily accessible to the entire team in a seamless fashion, even if a patient presents to the birth center unexpectedly [8, 16]. In the authors' institution, the PPC plan is part of the electronic medical record, so that it is easily accessible and can be integrated into the patient's history and physical documentation. We train birth center staff to make all staff and physicians aware of its location. In addition, an on-call member of the team is always available to clarify plans and/or to assist with implementation of the plan. When the patient presents to the birth center, the care coordinator and/or members of the NICU team visit regularly to ensure that the family feels comfortable with the implementation of the plan and to clarify questions. In the absence of electronic medical records, written copies of the care plan should be provided to the family, their care providers, and in-patient units. The prenatal care plan is not "written in stone;" it is a place for in-patient staff to validate goals and understand what conversations have already taken place [21]. This allows care providers new to the family to be able to say:

> *I've reviewed your care plan for Joanna and understand that you would like her to be placed on her chest as soon as she's born, so I'll get some warm blankets ready next to you. How are you feeling today, now that Joanna's delivery is so close?*

While the focus of PPC planning is on the parents, the written plan is also of significant importance to the care team, helping them to provide competent, supportive care. In the case of a LLFC, labor and delivery nurses report feeling inadequately prepared and want access to pre-hospitalization information related to the woman's care [32]. Specifically, they need to know plans for obstetric care such as the extent of monitoring and mode of delivery, but they also want written information regarding the diagnosis and prognosis, so they can be prepared for the physical appearance of the baby. They also appreciate knowing what went into the prenatal counseling and how the family came to their decisions [32]. For example, one labor and delivery nurse explained:

> *I think more information would help because when they come here, we don't know what they've already been told, what they've processed, what they've hung on to.*

Awareness of a palliative care plan allows care during the pregnancy to be congruent with the families' goals and may minimize disruptive or emotionally painful questions and actions from providers who interact with the family "as if a normal outcome was expected" [7, 8].

Many sample PPC birth plans have been previously published and are available online on sites such as www.perinatalhospice.org [33]. Most include some or all of the information in Table 15.4 (see Chap. 4 for further details on the decision-making process which will result in the final plan).

Table 15.4 Key components to a perinatal palliative care birth plan

Theme	Details	Considerations/examples
Family and team identification	Names Fetal diagnosis Care team members	Mother, father/partner, other family to be present, name of baby, baby's diagnosis, EDD, care coordinator
Location of birth	Location of birth center should facilitate necessary pediatric support. Can patient deliver at a community hospital or should she be at an academic medical center and/or children's hospital?	Geography, availability of family support, team/institution culture, experience/comfort of providers
Overall goals	Parents' crucial goals and wishes for their baby. This provides a quick overview of a guiding philosophy for their care	Goal examples: "Baby to be born alive for a chance to hold and comfort and baptize. Family desires fetal monitoring and full obstetric intervention" "A physician assessment with possible trial of therapy in NICU or allow natural death if the prenatal diagnosis and poor prognosis is confirmed" "A celebration of birth"
Care prior to delivery	Antepartum monitoring goals Legacy creating	Ultrasounds can be opportunities for prenatal memory-making even if they are not medically necessary. Some families are comforted by them while other families find them stressful. It can be helpful to point out what is developing normally with the baby, along with what is not developing as expected. If family desires a natural death and would decline a surgical delivery, intensive antepartum monitoring (such as biophysical profile ultrasounds) may not be medically necessary
Care during labor and delivery	Mode of delivery Fetal monitoring Timing of delivery	Examples: If the goal is a live birth, the family may choose continuous fetal monitoring during labor and may accept the risks of a cesarean section in the event of fetal distress. Other families may want to reduce the chance of a surgical delivery and thus would decline continuous fetal monitoring.

(continued)

Table 15.4 (continued)

Theme	Details	Considerations/examples
Care at birth	Goal discussions should include: Resuscitation preferences and extent of medical intervention to be provided Spiritual care to be provided Symptom management First moments with the baby	Examples: Allow natural processes (comfort care) vs. assessment and attempts at initial interventions Baptism or other ritual by family member, hospital chaplain, of family's clergy Morphine/Ativan/oxygen Hold in mother's arms vs go to warmer for assessment
Newborn care	Goals may include: Staying with family Transition to NICU for further assessment Transition to home hospice	Intervention examples may include: Dressing, bathing, feeding Set limitations on extent of attempts at curative therapies Determination of whether standard newborn medications and screening are necessary (example, newborn state screen, Vit K, etc.)
Care at the time of death	Anticipatory guidance and education should be provided by IDT to prepare family for care around the time of death What does death look like? What happens to the body after death? Options for accompaniment: Who does the family want to be with them? After death diagnostics? Altruism Funeral planning	Examples: Holding the baby while dying Options for legacy creation/memory-making Extended family, IDT members, or privacy Autopsy or genetic testing Organ, tissue, cord blood, or breast milk donation Options for rituals, memorial service, and extended family meeting the baby, accompany body to the morgue or home Cremation, burial

Support for the Interdisciplinary Care Team

Self-Care and Team Support

In some programs, the care coordinator continues involvement with the family through the provision of ongoing bereavement support, while in other programs, a family is referred to appropriate support groups and other resources. Families often value continued communication and relationships with their team, as those individuals were part of their baby's story. Continued bereavement support allows a relationship with the family for months and years after delivery and not only supports the family but can also be gratifying and important to the care team. When providing relationship-based care, providers must recognize the significance of the loss for themselves [15]. Hutti's research found that "nurses from the diverse specialty areas recognized that through their care of these families they actually became part of their patients' stories for life, birth, death, and grief" [34].

In becoming part of families' stories, providers must recognize that they are both positively and (potentially) negatively affected by the care they provide (see also Chap. 3, section "Moral Distress"). Just as families must determine the meaning of their loss, providers must also ask of themselves, "What does this mean to me?" They are influenced both by their relationship with the grieving family and by witnessing the suffering and distress of another.

Several studies have described potential negative effects of providing perinatal bereavement care: compassion fatigue can lead to feeling overwhelmed and incompetent, using alcohol to relax after work [34], and feeling burnout and depression. PCC providers are at increased risk for work-related psychological disorders [35].

On the other hand, providing compassionate care can also be incredibly gratifying and can provide immense job satisfaction. Hutti described that nurses were "privileged to provide care to women during fetal loss, but they also recognized that what nurses said and did as part of the care they provided would be remembered by these families" [34]. In a study of OB/GYN nursing professionals in Hong Kong, the majority reported positive attitudes toward bereavement care [36]. Much of the job satisfaction comes from being able to provide the best care to bereaved parents and make a difference to them [37]. Supporting the care team starts with not just formal acknowledgement of their contributions but also a deeper recognition of the powerful impact of relationship-based care on those who are suffering. Recognition is acknowledgment put into action. For example, after a death, providers can pause to remind themselves and their team members that they provided good care that "made a difference." Providers may recognize their value when they see that a family's goals were met during the birth and death of the baby and that the process helped to bring them peace. It is important to self-care that PPC providers take time to give such recognition to themselves, just as an effective manager takes the time to determine how each employee prefers to be recognized. An important source of recognition can also come from the PPC team, whose huge capacity for caring for others can and often does include team members. Self-care and other-care may look very different for each provider and may take different forms depending on the needs of the individual, the care team, and their organization.

Purposeful, intentional work by administrators and individuals to acknowledge and recognize the impact of PPC on providers is crucial to avoid counterproductive coping mechanisms. In a study of staff nurses caring for babies at the end-of-life, the respondents reported psycho-emotional response of chronic fatigue, decreased interest in exercise, irritability, and being overly critical [38]. The authors suggest numerous interventions to help care providers cope: exercise and mindfulness activities, prayer/faith, time with family, mutual support among care team members, support from formal and informal networks, and continuing education. Yet if the symptoms of physical and emotional stress make restorative self-care difficult, individuals can enter a vicious cycle leading to burnout. The very activities that may be supportive are the same activities in which providers experiencing burnout may lose interest. For example, if physical activity and social interaction are what these staff nurses need for restoration following their work, their actual symptoms of stress may be getting in the way in their remedies. Acknowledgment of this cycle is crucial for the individual PPC provider as well as for the team around him or her.

Organizational Support

While individual recognition, self-care, and team support are crucial, the stress of providing PPC is also reduced by organizational acknowledgement and recognition in the form of procedures that improve a provider's ability to provide good care to patients [8]. For many, it is not witnessing the distress of the family that is most stressful, rather it is the barriers to providing good care, such as:

- Inadequate staffing and inadequate access to resources.
- Lack of competence. Many providers report inadequate training on end-of-life care which leaves them feeling unprepared in critical situations. Continuing education may not always be widely accessible, and, when it is available, financial and other support may not be sufficient to allow providers to participate.
- Lack of a support system. Providers need professional mentors as well as a "safe place" to be able to debrief from difficult situations. In a study that described physicians' experiences when caring for families of children with sudden, acute life-threatening conditions, the physicians reported that they needed a place where they could speak freely among themselves and use humor to cope [39].

Just as personal recognition of the impact of providing PPC differs between individuals, organizational support for the IDT may take different forms depending on the nature of the program. No matter what form it takes, recognition validates that the care of the dying is just as important as care of the living. Table 15.5 lists a variety ways by which institutions can recognize the impact of their care and support their team members.

Institutional policies and procedures that effectively manage end-of-life care provide a framework for care provision as well as recognition for individuals and teams. In the research of Engler et al., "respondents from NICUs with bereavement/end-of-life policies in place were significantly more comfortable caring for the critically ill and/or dying infant and the infants' families, compared to respondents from NICUs without such policies. These findings underscore the importance of adequate administrative and educational support for RNs and APNs" [41].

An organization offers significant support to care team members by facilitating their development of competence. The receipt of frequent continuing education and networking relationships is an important opportunity for care providers. They want to feel competent to give exceptional care, not just adequate care. Education and communication also provide an opportunity for valuable feedback that can improve practice. In a comprehensive literature review to set guidelines for evidence-based neonatal bereavement care, Kendall and Guo concluded that hospitals should provide ongoing training for staff on grief and bereavement issues [44]. Studies of the experiences of nurses, midwives, and physicians who provide end-of-life care concur that their education for this kind of work was sparse and that continuing education through both formal trainings and professional mentorship is invaluable. Feeling competent in their provision of end-of-life care creates positive feelings in

Table 15.5 Institutional support for self-care in interdisciplinary perinatal palliative care teams

Activity	Comments
Formal or in-the-moment debriefing sessions	Provide an opportunity for storytelling as a method of coping as well as an opportunity to know that providers are not alone [40]
Support of work/life balance	Some hospitals offer the opportunity to take the next shift off after a nurse cares for a family after death
Not taking another patient or admission right after a death	Several studies [38, 41] have demonstrated that the time surrounding a newborn's death can be extremely tense and stressful for the nurses. Not only do practitioners want to provide exceptional care, there is pressure to perfect a once-in-a-lifetime opportunity to assist families in meeting their babies. While the patient may have given birth and her immediate medical needs have been met, her emotional needs are now the priority. Asking the nurse to take a new admission at this moment is a prime example of not acknowledging the importance of this work
Presence of management or other support staff and the availability of help	Many hospitals ensure that all staff are competent in end-of-life care and call in extra staff when a family experiences a loss. This practice has two effects: it ensures the development of many staff with consistent skills, and it encourages self-care to proactively protect against burnout. It also avoids letting any one provider become "the expert" and ensures that patients receive consistent care [42]
The practice of rituals	Rituals may take the form of prayer, formal and informal services, memory-making, or simply taking a "pause" to acknowledge a significant moment [43]
Opportunities to continue the relationship with bereaved family	Providers benefit from witnessing not only the suffering but also the healing of their patients

the care provider (e.g., "I know I can offer valuable assistance during this difficult time") and can also prevent a suboptimal experience for both provider and patient (e.g., "I'll admit I avoided going into their room because I was so worried that I would say or do the wrong thing"). Therefore, organizations providing PPC services should invest in continuing education, networking, and mentoring opportunities to help providers maintain competence in the field. For educational resources, including those on self care, see Chap. 17.

Conclusion

Interdisciplinary palliative care birth planning places care providers in a unique position to partner with families as they struggle to parent their babies following the diagnosis of a LLFC. Through relationship-based individualized planning, care coordinators surround families with a support team that understands their goals and needs, help them make difficult decisions, and guide them in designing a care plan that encompasses the pregnancy as well as the baby's care before, during, and after birth. This care plan gives parents the opportunity to regain some control, feel competent in their role, and be reassured that a written care plan will help communicate and guide decision-making. Interdisciplinary palliative care planning builds supportive relationships between parents and the PPC team, which helps the parents achieve their goal of being "a good parent" as they make decisions about the care of their baby.

References

1. Unintended Pregnancy Prevention|Unintended Pregnancy|Reproductive Health|CDC [Internet]. [cited 2019 Jan 29]. Available from: https://www.cdc.gov/reproductivehealth/unintendedpregnancy/index.htm
2. Gudex C, Nielsen BL, Madsen M. Why women want prenatal ultrasound in normal pregnancy. Ultrasound Obstet Gynecol. 2006;27(2):145–50.
3. Côté-Arsenault D, Denney-Koelsch E. "Have no regrets:" parents' experiences and developmental tasks in pregnancy with a lethal fetal diagnosis. Soc Sci Med 2016 154:100–109.
4. Abramsky L, Chapple J, editors. Prenatal Diagnosis: the human side. 2nd ed. Cheltenham: Nelson Thornes; 2003. p. 250.
5. Leuthner S, Jones EL. Fetal concerns program: a model for perinatal palliative care. Mcn Am J Matern Child Nurs. 2007;32(5):272–8.
6. Côté-Arsenault D, Denney-Koelsch E. "My baby is a person": parents' experiences with life-threatening fetal diagnosis. J Palliat Med. 2011;14(12):1302–8.
7. Lalor J, Begley CM, Galavan E. Recasting Hope: a process of adaptation following fetal anomaly diagnosis. Soc Sci Med. 2009;68(3):462–72. https://doi.org/10.1016/j.socscimed.2008.09.069.
8. Wool C. State of the science on perinatal palliative care. J Obstet Gynecol Neonatal Nurs. 2013;42(3):372–82; quiz E54–55
9. Parkes CM. Guidelines for conducting ethical bereavement research. Death Stud. 1995;19(2):171–81.
10. Limbo R, Kobler K, Levang E. Respectful disposition in early pregnancy loss. MCN Am J Matern Child Nurs. 2010;35(5):271–7; quiz 277–9
11. Cole JCM, Moldenhauer JS, Jones TR, Shaughnessy EA, Zarrin HE, Coursey AL, et al. A proposed model for perinatal palliative care. J Obstet Gynecol Neonatal Nurs. 2017;46(6):904–11.
12. Leuthner SR. Fetal palliative care. Clin Perinatol. 2004;31(3):649–65.
13. Wool C. Clinician perspectives of barriers in perinatal palliative care. MCN Am J Matern Child Nurs. 2015;40(1):44–50.
14. Tosello B, Dany L, Bétrémieux P, Le Coz P, Auquier P, Gire C, et al. Barriers in referring neonatal patients to perinatal palliative care: a French multicenter survey. PLoS One. 2015;10(5):e0126861.
15. Limbo R, Kobler K. The tie that binds: relationships in perinatal bereavement. MCN Am J Matern Child Nurs. 2010;35(6):316–21; quiz 321–3
16. Denney-Koelsch E, Black BP, Côté-Arsenault D, Wool C, Kim S, Kavanaugh KA. Survey of perinatal palliative care programs in the United States: structure, processes, and outcomes. J Palliat Med. 2016;19(10):1080–6.
17. Guon J, Wilfond BS, Farlow B, Brazg T, Janvier A. Our children are not a diagnosis: the experience of parents who continue their pregnancy after a prenatal diagnosis of trisomy 13 or 18. Am J Med Genet A. 2014;164A(2):308–18.
18. Kenner C, Press J, Ryan D. Recommendations for palliative and bereavement care in the NICU: a family-centered integrative approach. J Perinatol. 2015;35(Suppl 1):S19–23.
19. Catlin A, Carter B. Creation of a neonatal end-of-life palliative care protocol. J Perinatol. 2002;22(3):184–95.
20. Limbo R, Wool C. Perinatal Palliative Care. J Obstet Gynecol Neonatal Nurs. 2016;45(5):611–3.
21. Kobler K, Limbo R. Making a case: creating a perinatal palliative care service using a perinatal bereavement program model. J Perinat Neonatal Nurs. 2011;25(1):32–41; quiz 42–3
22. Denney-Koelsch E, Côté-Arsenault D, Hall WJ. Feeling cared for versus experience added burden: parents' interactions with health-care providers in pregnancy with a lethal fetal

diagnosis. Illn Crisis Loss. 2018;26(4):293–315. https://doi.org/10.1177/1054137316665817.
23. Pridham K, Limbo R, Schroedter M. Guided participation in pediatric nursing practice; relationship-based teaching and learning with parents, children, and adolescents. New York: Springer; 2018. p. 458.
24. Brosig CL, Pierucci RL, Kupst MJ, Leuthner SR. Infant end-of-life care: the parents' perspective. J Perinatol. 2007;27(8):510–6.
25. McKechnie AC, Pridham K, Tluczek A. Preparing heart and mind for becoming a parent following a diagnosis of fetal anomaly. Qual Health Res. 2015;25(9):1182–98.
26. Winn P, Acharya K, Peterson E, Leuthner S. Prenatal counseling and parental decision-making following a fetal diagnosis of trisomy 13 or 18. J Perinatol. 2018;38(7):788–96.
27. Hill DL, Miller V, Walter JK, Carroll KW, Morrison WE, Munson DA, et al. Regoaling: a conceptual model of how parents of children with serious illness change medical care goals. BMC Palliat Care. 2014;13(1):9.
28. PLIDA_PositionStatement_OffertheBabytoBereavedParents.pdf [Internet]. [cited 2018 Jun 14]. Available from: https://plida.org/wp-content/uploads/2012/01/PLIDA_PositionStatement_OffertheBabytoBereavedParents.pdf
29. Tucker Edmonds B, McKenzie F, Panoch JE, White DB, Barnato AEA. Pilot study of neonatologists' decision-making roles in delivery room resuscitation counseling for Periviable births. AJOB Empir Bioeth. 2016;7(3):175–82.
30. PLIDA_PregnancyAfterPerinatalLossRequiresUniqueCare.pdf [Internet]. [cited 2018 Jun 19]. Available from: https://plida.org/wp-content/uploads/2012/01/PLIDA_PregnancyAfterPerinatalLossRequiresUniqueCare.pdf
31. PLIDA_PregnancyTerminationFollowingAdverseFetalorMaternalDiagnosis.pdf [Internet]. [cited 2018 Jun 14]. Available from: https://plida.org/wp-content/uploads/2012/01/PLIDA_PregnancyTerminationFollowingAdverseFetalorMaternalDiagnosis.pdf
32. Parker A, Swanson H, Frunchak V. Needs of labor and delivery nurses caring for women undergoing pregnancy termination. J Obstet Gynecol Neonatal Nurs. 2014;43(4):478–87.
33. PPC birth plans (n.d.). www.perinatalhospice.org. Accessed 5 Mar 2019.
34. Hutti MH, Polivka B, White S, Hill J, Clark P, Cooke C, et al. Experiences of nurses who care for women after fetal loss. J Obstet Gynecol Neonatal Nurs. 2016;45(1):17–27.
35. Leinweber J, Rowe HJ. The costs of "being with the woman": secondary traumatic stress in midwifery. Midwifery. 2010;26(1):76–87.
36. Chan MF, Chan SH, Day MC. Nurses' attitudes towards perinatal bereavement support in Hong Kong: a pilot study. J Clin Nurs. 2003;12(4):536–43.
37. Martel S, Nurses I-BL. Experiences of end-of-life photography in NICU bereavement support. J Pediatr Nurs. 2018;42:e38–44.
38. Downey V, Bengiamin M, Heuer L, Juhl N. Dying babies and associated stress in NICU nurses. Neonatal Netw. 1995;14(1):41–6.
39. Bartel DA, Engler AJ, Natale JE, Misra V, Lewin AB, Joseph JG. Working with families of suddenly and critically ill children: physician experiences. Arch Pediatr Adolesc Med. 2000;154(11):1127–33.
40. Lindsay G, Cross N, Ives-Baine L. Narratives of neonatal intensive care unit nurses: Experience with End-of-Life Care. Illness Crisis Loss. 2012;20(3):239–53.
41. Engler AJ, Cusson RM, Brockett RT, Cannon-Heinrich C, Goldberg MA, West MG, et al. Neonatal staff and advanced practice nurses' perceptions of bereavement/end-of-life care of families of critically ill and/or dying infants. Am J Crit Care. 2004;13(6):489–98.
42. Foreman S. Developing a process to support perinatal nurses after a critical event. Nurs Womens Health. 2014;18(1):61–5.
43. Kapoor S, Morgan CK, Siddique MA, Guntupalli KK. "Sacred pause" in the ICU: evaluation of a ritual and intervention to lower distress and burnout. Am J Hosp Palliat Care. 2018;35(10):1337–41.
44. Kendall A, Guo W. Evidence-based neonatal bereavement care. Newborn Infant Nurs Rev. 2008;8(3):131–5.

Part IV

Special Considerations for the Field of Perinatal Palliative Care

16 Considerations in Unique Populations in Perinatal Palliative Care: From Culture, Race, Infertility, and Beyond

Natalia Henner, Danuta M. Wojnar, and Erin M. Denney-Koelsch

Underserved and Minority Populations

Case 16.1
Tricia is a 25-year-old African-American woman, expecting a third baby, now at 34 weeks gestation. She is seeking a second opinion for management of a pregnancy affected by a fetal diagnosis of body-stalk anomaly (giant omphalocele, severe scoliosis and resultant pulmonary hypoplasia, short umbilical cord, myelomeningocele, suspected caudal regression). Her prior maternal-fetal medicine (MFM) and neonatology teams counseled that her fetus has a lethal anomaly, and fetal magnetic resonance imaging (MRI) confirmed the diagnosis. Tricia requested a trial of therapies for the baby as well as scheduled cesarean section with a hope to optimize perinatal transition and avoid umbilical cord rupture. The team suggested that such interventions are futile and requested assistance of the ethics consultation service. Tricia is now transferring her care in order to get a second opinion.

N. Henner (✉)
Divisions of Neonatology and Palliative Care, Ann and Robert H. Lurie Children's Hospital of Chicago, Northwestern University, Feinberg School of Medicine, Department of Pediatrics, Chicago, IL, USA
e-mail: nhenner@luriechildrens.org

D. M. Wojnar
Seattle University, College of Nursing, Seattle, WA, USA

E. M. Denney-Koelsch
University of Rochester Medical Center/Strong Memorial Hospital, Department of Medicine, Division of Palliative Care, Rochester, NY, USA

E. M. Denney-Koelsch, D. Côté-Arsenault (eds.), *Perinatal Palliative Care*,
https://doi.org/10.1007/978-3-030-34751-2_16

Tricia was seen in a joint consultation with MFM and perinatal palliative care teams. She shared her frustrations with the care previously received, and her perception of being devalued, dismissed, and labelled "a difficult patient." She was angry and at times used profanities. She explained her deep mistrust of the medical system (based on her and her family's prior experiences) and pointed to discrepancies in fetal ultrasounds and MRI as evidence of healthcare providers being uncertain about the extent of fetal malformations. She wanted a trial of therapies on behalf of her unborn baby girl and didn't want "to give up."

Tricia cited her faith as a guiding force in her life. She shared that she doesn't agree with the concept of "making decisions," as she believes that her baby's fate is predetermined. She was angered by the idea that medical therapies can be withheld from her and her child based on a notion of futility with which she did not agree. Tricia also revealed multiple concurrent life stressors, including a strained relationship with her mother, history of domestic violence, a complex relationship with her partner, and significant financial stressors. She also shared recent experiences of loss of several family members, some after discontinuation of life-sustaining therapies in the ICU and in hospice.

Following a more detailed discussion of Tricia's approaches to decision-making and goals, she and the teams acknowledged that her baby had a very low chance of surviving perinatal transition. However, a chance of meeting her baby alive and seeing an effort on behalf of the medical teams was paramount to Tricia's well-being and ongoing partnership with the healthcare system. A multidisciplinary team of providers from maternal-fetal medicine, neonatology, palliative care, social work, spiritual care, and nursing developed a comprehensive care plan which included cesarean section to optimize fetal health, an attempt at neonatal resuscitation including noninvasive ventilation, and prioritizing mom's and baby's time together following a resuscitation attempt.

Baby Hope was born at 35 weeks gestation, with a body-stalk anomaly. The neonatology team provided limited neonatal resuscitation including face-mask positive-pressure ventilation, and Hope was able to maintain spontaneous respirations for about 10 minutes, which she spent on her mother's chest (accommodations were made during the cesarean section to allow for that). She was baptized, and her grandmother was able to hold her. Tricia later acknowledged that her mistrust in healthcare providers, her perception of a collective bias against her and dismissal of her values, as well as her life stressors all affected her interactions with her previous team and "made her want to fight." She was grateful for an opportunity to meet her baby and felt that her baby's life had value and was a lesson from God. She accepted counseling from perinatal loss team, as well as a referral to a mental health provider for depression and anxiety screening.

Racial and Ethnic Disparities in Perinatal Care and Outcomes

One of the goals of PPC as a field is to provide expert care for a vulnerable patient population, namely, those mothers and families facing unconventional and complex healthcare decisions. While many important advances have been made, significant barriers to care provision remain, especially for racial and ethnic minority patients.

There is a paucity of data assessing minorities' views on PPC provision and the needs of minority patient populations. Frequently cited limitations in studies of pediatric palliative care and parental communication preferences are homogeneity of participants' race, culture, and language [1]. Few studies include >20% of non-White participants, and most of the studies of parental attitudes require participants to speak English. Therefore, minority patients seeking access to perinatal palliative care are likely under-represented in studies of this emerging field, and sparse data from pediatric palliative care studies are used to provide guidance.

Racial disparities in perinatal care and outcomes persist despite important public health efforts [2]. Racial minority women experience higher rates of perinatal death, intrauterine growth restriction, preeclampsia, preterm birth, cesarean delivery, and other perinatal complications. These differences persist even when controlled for early access to prenatal care [3], suggesting a more complex problem. It is becoming clear that implicit and explicit societal racism, physiologic stress, and healthcare bias are contributing to higher perinatal and maternal mortality [4, 5]. Healthcare professionals also contribute to the problem, by dismissing or minimizing symptoms and stereotyping behaviors [6].

Views on Advanced Care Planning and Decision-Making

Part of expert PPC provision is assessment of patients' views on advanced care planning and decision-making. While there are no studies of racial and ethnic minority patients' views on prenatal decision-making, pediatric and adult data can provide important insight. Many adult patients in the African-American community perceive that advanced care planning can be helpful; however, there are important barriers to consider [7]. Lack of knowledge about palliative care contributes to a common mistrust of the field. Fears that palliative care involvement may hasten death or cause providers to deliver inadequate care are common [7]. Palliative care interventions, specifically advanced care planning, may be perceived in conflict with faith and religious beliefs, and a notion of "giving up" in the face of God's powers to heal may be a barrier to end-of-life care planning. In contrast, Hispanic parents engage with palliative care services less hesitantly and are more open to discussions of advanced directives and hospice enrollment for their terminally ill children compared to other racial/ethnic groups [8–11].

Perhaps in the face of cultural sensitivity (but more likely due to biases), providers tend to misjudge parental preferences regarding prognostic information sharing among racial minority patients. One study highlighted physicians' beliefs that African-American and Hispanic parents want less prognostic information and less information about likelihood of cure and prefer a more passive decision-making role [12]. However, there was no difference by race/ethnicity in how much prognostic information parents of children with cancer want, their desire for information about likelihood of cure, prevalence of a highly distressed emotional response, or preference for passive decision-making. These data are similar to those described by Feudtner, where informed decision-making was viewed as a core attribute of being a good parent, regardless of race [13]. It is possible that some of these misperceptions are based on findings in adult minority patients who are less likely to want prognostic information about their illness [14]. This highlights the need for further perinatal and pediatric palliative care research on minority parents' approaches to advanced care planning, rather than extrapolation from adult data.

Parental Decision-Making

Little is known about approaches to complex perinatal decision-making among racial and ethnic minority parents. Pediatric data suggest that, compared to Caucasian parents, Black and Latino parents report less effective decision-making, less support in decision-making, greater uncertainty in choosing options, and less clarity when discussing and addressing their values [15]. Importantly, parents have less clarity regarding choices for children who were diagnosed with a life-limiting condition at birth as compared to those diagnosed later in life, highlighting further complexities of PPC planning for minority groups. Some Mexican American families of seriously ill children report healthcare-related discrimination based on ethnicity, poverty and insurance status, and physical appearance [16], all likely contributing to decisional conflicts. Unsurprisingly, parents whose primary language is not English report greater uncertainty in choosing options, and language is a huge barrier in understanding information [16]. It is evident that further efforts are needed to decrease mistrust and miscommunication in order to improve PPC delivery to minority patients. It is also crucial to use in-person professional medical interpreters whenever possible (as opposed to relying on family or friends) and to carefully consider an altered dynamic of the conversation. Ideally, an interpreter is briefed on the clinical context and goals of the conversation in order to be prepared for the interaction and best assist the family. The provider leading the conversation should address the family directly, ask interpreter for language clarifications when necessary, and pay attention to nonverbal cues from all parties in the room.

Racial and Ethnic Disparities in End-of-Life Care Planning

An important aspect of PPC is planning for a possible transition to home hospice care. Pediatric palliative care data suggest that there are significant racial and ethnic disparities in children's location of death [17]. One study suggests that 70% of parents want their terminally ill children with cancer to die at home, with no significant differences between White and non-White parents [18]. However, of children with cancer of all age groups, White non-Hispanic children are consistently more likely to die at home, while minority pediatric patients receive more intensive care at the end-of-life and are more likely to die in the hospital [19]. There are several possible contributors to this disparity, including socioeconomic status of minority parents affecting their choices, healthcare coverage, and access to home nursing. Adult data also suggest that terminally ill patients who are supported by religious communities access hospice care less and use more aggressive medical interventions [20]. These are all important considerations for PPC providers as they strive to meet the needs of racially and ethnically diverse families.

Access to pediatric home palliative and hospice care remains sparse in many parts of the country. However, it is critical to take into consideration end-of-life care locations and preferences for neonates and children with life-limiting conditions [9, 10]. Hospice enrollment is higher when there is pediatric hospice accessibility, in conjunction with institutional and state palliative care policies. Pertinent to PPC, enrollment in hospice is higher for children with congenital anomalies, many of whom are diagnosed in the perinatal period [9].

There are important cultural considerations in approaching home hospice care for perinatal and pediatric patients. While mistrust of the healthcare system and perceived conflicts of palliative care with faith and religious beliefs may be more common among African-American parents, there is some evidence that Spanish speakers stress the importance of community and being home for end-of-life care [9, 10, 21]. However, Latino families may be facing additional difficulties of geographic separation from their support networks, transportation issues, and complex immigration status [22]. There may also be additional stressors and cultural differences in how to communicate with the sick child and siblings. However, there seems to be less distress over issues of symptom management at the end-of-life among Spanish-speaking parents caring for their terminally ill children, and few reports of difficulties with doing bedside nursing care at home [10]. Importantly, hospice is somctimes understood as a place and not a service by some Hispanic families, and more detailed clarifications of services may be helpful [23]. In summary, providers should be aware of differences in how families access palliative care and interact with palliative care providers. Attention should be paid to addressing biases and encouraging open communication about treatment preferences.

Cultural Perspectives on Perinatal Palliative Care

Ethnic Differences in Responding to Perinatal Loss

Perinatal loss is a uniquely challenging experience for women. Despite efforts to bring attention to this topic, many women continue to feel isolated and inadequately supported when they experience such losses. Although no studies currently exist, our and our PPC colleagues' experience suggests that fewer African-American and Hispanic patients seek support of PPC services compared to White patients.

Perinatal palliative care and obstetric providers may be contributing to the gaps in care to ethnic minority women experiencing perinatal loss due to incomplete understanding of issues faced by this patient group.

African-American mothers commonly experience feelings of guilt in the setting of pregnancy complications and not being able to access healthcare in a prescribed way [24]. Thus, a sensitive approach to late referrals and timely delivery of PPC is key in these situations. It is more common for expectant African-American mothers to deal with concurrent or frequent stressful life events, such as persistent economic hardships, death of close family members, substance abuse, incarceration of family members, unemployment, and housing instability [25–27]. Minority patients have less access to mental health services, which are often critical to ensure physical and emotional well-being during a challenging pregnancy affected by a life-limiting fetal diagnosis. Perception of unfair treatment due to insurance status may also be common, further alienating providers and families [28].

Less frequent interactions with PPC services among African-American families may be partly explained by preferences for aggressive postnatal therapies and advocacy for such therapies in the setting of long-standing mistrust of healthcare system. It may also be an effect of more prevalent spiritual/religious beliefs guiding attitudes on therapies, not perceiving "choices" in view of God's plans, and ongoing miracle-based beliefs even when preparing for perinatal death [29]. It is also possible that various experiences with other sick family members who got better despite poor prognosis, and more frequent experiences with death of family members, frame perceptions and interactions with PPC providers [25]. This further highlights the need for balanced and culturally competent perinatal counseling, ongoing prognostic humility, and support of families through concurrent palliative and cure-directed therapies.

Clear ethnic differences in responding to perinatal loss exist. Fewer ethnic minority women attend support groups, which can be explained by financial and language barriers, role of family support, role of spirituality as primary source of support, and importance of church-based community [24]. There may also exist a cultural value of "being strong," with many competing life challenges that pose as barriers to grieving in a social context [24, 25, 28]. One study of Arab women who experienced perinatal loss showed many were distressed by common acts of consolation such as pictures and footprints [30], highlighting the likely difference in emotional support preferences and expressions of grief between varied cultural traditions. Importantly, more ethnic minority women have higher detachment scores (defined as avoiding others and feeling withdrawn) following perinatal loss [31], and special attention must be paid to bereavement support and provision of access to mental health screening for women and families at risk [32].

Social and Cultural Considerations in Pregnancy Loss, Stillbirth, and Pregnancy Termination

Cultural considerations influence families' perspectives of pregnancy loss and stillbirth, and PPC providers should be aware of these important social concepts in order to provide most optimal care. The social value of an unborn infant differs among cultures, as well as within culturally similar groups of patients. Varying religious and cultural notions of personhood and/or provisional personhood of a fetus or a neonate may affect how families grieve, express grief, and discuss the loss with family members and healthcare providers [33]. Of note, perinatal death is more common in developing nations, and parents from these societies may express feelings about perinatal loss differently. While it may be described as "God's will," most women experience intense loss regardless of societal expectations for their grief and should be supported accordingly. In addition, there are important considerations for naming and burial practices, with which PPC and obstetric providers may not be familiar. Religious views also influence postmortem examination practices [33, 34] which may be relevant to perinatal planning discussions.

Intersection of PPC and abortion care is complex, but it is not uncommon for PPC providers to assist families making difficult decisions regarding pregnancy termination versus continuation in the setting of life-limiting fetal anomalies. Views on pregnancy termination in the setting of congenital anomalies differ significantly among social and cultural groups, as well as among individual women within those groups. While some women consider the notion of pregnancy termination unacceptable regardless of severities of fetal anomalies, others may appreciate a discussion of this option as part of advanced care planning that falls within the spectrum of PPC. There may be significant cultural and societal variations in what constitutes a "lethal" or "severely life-limiting" fetal anomaly [35–38]. This may lead some women to seek pregnancy termination or request non-interventions for a live born neonate that may fall outside established medical norms in the United States, prompting conflict between families and providers. In such cases, respectful multidisciplinary collaborations are critical to ensure adherence to ethical standards of perinatal care delivery. Much can be learned from women who described their isolation, guilt, and a concept of "chosen loss" after undergoing pregnancy termination in the setting of fetal anomalies [39, 40]. A better understanding of this healthcare decision may guide more nuanced PPC approaches.

Religious and Cultural Considerations for Perinatal End-of-Life Care Planning

Religious considerations shape many families' attitudes and practices surrounding PPC planning. For example, provision or withholding of nutrition and hydration at the end-of-life may be highly dependent on families' religious and cultural views, which are important to address if planning to care for an infant who is unable to eat by mouth [41, 42]. A position paper of the American Society for Parenteral and Enteral Nutrition calls for respect of patients' religious views [43], but particularities of newborn care may further complicate perinatal planning given various interpretations of religious practices. For example, in Islamic tradition, if withholding medical therapies would lead to a child's death, it is considered passive euthanasia, which is not allowed, though discontinuation of therapies when death is imminent is permitted [44]. Families may seek support of their religious community leaders in clarifying their options, and such support should be offered and encouraged. In some instances, it may also be important to assess family's views on brain death versus death after cardiac cessation of activity in order to best prepare for complex decision-making if a trial of life-sustaining therapies is pursued. It is critical to not assume patients' preferences in the context of their religious views, as significant variation in attitudes on withdrawing of mechanical support and brain death exist within Judaism, Christianity, Islam, and Eastern religions [45]. (See also Chap. 11)

Additional practices surrounding presence with the body, burials and cremations, and commemorative ceremonies may be guided by religious considerations. For example, Judaic tradition demands that the body cannot be left alone and a family member must accompany it at all times [34]. Death rituals for Muslim children include ritual bathing, anointment, and burial within 24 hours of death, and these acts are performed on aborted and premature infants as well [44, 46]. Such considerations require accommodations for family members in labor and delivery or postpartum wards, as well as expedited coordination of care and communication between providers, the morgue, and the funeral home. Religious considerations surrounding organ and tissue donation must be considered as part of PPC planning for those families interested in this option.

Some religious traditions (Judaism, Islam) view suffering as a test of faith, and it is important for PPC providers to understand families' narratives even if they are counter to commonly prescribed practices (bereavement support, mental health support, etc.). Patients and caregivers may find meaning in pain, which may significantly affect decision-making as well as pain management at the end-of-life [34, 47], and proactive exploration of these views may significantly improve postnatal care delivery. Some Latino families share a fatalistic ideology or a view that fate is predetermined and may have difficulties with a concept of perinatal advanced care planning and decision-making [48].

PPC teams often provide consultations not just to a pregnant woman but to her partner and sometimes extended family. While each family is unique, there are certain cultural considerations that should be taken into account in order to provide most optimal care. For example, gender roles in Latino families may be highly defined, with mothers the likely caretakers and facilitators of health-seeking behavior and fathers as lead decision-makers who are not as engaged in daily caregiving [48]. Sharing feelings or concerns about illness may not be acceptable to some men, which may present as detachment and lead to judgment from providers. Of course, these notions do not solely apply to Latino families, and special attention should be paid to paternal expressions of grief and communication preferences. Extended family often plays a role in decision-making, and inclusion of extended family may increase Latina women's engagement with PPC services. In addition, such cultural concepts as "respeto" (ways of interaction with authority and elders) may influence a parent-physician relationship and further complicate communication for families in tragic and unfamiliar circumstances [48].

In summary, perinatal loss is a unique experience for every woman and family. Providers need to practice cultural humility, not make assumptions about end-of-life care preferences, and tailor birth plans in accordance with cultural traditions.

Multiples

Case 16.2

Samantha is a 35-year-old Caucasian woman, expecting monochorionic-diamniotic twins, now at 26 weeks gestation. This is Samantha's second pregnancy, and she and her husband Tim have a healthy 3-year-old boy. This pregnancy is complicated by baby A (Peter) having Trisomy 13, with holoprosencephaly, cleft lip and palate, VSD, and intrauterine growth restriction. Baby B (John) does not have any fetal anomalies and is growing adequately. Samantha is being referred for a perinatal palliative care consultation by her obstetric provider.

Samantha and Tim have done extensive online research on Trisomy 13 and have connected with several families through a Facebook page. They met with a genetic counselor, and Samantha has transferred care to an MFM provider. They have decided to continue the pregnancy in light of their religious beliefs and a fear of losing a healthy twin if Samantha were to undergo a selective reduction of an affected twin.

In a multidisciplinary consultation with neonatology, PPC, MFM, and social work, Samantha and Tim shared that they have accepted the risk of Peter's intrauterine fetal death (IUFD) and likely short life if he were to be born alive. Given their personal beliefs and attitudes, they do not desire any postnatal interventions that would prolong Peter's life at a cost of being separated from his family and his brother and want to prioritize John's health and Peter's comfort at the time of delivery.

Given complexities of twin gestation, high risk of IUFD of an affected twin, and risk of preterm delivery of both twins, various considerations for care were discussed. Careful consideration was given to issues of fetal monitoring and mode of delivery (cesarean section for fetal distress was deemed to be necessary as it would be difficult to differentiate the twins' heart rates prenatally). The PPC team discussed possible noninvasive steps to optimize Peter's perinatal transition as consistent with parental goals. They considered a possibility that both twins might be born preterm or that John has a difficult perinatal transition regardless of his brother's state, which would necessitate an admission of both twins to the NICU (albeit with different modes of mechanical support) to allow family cohesiveness. The team also considered a possibility that both boys would be able to go home and logistics of home hospice admission while caring for a healthy newborn. They met with the family several times and helped them draft a birth plan.

Peter and John were born at 36 weeks gestation. Peter underwent noninvasive resuscitation in the delivery room (suctioning, positive-pressure ventilation) and lived for 36 hours. He stayed in the room with his mother the entire time, under the care of the NICU team and postpartum/neonatal nursing teams; he was able to drink a few drops of milk and remained comfortable until he died of what appeared to be worsening central apnea. John received routine newborn care in the nursery and in his mother's room. Child life service facilitated sibling's visits and provided intensive support for the family, as did the social work team and spiritual care services.

Perinatal Palliative Care Planning in Cases of Multiple Gestation Pregnancies and Births

Multiple gestation pregnancies when one or both fetuses have a life-limiting condition present many unique challenges for providers. Due to many nuances of obstetric care of multiple gestation pregnancies, the risk of preterm labor, and possibly varying goals for each individual fetus and baby, PPC teams must closely collaborate with obstetric and neonatal providers. Selective reduction from triplets to twins or from twins to singleton may be of important consideration in these cases, and a close look at risks/benefits to the mother and the remaining fetus(s) must be carefully weighed by all providers.

Providers' and families' attitudes regarding fetal monitoring and mode of delivery for infants with life-limiting conditions have been evolving in the past decade largely due to emerging neonatal outcomes data and parental perspectives. While some women may want to avoid cesarean section for fetal distress, it may be necessary in the setting of twin gestation in order to optimize outcomes for the healthy twin (as fetal monitoring of twins may be more challenging). In such cases, all teams must be prepared to provide routine or resuscitative care to one infant and possibly end-of-life care to another infant in the operating room.

Twin or multiple gestation births in which one baby has life-limiting fetal anomalies pose unique challenges for families. There are several more possibilities to consider; careful attention must be given to timing of delivery, locations of care for both babies, team staffing models, discharge planning, and family support. If intrauterine death of a sick twin is anticipated and efforts to avoid it are not pursued, the implications (both emotional and physiologic) of carrying the deceased twin while still pregnant with a healthy twin must be considered. Timing of delivery may be affected by in utero death of one twin and may lead to preterm delivery of a healthy twin. If both twins are born alive, considerations of care location become important. In case a healthier twin is admitted to the NICU, it may be prudent to discuss care locations for the twin with life-limiting anomalies, as some families would prefer to have twins in the same unit or hospital. If both twins are able to stay with the family after birth, nursing staffing models have to be taken into account in order to provide simultaneous routine newborn care and end-of-life care. Early engagement of home hospice services and a pediatrician may be important if both twins are able to leave the hospital 1–2 days after birth and if getting them home together is a priority for the family.

Challenges of the Perinatal Loss of a Co-twin

There is growing recognition of the effects of perinatal loss on women and families. In cases of twin or higher order pregnancies, decisions, as well as support needs, may be more nuanced, and PPC services may be helpful in both patient care and staff education. Bereavement support for families who have lost a co-twin is complex and is often overshadowed by the needs of a surviving twin. Some mothers share diminished opportunity to express grief as they are focusing on the health of a surviving co-twin [49]. Others put decisions about funeral planning on hold and regret some of those decisions at a later time, which highlights importance of anticipatory guidance if a death of a co-twin is expected [50]. Families share importance of strong connections with the healthcare providers and ongoing appreciation of the challenges of a co-twin's death. Reminders to feel "grateful" for the surviving twin are certainly not appreciated. Families have heightened anxiety about surviving twin's care and well-being and express the need for better continuity of care when the baby is in the NICU [51].

Families often express the challenges of feeling simultaneous joy and grief, and not knowing how to express both emotions. Perhaps that's one of the reasons many need ongoing identification of the surviving twin as a twin, and validation of the personhood of the deceased twin [49]. Many nurseries and NICUs offer symbolic designation on the surviving twin's door or a chart (butterfly, star), and it is prudent to ask parents whether this practice is in line with their wishes. Some families could benefit from special accommodations while receiving care in the hospital, so as to not be surrounded by other healthy multiples in the nursery. Practical considerations for legacy-making may include twin photography or, if unavailable, paintings from photographs of a deceased co-twin. Lastly, given the unique nature of this loss, dedicated support groups may be helpful for some families and may include local hospital groups and online groups such as Twinless Twin and Center for Loss in Multiple Births [52, 53].

In summary, perinatal palliative care for twin gestation needs to focus on many competing priorities and emotions. Multidisciplinary collaborations are key, with added need for flexibility of birth plans and sensitivity to this unique loss.

Infants at the Border of Viability

Perinatal Palliative Care in the Setting of Preterm Delivery

In addition to the usual prematurity risks, many infants with life-limiting anomalies are at risk of being born preterm. Premature birth of an infant with life-limiting anomalies may further complicate PPC planning for families and providers. There are some conditions where preterm delivery can be anticipated, such as those associated with significant polyhydramnios, multiples, and certain genetic anomalies. Other conditions may pose a higher risk to the mother if pregnancy continues, necessitating preterm delivery (e.g., preeclampsia, mirror syndrome in the setting of worsening hydrops). It's important to consider that if delivering a live born baby is the main priority for the family, prematurity may be a necessary trade-off, even in the face of likely shortened survival. Prenatal counseling of families is extensively discussed in Chap. 7.

If preterm delivery of an infant with life-limiting anomalies is likely, expectations about possibly getting home with hospice would have to be adjusted. Emotional differences may surface among women and their partners, as some may welcome a preterm delivery as relief from further anticipatory grief, while others may feel robbed of their time with the baby. It is important for providers to explore and to validate these feelings and to not make assumptions. It is also important to proactively address diminishing options for interventions (such as some surgical interventions or extracorporeal membrane oxygenation (ECMO)) for infants with known congenital anomalies who may be born extremely preterm. Early discussions of how prematurity may affect decision-making and outcomes may spare some families anguish of being denied therapies they were hoping for.

Perinatal Palliative Care of Infants at the Border of Viability

Infrequently, women who undergo pregnancy termination in the setting of LLFC may request induction of labor without KCl injection prior to 24th week of fetal gestation [54], with no neonatal resuscitation to follow. As it's a relatively uncommon practice, PPC providers may be asked to weigh in with considerations of ethics, neonatal comfort, staff support, and bereavement care. Further collaborations with obstetricians, abortion providers, and neonatologists may be necessary in order to provide most comprehensive care to this unique patient population.

Primary palliative care in the delivery room for infants at the border of viability (with or without congenital anomalies) can be challenging. There are no relevant pain scales to use in this patient population, and assessments of comfort are highly subjective. Gasping is common, for which some but not all babies receive opioids [55]. Age at death varies, and parents need to be prepared for a possibly longer ongoing survival than commonly expected. Most neonatologists are highly skilled in providing end-of-life care to peri-viable infants in the delivery room, but some nuances of care (ethics, communication, symptom support) may remain challenging [56], and consistent training during fellowship is needed (see also Chaps. 8 and 9).

In summary, prematurity adds another dimension to the birth and care of babies with life-limiting anomalies. Sometimes prematurity may further limit treatment options, for which parents should be prepared.

Perinatal Loss with Parents Who Have Struggled to Conceive

Case 16.3

Andrea recounted unique experiences of pregnancy planning, the heartbreak of infertility, the joy of pregnancy, and the subsequent devastation of miscarriage through the lens of being a prospective nonbiological lesbian mother in a phenomenological investigation of lesbian couples' miscarriage [57].

It took Andrea and her partner Jackie nearly 5 years to arrive at the decision to pursue biological parenthood. Because Jackie's age was more suitable to become pregnant than Andrea's, the couple decided Jackie would become the biological parent. Once the decision was made, the couple spent considerable time discerning who would be the right sperm donor for their future child. After many conversations, Andrea and Jackie decided to approach a friend they thought would be "just the right person for this." During the study interview, Andrea recalled having a great fear of rejection followed by a sense of relief when the couple's friend/prospective donor and his partner agreed to assist them with becoming pregnant. Andrea stated, "from that moment on we were all in it together." Unfortunately, after a year of failed attempts to conceive, Jackie was officially diagnosed with infertility and Andrea along with the donor-friend and his partner gradually became less enthusiastic about pursuing biological parenthood altogether.

Although they were all ecstatic when Jackie conceived after several rounds of infertility treatments, once she suffered a miscarriage, they collectively withdrew their support for more pregnancy attempts. Andrea recounted how difficult it was to go back to "square one" after each failed attempt to conceive and how devastating it was to experience pregnancy loss. It was equally difficult for Andrea to witness Jackie's gradual descent to becoming self-absorbed, anxious, and absent-minded completely consumed by the process of becoming pregnant. Andrea remembered, "It was a very difficult time for me; I missed my old partner and I wanted her back." After the miscarriage Andrea felt she had to be strong for Jackie and to deal with her own grief in solitude. She recalled, "I expressed my feelings openly mainly in the shower where nobody could see or hear my sobbing. Because I wasn't the one who carried the baby and I didn't have any role models to know how to be a co-mother in this situation, I didn't feel entitled to grieve openly." She also remembered, "the whole process of becoming pregnant brought a lot of stress for all of us; it was like being on a roller coaster ride all the way up and down, over and over again, with no end in sight and it was emotionally draining." Andrea's decision to withdraw her support for Jackie's attempts to become pregnant left Jackie heartbroken and clinically depressed in spite of the loving support consistently offered by Andrea. By Andrea's own account, she became argumentative and emotionally distant from Jackie to the point of needing to seek couple's counseling. Although professional assistance offered by a skillful therapist eventually brought the love back to Andrea and Jackie's relationship, Andrea concluded that "no one can really understand how devastating the whole process of dealing with infertility, attempting pregnancy, becoming pregnant and subsequently going through the loss of planned and much wanted pregnancy can be unless someone actually lives through the experience."

The Experience of Infertility

Grief and bereavement are considered universal human experiences of dealing with and adjusting to death of the loved one. Experts on loss and grief have long recognized the active nature of grief during which the survivors navigate through the myriad of complex emotions while attempting to reestablish themselves as individuals without the loved one they lost [58]. In some situations, people may experience grief over something they strongly desired to have or achieve but were unable to, such as the many individuals and couples who desire biological parenthood but suffer from infertility or recurrent pregnancy loss and, thus, never become parents. Most of these losses are invisible, often experienced in isolation, hidden even from close family and friends. Some authors refer to these life experiences as reproductive traumas [59, 60] that elicit emotional distress, social isolation, low self-esteem, and loss of control [61]. Peel [62], in the study of pregnancy loss among lesbian and bisexual women, asserts that the psychological distress of infertility may be more profound in lesbian and bisexual women than the general population because of the heterosexist monopoly of human reproduction, the difficulties associated with conception for sexual minority women, and the overall silencing of fertility issues for sexual minorities. Others [63, 64] suggest that the incidence of infertility may be higher in lesbian than the general population because lesbians generally attempt pregnancy later in life, once they discern that biological parenthood is something they want to pursue in spite the existing homophobic and heterosexist attitudes in society.

Clinicians caring for individuals, couples, and small groups of prospective parents facing infertility or perinatal loss (like the two couples who attempted pregnancy together in the case study) must be mindful of the negative emotions associated with infertility [61], the grief associated with perinatal loss [57], and the life contexts of the patients [63] they care for. Most of the investigations examining the issue of infertility are limited by cross-sectional design. Individuals and couples seeking infertility treatments, regardless of their sexual orientation, tend to have higher levels of emotional distress than people who are not in treatment because of the invasive nature of infertility treatments and the associated time and financial investment [65]. It is also important to note the importance of social support for those individuals and couples to create a buffer against anxiety and depression frequently resulting from infertility [66]. Lastly, the impact of infertility on couples' relationships cannot be underestimated. Although studies show that the majority of partners with infertility are emotionally supportive of each other at the beginning of infertility treatment [67] within a few years of unsuccessful attempts to conceive, emotional closeness and sexual desire greatly decline [68].

In summary, infertility can have negative ramifications on the emotional well-being and social relationships for individuals and couples. Compassionate care and support, ongoing assessment, and supportive interventions may reduce emotional distress for infertile patients and make their journey toward biological parenthood less stressful.

Pregnancy Loss After Infertility

A life-limiting fetal diagnosis or any unexpected pregnancy loss for individuals and couples with the history of infertility may add to the complexity of the already stressful experience. As discussed in the preceding section, the experience of infertility is similar for individuals and couples from various walks of life and sexual orientations. There are also many similarities between the lesbian and heterosexual women experiences of pregnancy loss after infertility [57, 69]. Heterosexual women who miscarry after infertility tend to feel they have already been through so much to get pregnant that it is highly unfair they have to go back to not being pregnant and going back to infertility, which often involves launching another series of treatments, figuring out how to pay for these treatments, and experiencing anger, sadness, and social isolation [69]. Likewise, lesbians who experience pregnancy loss may feel frustrated with having to resume insemination process as well as feel isolated and misunderstood by others [57]. In many ways research describing everyday experience of lesbian miscarriage is similar to the experience of heterosexual women with infertility.

LGBTQ Community and Perinatal Loss

Like all other members of society LGBTQ individuals and their partners often seek biological parenthood. Yet, becoming parents as members of LGBTQ community involves complex biological, social, and legal challenges that are not part of heterosexual experience [64]. Because childbearing is not an expectation of individuals self-identified as LGBTQ, the support they receive from the family of origin and friends may also be limited. Moreover, many members of the LGBTQ community experience multiple barriers to care in the area of reproductive health [70]. Well-meaning but ill-informed providers may constrain rather than support the individuals' childbearing or parenting efforts. Therefore, seeking biological parenthood requires strong will and desire to parent by the LGBTQ community members in spite of significant life constraints [71].

In a grounded theory study, Ellis and colleagues [70] reported that male-identified and gender-variant gestational parents experienced loneliness that permeated all participants' experiences, social interactions, and emotional responses during every stage of seeking and achieving biological parenthood. The preconception period was seen by the participants as the most stressful time and when they had the least involvement with healthcare. In the Ellis et al. study, similar to gay, lesbian, and bisexual parents [57, 62, 63], some gender variant participants felt comfortable with themselves as biological parents, while others felt constrained by the lack of social support and access to equitable public policies and resources. Therefore, in the context of complex circumstances surrounding the conception, pregnancy, and childbirth for the LGBTQ community, their reproductive loss experience may become more stressful and traumatic than for the general population. The intensity of loss and grief may be exacerbated by the internal complexities of the couple's relationship, the lack of social support, and the time and energy spent to plan and achieve pregnancy, especially where the requirement of seeking a donor external to the intimate couple's relationship and/or reproductive care to conceive are in order.

Just like heterosexuals, most individuals who self-identify as LGBTQ and experience pregnancy loss, require interactions with the healthcare team. The traumas they already suffered may be intensified if the non-pregnant partner is treated as if they do not matter or they have no right to the baby [57, 62, 63, 71, 72].

In summary, there is much evidence that achieving pregnancy and experiencing pregnancy or perinatal loss is associated with universal experiences regardless of parents' sexual identity or gender. However, prospective parents who identify as members of LGBTQ community face additional stressors and barriers associated with parenthood and perinatal loss that are not the part of heterosexual experience. Therefore, they may have additional or different care needs than heterosexual parents and may be at heightened risk for prolonged or chronic grief. Through integrating careful examination of the important grief issues of LGBTQ individuals into routine clinical practice after the loss, providers may develop skills to avoid heteronormative assumptions and be enabled to deliver compassionate, holistic care. This may include avoiding assumptions, seeking alternative resources, and moving away from the traditional understanding of what constitutes family. It is also imperative for providers to be knowledgeable about the cultural and historical contexts that may prevent the individuals and couples from disclosing their identity. Finally, creating an environment of inclusiveness and unconditional support may create an environment of high-quality supportive care offered to all bereaved parents ranging from the heterosexuals to the members of LGBTQ community.

When the Mother Is the One Who Is Seriously Ill

Case 16.4

Karlie and John were pregnant with their first baby. Pregnancy was going smoothly at first. Karlie began having a lot of pelvic pain and saw her obstetrician, who felt that it was normal early-pregnancy stretching of the uterus and round ligament pain. However, the pain escalated to the point that Karlie was having difficulty walking and her right hip was very painful to move. In the first half of the pregnancy, her obstetrician was hesitant to do a CT scan due to concern for fetal exposure to radiation, but at 23 weeks gestation, Karlie and her physician felt that it was important to know what was going on. Sadly, the CT showed a large pelvic mass which was invading her iliac crest and right hip join. She was admitted to the hospital for pain control and a biopsy, which showed a rare form of bone tumor. Karlie and John met with a multidisciplinary team that included maternal-fetal medicine, neonatology, medical oncology, radiation oncology, palliative care, nursing, and social work. They discussed the complex decision-making the couple faced: whether to begin treatment for Karlie (radiation and chemotherapy) which would improve her chances of survival but put the baby at risk or to postpone treatment until the baby was further along in gestation. They considered all their options and elected to carry the pregnancy until 28 weeks, postponing treatment for Karlie by 5 weeks, to allow the baby to reach a gestational age with better long-term outcomes. Baby Bella was delivered by C-section due to mother's pelvic mass and brought to the NICU, where she did very well overall. Karlie was transferred to the cancer center where she began radiation and chemo about a week later. Karlie's disease initially responded to treatment with reduction in pain and many months of good-quality time with Bella. After 6 months, her disease progressed despite treatment, and she elected to stop treatment and pursue hospice care at home. Karlie, John, Bella, and Karlie's family surrounded her as she died peacefully at home.

A challenging situation sometimes faced by PPC teams is when the mother is diagnosed with a serious illness or injury during pregnancy. Medical decision-making in this case must concern the combined health of the maternal-fetal dyad. Pregnancy management and its effect on the fetus must both be considered. A challenging example of this is the mother described in Case 16.4, who is diagnosed with an advanced malignancy during her pregnancy and must make difficult decisions about whether to deliver early in order to allow cancer-directed treatments that would be highly risky for the fetus (e.g., chemotherapy or radiation). As in this case, these decisions are always heart-wrenching and require sensitive discussions that include the risk to the mother to delay treatment and the risk to the baby being born prematurely.

There was a high-profile case recently in which a mother who was 8 weeks pregnant and found out that she had a recurrent brain tumor. The family felt very strongly that termination was not possible based on their religious beliefs and chose to carry the pregnancy as long as possible. She delivered by C-section at 24 weeks since she was dying. Sadly the baby also died a few days later due to of complications of prematurity.

There are innumerable medical challenges to caring for a critically ill mother who is pregnant, with concerns for fetal effects of hypotension, use of vasopressors, oxygenation, radiation exposure due to imaging procedures, and teratogenic drugs

[73]. These should be considered when counseling families, but management recommendations are beyond the scope of this book. There have been cases of a mother having a severe traumatic brain injury resulting in brain death, but successful delivery of the neonate occurred after a mother was kept alive for a prolonged period (110 days in this case) at the family's request [74].

The ethical and legal complexities of any situation in which there is conflict between the best interests of the mother and the fetus are inherently challenging. In general, however, when continuing a pregnancy threatens mother's life, many years of precedent and ethical teachings indicate that the priority must be to protect the mother's life over fetal survival [75] (see also Chap. 3). These cases are always very challenging and emotionally fraught for both the family and care providers. A palliative care team's role in these issues would be to assist communication between family and multiple provider teams to ensure all information is understood and that parents understand the risk-benefit analysis involved in decision-making. When conflict endures, an ethics consultation should be obtained.

Another role of PPC may be symptom management for the mother, including balancing the risks of medications such as opioids for the mother that may have effects on fetal development. In general, opioids can be used safely and effectively in pregnancy, though the infant must be monitored for neonatal abstinence syndrome after birth (see Chap. 9). Pharmacists can be consulted for advice for the best symptom management medications in pregnancy.

Conclusion

The intent of this chapter was to provide an overview of current research and to share insights from the authors' clinical practice regarding the experiences of perinatal loss for specific unique and potentially underserved populations of parents. Research demonstrates that perinatal loss can have devastating effects on the mental health of women and their partners. It is a time of intense emotions for individuals and couples regardless of their socioeconomic background, cultural or ethnic belonging, gender, religious affiliation, or sexual orientation. Grief, anxiety, and depression are common emotional responses to perinatal loss cited in the literature. Still, the levels of parental-fetal attachment vary at different stages of pregnancy and for different individuals making it difficult to make accurate predictions regarding the immediate, short-term, and long-term consequences of perinatal losses on individuals and couples.

The experience families face when the mother is the one who is seriously ill leads to a very different and heart-wrenching struggle in decision-making. Knowing the experiences and needs of the family is essential for the healthcare team to consider, as they strive to provide the most compassionate and supportive care. In other words, it is important for the members of the healthcare team to offer compassionate care and support regardless of the individual parents' responses to loss, socioeconomic or cultural background, or varied life experiences. It is imperative to take the time to explore the context in which the pregnancy was conceived, the stakes it had for the parents, and the meaning attributed to loss. Likewise, it is important for members of the care team to acknowledge the loss. The need for information and anticipatory guidance cannot be underestimated. While the individual experiences, cultures, racial and ethnic backgrounds, and therefore unique needs of parents may vary, supportive interventions such as active listening, providing evidence based information, and offering referrals to professional counseling and/or the perinatal loss support groups have been proven effective.

References

1. Davies B, Contro N, Larson J, Widger K. Culturally-sensitive information-sharing in pediatric palliative care. Pediatrics. 2010;125:e859–65. peds-2009.
2. Arias E, MacDorman MF, Strobino DM, Guyer B. Annual summary of vital statistics – 2002. Pediatrics. 2003;112(6):1215–30.
3. Healy AJ, Malone FD, Sullivan LM, Porter TF, Luthy DA, Comstock CH, et al. Early access to prenatal care: implications for racial disparity in perinatal mortality. Obstet Gynecol. 2006;107(3):625–31.
4. Nelson A. Unequal treatment: confronting racial and ethnic disparities in health care. J Nat Med Assoc. 2002;94(8):666.
5. Geronimus AT, Hicken M, Keene D, Bound J. "Weathering" and age patterns of allostatic load scores among blacks and whites in the United States. Am J Public Health. 2006;96(5): 826–33.
6. Kramer MR, Hogue CR. What causes racial disparities in very preterm birth? A biosocial perspective. Epidemiolog Rev. 2009;31(1):84–98.
7. Rhodes RL, Elwood B, Lee SC, Tiro JA, Halm EA, Skinner CS. The desires of their hearts: the multidisciplinary perspectives of African Americans on end-of-life care in the African American community. Am J Hospice Palliative Med®. 2017;34(6):510–7.
8. Thienprayoon R, Lee SC, Leonard D, Winick N. Racial and ethnic differences in hospice enrollment among children with cancer. Pediatr Blood Cancer. 2013 Oct;60(10):1662–6.
9. Lindley LC, Trujillo LV. End-of-life care for Hispanic children: a study of California Medicaid beneficiaries. Hispanic Health Care Int. 2016;14(4):164–9.
10. Thienprayoon R, Marks E, Funes M, Martinez-Puente LM, Winick N, Lee SC. Perceptions of the pediatric hospice experience among English-and Spanish-speaking families. J Palliat Med. 2016;19(1):30–41.
11. Liberman DB, Pham PK, Nager AL. Pediatric advance directives: parents' knowledge, experience, and preferences. Pediatrics. 2014: peds-2013.
12. Ilowite MF, Cronin AM, Kang TI, Mack JW. Disparities in prognosis communication among parents of children with cancer: the impact of race and ethnicity. Cancer. 2017 Oct 15;123(20):3995–4003.
13. Feudtner C, Walter JK, Faerber JA, Hill DL, Carroll KW, Mollen CJ, Miller VA, Morrison WE, Munson D, Kang TI, Hinds PS. Good-parent beliefs of parents of seriously ill children. JAMA Pediatr. 2015 Jan 1;169(1):39–47.
14. Blackhall LJ, Murphy ST, Frank G, Michel V, Azen S. Ethnicity and attitudes toward patient autonomy. JAMA. 1995 Sep 13;274(10):820–5.
15. Knapp C, Sberna-Hinojosa M, Baron-Lee J, Curtis C, Huang IC. Does decisional conflict differ across race and ethnicity groups? A study of parents whose children have a life-threatening illness. J Palliat Med. 2014 May 1;17(5):559–67.
16. Davies B, Larson J, Contro N, Cabrera AP. Perceptions of discrimination among Mexican American families of seriously ill children. J Palliat Med. 2011 Jan 1;14(1):71–6.
17. Cawkwell PB, Gardner SL, Weitzman M. Persistent racial and ethnic differences in location of death for children with cancer. Pediatr Blood Cancer. 2015 Aug;62(8):1403–8.

18. Kassam A, Skiadaresis J, Alexander S, Wolfe J. Parent and clinician preferences for location of end-of-life care: home, hospital or freestanding hospice? Pediatr Blood Cancer. 2014;61(5):859–64.
19. Johnston EE, Alvarez E, Saynina O, Sanders L, Bhatia S, Chamberlain LJ. Disparities in the intensity of end-of-life care for children with cancer. Pediatrics. 2017;140:e20170671.
20. Balboni TA, Balboni M, Enzinger AC, Gallivan K, Paulk ME, Wright A, et al. Provision of spiritual support to patients with advanced cancer by religious communities and associations with medical care at the end of life. JAMA Internal Med. 2013;173(12):1109–17.
21. O'mara SK, Zborovskaya Y. End-of-life care in the Hispanic community. J Hospice Palliat Nurs. 2016;18(1):53–9.
22. Periyakoil VS, Neri E, Kraemer H. Patient-reported barriers to high-quality, end-of-life care: a multiethnic, multilingual, mixed-methods study. J Palliat Med. 2016;19(4):373–9.
23. Cruz-Oliver DM, Sanchez-Reilly S. Barriers to quality end-of-life Care for Latinos: hospice health care professionals' perspective. J Hospice Palliat Nurs. 2016;18(6):505–11.
24. Van P, Meleis AI. Coping with grief after involuntary pregnancy loss: perspectives of African American women. J Obstet Gynecolog Neonatal Nurs. 2003;32(1):28–39.
25. Kavanaugh K, Hershberger P. Perinatal loss in low-income African American parents. J Obstet Gynecolog Neonatal Nurs. 2005;34(5):595–605.
26. Brodsky AE. "Making it": the components and process of resilience among urban, African-American, single mothers. Am J Orthopsychiatry. 1999;69(2):148–60.
27. Schulz A, Israel B, Williams D, Parker E, Becker A, James S. Social inequalities, stressors and self-reported health status among African American and white women in the Detroit metropolitan area. Soc Sci Med. 2000;51(11):1639–53.
28. Boyden JY, Kavanaugh K, Issel LM, Eldeirawi K, Meert KL. Experiences of African American parents following perinatal or pediatric death: a literature review. Death Stud. 2014;38(6):374–80.
29. Wilson SM, Miles MS. Spirituality in African-American mothers coping with a seriously ill infant. J Specialists Pediat Nurs. 2001;6(3):116–22.
30. Lundqvist A, Nilstun T, Dykes AK. Neonatal end-of-life care in Sweden. Nurs Crit Care Res. 2003;8(5):197–202.
31. Dimarco MA, Menke EM, Mcnamara T. Evaluating a support group for perinatal loss. MCN: Am J Maternal/Child Nurs. 2001;26(3):135–40.
32. Laurie A, Neimeyer RA. African Americans in bereavement: grief as a function of ethnicity. Omega-J Death Dying. 2008;57(2):173–93.
33. Shaw A. Rituals of infant death: defining life and Islamic personhood. Bioethics. 2014;28(2):84–95.
34. Hurwitz PJ, Picard J, Steinberg A, editors. Jewish ethics and the care of end-of-life patients: a collection of rabbinical, bioethical, philosophical, and juristic opinions. Jersey City: KTAV Publishing House, Inc.; 2006.
35. Dommergues M, Mandelbrot L, Mahieu-Caputo D, Boudjema N, Durand-Zaleski I. ICI Group-Club de médecine foetale. Termination of pregnancy following prenatal diagnosis in France: how severe are the foetal anomalies? Prenat Diagn. 2010;30(6):531–9.
36. Bourdens M, Tadonnet J, Hostalery L, Renesme L, Tosello B. Severe fetal abnormality and outcomes of continued pregnancies: a French multicenter retrospective study. Maternal Child Health J. 2017;21(10):1901–10.
37. Usui N, Kanagawa T, Kamiyama M, Tani G, Kinugasa-Taniguchi Y, Kimura T, Fukuzawa M. Current status of negative treatment decision-making for fetuses with a prenatal diagnosis of neonatal surgical disease at a single Japanese institution. J Pediatr Surg. 2010;45(12):2328–33.
38. Mehler K, Gottschalk I, Burgmaier K, Volland R, Büscher AK, Feldkötter M, et al. Prenatal parental decision-making and postnatal outcome in renal oligohydramnios. Pediatr Nephrol. 2018;33(4):651–9.
39. Wool C. Systematic review of the literature: parental outcomes after diagnosis of fetal anomaly. Adv Neonatal Care. 2011;11(3):182–92.

40. Lotto R, Armstrong N, Smith LK. Care provision during termination of pregnancy following diagnosis of a severe congenital anomaly–a qualitative study of what is important to parents. Midwifery. 2016;43:14–20.
41. Chichester M, Wool C. The meaning of food and multicultural implications for perinatal palliative care. Nurs Womens Health. 2015;19(3):224–35.
42. Alsolamy S. Islamic views on artificial nutrition and hydration in terminally ill patients. Bioethics. 2014;28(2):96–9.
43. ASPEN Ethics Position Paper Task Force, Barrocas A, Geppert C, Durfee SM, Maillet JO, Monturo C, Mueller C, Stratton K, Valentine C, ASPEN Board of Directors. ASPEN ethics position paper. Nutrition Clin Pract. 2010;25(6):672–9.
44. Hedayat K. When the spirit leaves: childhood death, grieving, and bereavement in Islam. J Palliat Med. 2006;9(6):1282–91.
45. Setta SM, Shemie SD. An explanation and analysis of how world religions formulate their ethical decisions on withdrawing treatment and determining death. Philos Ethics Humanit Med. 2015;10(1):6.
46. Leong M, Olnick S, Akmal T, Copenhaver A, Razzak R. How Islam influences end-of-life care: education for palliative care clinicians. J Pain Symptom Manag. 2016;52(6):771–4.
47. Mendieta M, Buckingham RW. A review of palliative and hospice Care in the Context of Islam: dying with faith and family. J Palliat Med. 2017;20(11):1284–90.
48. Muñoz-Blanco S, Raisanen JC, Donohue PK, Boss RD. Enhancing pediatric palliative care for Latino Children and their families: a review of the literature and recommendations for research and practice in the United States. Children. 2017;5(1):2.
49. Meaney S, Corcoran P, O'Donoghue K. Death of one twin during the perinatal period: an interpretative phenomenological analysis. J Palliat Med. 2017;20(3):290–3.
50. Pector EA. Views of bereaved multiple-birth parents on life support decisions, the dying process, and discussions surrounding death. J Perinatol. 2004;24(1):4.
51. Richards J, Graham R, Embleton ND, Campbell C, Rankin J. Mothers' perspectives on the perinatal loss of a co-twin: a qualitative study. BMC Pregnancy Childbirth. 2015;15(1):143.
52. Twinless Twin Support Group. (n.d.), http://www.twinlesstwins.org.
53. Center for Loss in Multiple Births, Inc. (n.d.). (CLIMB), http://www.climb-support.org
54. Chappé H, Bétrémieux P, Morel V, Huillery ML, Le GB. Termination of pregnancy without feticide: a French national survey. Journal de gynecologie, obstetrique et biologie de la reproduction. 2016;45(6):619–25.
55. Durrmeyer X, Scholer-Lascourrèges C, Boujenah L, Bétrémieux P, Claris O, Garel M, et al. Delivery room deaths of extremely preterm babies: an observational study. Arch Dis Child Fetal Neonatal Ed. 2016: fetalneonatal-2016.
56. Garten L, Glöckner S, Siedentopf JP, Bührer C. Primary palliative care in the delivery room: patients' and medical personnel's perspectives. J Perinatol. 2015;35(12):1000.
57. Wojnar D. Miscarriage experiences of lesbian couples. J Midwifery Womens Health. 2007;52(5):479–85.
58. Stroebe M, Schut H. The dual process model of coping with bereavement: rationale and description. Death Stud. 1999;23(3):197–224.
59. Boivin J, Bunting L, Collins JA, Nygren KG. International estimates of infertility prevalence and treatment-seeking: potential need and demand for infertility medical care. Hum Reprod. 2007;22(6):1506–12.
60. Jaffe J. Reproductive trauma: psychotherapy for pregnancy loss and infertility clients from a reproductive story perspective. Psychotherapy. 2017;54(4):380–5.
61. Wirtberg I, Moller A, Hogstrom L, Tronstad S-E, Lalos A. Life 20 years after unsuccessful infertility treatment. Hum Reprod. 2007;22(2):598–604.
62. Peel E. Pregnancy loss in lesbian and bisexual women: an online survey of experiences. Hum Reprod. 2009;25(3):721–7.
63. Wojnar DM, Katzenmyer A. Experiences of preconception, pregnancy, and new motherhood for lesbian nonbiological mothers. J Obstet Gynecol Neonatal Nurs. 2014;43(1):50–60.

64. Wojnar DM, Swanson KM. Why shouldn't lesbian miscarriage receive equal consideration? J GLBT Fam Stud. 2006;2(1):1–12.
65. Greil AL, McQuillan J, Lowry M, Shreffler KM. Infertility treatment and fertility-specific distress; a longitudinal analysis of a population – based sample of US women. Soc Sci Med. 2011;73(1):84–94.
66. Rockliff HE, Lightman SL, Rhidian E, Buchanan H, Gordon U, Vehara K. A systematic review of psychosocial factors associated with emotional adjustment in in-vitro fertilization patients. Hum Reprod Update. 2014;20(4):594–613.
67. Schanz S, Reimer T, Eichner M, Hautzinger M, Hafner H-M, Frielbeck G. Long-term life and partnership satisfaction in infertile patients: a 5 –year longitudinal study. Fert Steril. 2011;96(2):416–21.
68. Marci R, Graziano A, Piva I, Monte GL, Soave I, Giughliano E, et al. Procreative sex in infertile couples: the decay of pleasure? Health Qual Life Outcomes. 2012;10(1):140–7.
69. Freda MC, Semelsberger C. Miscarriage after infertility: a woman's guide to coping. Minneapolis: Fairview Press; 2003.
70. Ellis SA, Wojnar DM, Pettinato M. Conception, pregnancy, and birth experiences of male and gender variant gestational parents: it is how we could have a family. J Midwifery Womens Health. 2015;60(1):62–9.
71. Black BP, Fields WS. Context of reproductive loss in lesbian couples. MCN Am J Matern Child Nurs. 2014;39(3):157–62.
72. Grant J, Mottet L, Tanis J. National transgender discrimination survey report on health and healthcare. Washington, DC: National Center for Transgender Equality and the National Gay and Lesbian taskforce; 2010.
73. Kazuyoshi A, Gareth Seaward P, Lapinsky SE. Fetal outcome in the critically ill pregnant woman. Crit Care. 2014;18:307.
74. Said A, Amer AJ, Masood UR, Dirar A, Faris C. A brain-dead pregnant woman with prolonged somatic support and successful neonatal outcome: a grand rounds case with a detailed review of literature and ethical considerations. Int J Crit Illn Inj Sci. 2013;3(3):220–4.
75. Maternal-Fetal-Conflict. (n.d.). Ethics in Medicine. University of Washington School of Medicine. https://depts.washington.edu/bioethx/topics/matern.html. Accessed 15 Aug 2018.

Education in Perinatal Palliative Care for Nurses, Physicians, and Other Health Professionals

17

Rana Limbo and Erin M. Denney-Koelsch

Key Points

- Guided participation teaching/learning theory consists of processes, competencies, and issues, providing a firm foundation for the development of educational curricula for other professionals.
- Relationship-based care includes competencies such as *being with* and *knowing and relating to the other as a person.*
- Teaching communication and empathy skills requires knowledge of specific skills, how each is conveyed between teacher and learner, and the expected outcomes associated with the skills.
- Inclusion of *bereaved parents as educators* in perinatal palliative care education can make a lasting impact on learners.
- Certifications for physicians and nurses are available through several organizations.

Introduction

According to dictionary definitions (www.merriamwebster.com), teaching is the act of showing or explaining how to do something; learning is the acquisition of knowledge or skills through experience or study or by being taught; and education is the process of receiving or giving systematic instruction that can include the theory and practice of teaching through sound educational practice theory and practice (i.e., pedagogy).

Educational theories or models aim to describe learning styles, methods of teaching and learning, and how to ensure that educational methods successfully lead to

R. Limbo (✉)
Resolve Through Sharing®, Gundersen Medical Foundation, La Crosse, WI, USA

E. M. Denney-Koelsch
University of Rochester Medical Center/Strong Memorial Hospital, Department of Medicine, Division of Palliative Care, Rochester, NY, USA

E. M. Denney-Koelsch, D. Côté-Arsenault (eds.), *Perinatal Palliative Care*,
https://doi.org/10.1007/978-3-030-34751-2_17

learning. The publication *From Sage on the Stage to Guide on the Side* [1] contrasts two types of pedagogy. The "sage" (a teacher who primarily lectures) is contrasted with the "guide" (a teacher who helps a learner discover knowledge through supportive guidance). Guided participation (GP) [2], the central theory of teaching and learning in this chapter, is a framework for how to enhance education through *co-creation* of knowledge with both teacher and learner as central. The learner's "empty" mind is not filled with information, skill, or expertise given by another; rather, the teacher and learner *jointly participate* (also referred to as co-creation) [3] in teaching and learning through being in relationship with each other as they attend to the education needs at hand. GP is reciprocal in nature – that is, both the expert (or guide) and the learner teach and learn, as the guide facilitates the learning. The teaching and learning that occur may involve a healthcare provider (HCP) and patient, or an HCP guide and other HCP learners. The patient may also serve as a teacher in absentia through case studies, synopses of patient encounters, and videotaped narratives.

While this entire book lays out many topics that could become content of PPC education (e.g., pain and symptom management, strategies for working with a family to develop a birth plan), this chapter focuses on the *how* of teaching the challenging concepts of PPC education – particularly the difficult skills of communication and empathy. We offer (1) the framework Guided Participation Theory and Relationship-Based Care and Education for teaching/learning, (2) specific teaching methodologies, and (3) information about programs and conferences that offer additional training, certifications, and fellowships. For a list of content resources, see "Appendix." The purpose of this chapter is to help grow the field of PPC by providing educational strategies for relationship-based education that is based on sound theory, evidence-based content, and the authors' experiences as educators that address the learning needs of PPC providers.

The Foundations of PPC Education: Guided Participation Theory and Relationship-Based Care

Relationship-based care is based on the centrality of provider relationships – with patient and family, with self, and with colleagues [4]. The care model was designed to strengthen or transform these critical relationships within an organization. Fundamental to relationships is caring [5] (see Chap. 2 for more about Swanson's middle-range theory of caring). Relationships that are based on the fundamental belief in the worth of the person and his or her ability to make it through a situation (or a learning opportunity) is philosophically foundational for the provider (teacher) connecting in a genuine way. Relationship-based care and education require a caring philosophy and approach and are consistent with the GP theory for teaching and learning. With a teacher who is an expert practitioner who approaches each learner with hope, respect, and care, a relationship can be entered that promotes experiential learning. Learning about providing PPC requires both *education* and *experience.* For example, mentoring by an experienced practitioner that is based on relationship-based education will keep the mentor's skills grounded in sound evidence and effectively transfer those skills to the mentee.

GP theory focuses on developing a *process for teaching/learning* that brings together ideas of participatory learning, learning in a social context, and relationship-based teaching and learning [6]. The focus of the process is interactions between a more experienced teacher and a less experienced learner, with each being resourceful and motivated. This chapter will focus on the three elements of GP: competencies, processes, and issues (Fig. 17.1) [7]. The GP *competencies* needed by the teacher are (a) being with, (b) knowing and relating, (c) communicating and engaging, (d) doing the task, (e) problem solving and decision making, and (f) regulating emotion. The GP *processes* for how to teach include (a) getting and staying connected, (b) joining and maintaining attention, (c) sharing understanding, (d) bridging, (e) structuring the task/learning, and (f) transferring responsibility. A GP *issue* is a problem needing a solution, often a topic or skill that needs to be understood or acquired, which may be identified by either the guide or the learner. The case studies presented will provide examples of strategies for working to solve issues by the application of problem-solving and decision-making competencies.

GP is designed to assist PPC educators in transferring relationship-based educational experiences into a relationship-based PPC practice, with the goal of providing care that is grounded in quality and high-level communication skills. Because of

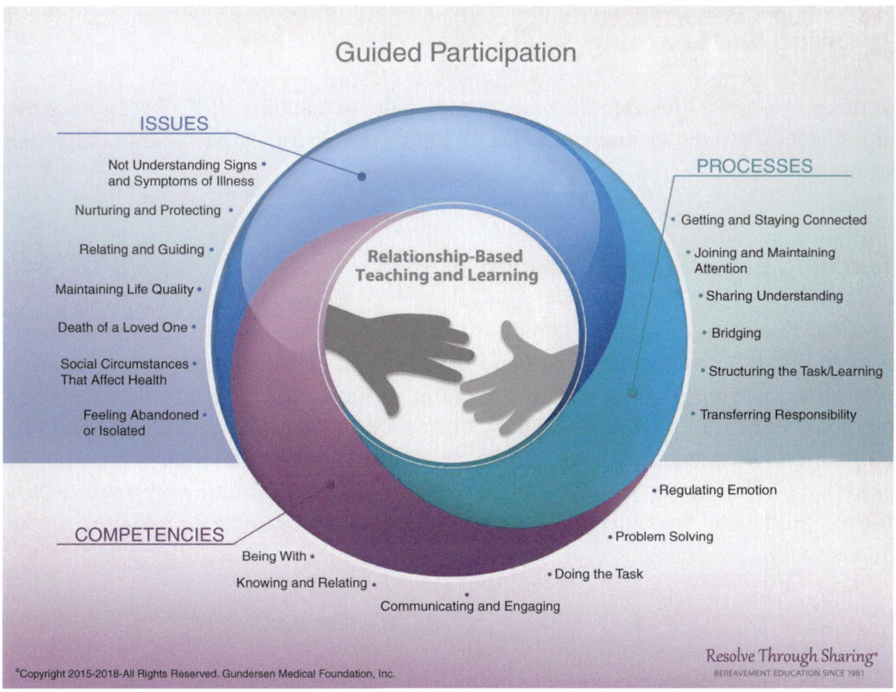

Fig. 17.1 Diagram of guided participation theory: processes, competencies, and issues. (Copyright Gundersen Lutheran Medical Foundation. 2017. Resolve Through Sharing. Used with permission. Guided Participation language from Karen F. Pridham, PhD, RN, FAAN [2, 7])

these core principles, GP is particularly appropriate for palliative care education. ***Good communication*** is foundational to relationship-based care, the kind of care that patients remember long after their interactions with care providers. In addition to good communication, relationship-based care includes ***compassion, empathy, integrity, and trust***.

In the context of this chapter, we aim to assist the reader in developing a PPC practice with a relationship-based pedagogy [8]. Transferring relationship-based educational experiences into a relationship-based practice creates care that is grounded in quality and high-level communication skills and skills that demonstrate *joint attention* – that is, the guide and learner talk *with* each other. The communication is reciprocal, with careful listening exhibited by both. Joint attention is the opposite of talking *at* another; instead, it shows engagement in the matter at hand [9]. Thoughts, ideas, and understandings are in alliance.

In the next sections, we discuss several teaching strategies and the types of topics that can best be taught using each strategy with an overarching relationship-based pedagogy [8]. We list the GP competencies relevant to each learning method at the end of each section. We encourage readers to consider their past education experiences that may have been based on the same strategies to deepen their insight into potential applications to their own teaching and learning.

Teaching and Learning Strategies

In this section, we illustrate the main components of teaching PPC. We discuss several teaching strategies and the types of topics that can best be taught using each strategy.

Teaching Basic Clinical Knowledge

Clinical knowledge, such as symptom management strategies (e.g., pain, shortness of breath), common diseases and their natural histories, and prognostication can often best be learned through reading, online modules, and lecture-based methods. For example, there are many online lectures, articles, and texts available on neonatal pain management. This type of "cognitive knowledge" can often be done by clinicians separately from an interactive session and may require less formal guidance. Structuring the task/learning is an appropriate GP process for this activity.

Case 17.1

An educator is asked to speak to an interdisciplinary group of learners about neonatal pain management. She considers the learning objectives of the learners. She searches the latest literature on neonatal pain perception, opioid use in the NICU, risks of opioid exposure in neonates, alternatives to opioids, and nonpharmacologic pain management. She prepares a set of slides covering these basic topics with supplemental readings. She uses her clinical expertise to provide relevant case examples in which the baby, family, and care team have challenges in pain management. A brief survey at the end of the session asked the participants about their perceived self-competency in managing neonatal pain in their patients. The slides can then be put online for future use.

Parents as Educators: The Richness of Parent Storytelling

Parent storytelling [10] is often described as the most memorable portion of a workshop, training, or conference. The time spent with parents often brings forth an emotional response, both from the audience and the parents themselves. With few exceptions, education for PPC providers should include parents telling their own stories, whether in person or on video. Adams and colleagues [10] found that parents experienced a sense of purpose from participating in this way and that learning was mutual among parents and caregivers. Both groups were able to offer solutions to challenges in using parents as educators, such as ways to avoid having the parents or learners overwhelmed by the intensity of end-of-life care.

When inviting parent panel members, educators should be sensitive to parental vulnerability. Most parents are driven by altruism to participate; nonetheless, they usually spend many days thinking about what they are going to say, concerned that their emotions will overwhelm them and interfere with their ability to speak. If possible, a provider known to the parents is in the best position to share the handwritten or email invitation, which should always include written guidelines (See "Appendix" at end of chapter). It is helpful to let them know exactly what is expected, who will comprise the audience, that there will be a time for audience questions and that tissues will be available. Include specifics about an honorarium, if applicable.

To prepare, you should consider: How long do you want them to speak? Should they bring keepsakes, photos, or other mementoes to share with participants? Will they be the only parents, or will the panel include others? How many? What type of loss did they have? How long ago was the loss? What specific information would you like them to address? Will other parents on the panel be upset hearing the stories of other families? Focal points are often different for each parent so that participants hear multiple perspectives.

Two GP processes that are most relevant to "parents as educators" as an educational strategy are *bridging* and *structuring the task/learning*.

Bridging

Bridging happens when a moderator makes connections to new ideas after a panel discussion. For example, he or she may refer back to a point made by the parent and then share a related idea to build on that information (Case 17.2).

By bridging, that is, by connecting the parent participant's storytelling with her prior similar clinical experience, the resident learned several key points: (a) check with the learner to determine what is going on for her when she was on her phone and (b) express empathy by using relational language.

Case 17.2

A same-sex couple, Janae and Crystal, married for 5 years, share a painful memory of learning 18 weeks into Janae's pregnancy that their baby boy, Jamal, has renal agenesis: The partners are devastated and describe their individual responses to the news. Janae sobbed as she heard the news from her maternal/fetal medicine (MFM) physician. Crystal, in a state of self-described shock, sat at Janae's side while sending a text to their strongest supports, their mothers.

In sharing their story with participants in PPC workshop, an MFM resident is taken back to a similar situation. She remembers thinking, "The partner seems oblivious to what is happening, as if none of this really matters. What is the matter with her?"

Through bridging (GP process), the resident reconsidered her initial impression and wondered to herself, "I decided she was not interested and was on her phone instead of supporting her partner. I wonder if the truth is far more complex. She may have been reaching out for help for both of them."

The next time, she may say instead, "You are being so helpful to Janae by reaching out for support," and "Janae, is there anything else that I could do to keep you connected with your loved ones during this time of suffering and uncertainty?"

Structuring the Task and Learning

The second process, called structuring the task/learning, is used by the guide who makes explicit connections between the parent comments to educational objectives of the activity and carefully planning the content and flow of the workshop agenda.

Using Videos

Video clips are an effective way of storytelling that do not require face-to-face. To decide which families to interview for a videotape, you may want to record an event that is either (a) common to most families having a baby with a life-threatening condition or (b) uncommon, yet potentially very useful for participants to apply in their clinical practice. When you require a high-quality video, consider engaging a professional videographer and editor, but simple videos can now be made on cell phones and other personal devices. It is essential to get parent consent for video recording and to be clear how the video will be used.

The power of storytelling is that it conveys a complex situation within a relatable context to other parents whose circumstances are different but who face the same decision and task. You can guide learners in understanding the story by bridging from your educational session to a clinical practice opportunity.

Guided participation competencies likely to be enhanced through parent storytelling are *doing the task, problem solving/decision making,* and *regulating emotion.*

Teaching How to Give Bad News

Many clinicians find that the most difficult part of caring for patients with serious medical problems is having to be the one to give the family "bad news." Bad news can be anything from something very serious (e.g., a lethal fetal condition in a long-desired baby) to something frustrating to their life (e.g., having to stay an extra day in the hospital for a complication). Although the emotional weight of these tasks is different, the necessary skills to execute the task are the same. The most common method for giving bad news is the SPIKES pneumonic [11], which includes the following six steps:

- *SETTING UP* the interview (preparation)
- Assessing the patient's *PERCEPTION* (patient's understanding of the condition)
- Obtaining the patient's *INVITATION* (permission to proceed with the medical information)
- Giving *KNOWLEDGE* and information to the patient (without jargon)
- Addressing the patient's *EMOTIONS* with *EMPATHIC* responses
- *STRATEGY* and *SUMMARY* (follow-up plan).

This is usually taught in an interactive workshop using role play (can be done in pairs or small groups) or with standardized patient actors (see also Chap. 5, Table 5.1). Case 17.3 shows the distinction between an ineffective and effective "giving bad news scenario."

Case 17.3

An educator is asked to teach "Giving Bad News" to a group of Ob/Gyn residents. She knows that the best way to teach communication skills is through GP. She works with a videographer to create a sample video using actors playing the roles of physician, nurse, and parent(s) with two parts: (a) delivering bad news poorly and (b) delivering bad news in a skilled way.

Example Video Scenario 1

Take 1: *The physician does not turn off her pager. As she attempts to consider the parents' emotions and demonstrate empathy, her pager goes off, causing a disrupted and awkward situation.*

Take 2: *The pager is on silent, allowing the physician to remain focused on the patient's tearfulness and shock.*

Example Video Scenario 2

Take 1: *The physician remains standing, provides no time to allow the patient to express his or her perception, and moves forward with delivering the bad news as the patient looks at the floor in a dazed state and is given no opportunity to ask or respond to questions.*

Take 2: *The physician is conscious of the relationship between herself and the parent from the moment she enters the room. She makes eye contact, enters slowly, and says, "May I sit here in the chair next to you?" Then she asks what the parent has been told about the results of the ultrasound examination. The physician waits, giving the parent time to gather his or her thoughts and time to respond, even though the parent may be crying and answering in a halting manner.*

Role Play

After discussing the two example scenarios as a group, each small group then practices what they have just seen with the actors. Each small group has an experienced observer who knows how to give professional feedback, including asking for feedback from each of the actors (e.g., "What was it like for you when the physician began telling you the test results before you had an opportunity to ask questions or introduce yourself?")

After all role plays are complete (ideally completed in small, private rooms for each group), the groups come together again to review what each person has learned. It is critical that the physician, parent, and observer all provide feedback. The observer should have a critique sheet, allowing for key observations and questions to be recorded. This demonstrates the core concept of the theory of GP, teaching and learning in an interactive setting with a guide who is experienced, has expertise in teaching empathy, and is comfortable developing trust among all participants.

Teaching Empathy: Creating Intimate Moments and Fostering Connectedness

Empathy is a key component of any difficult interaction. Teaching empathy is one of the most challenging tasks, "because, rather than falling into Bloom's cognitive or psychomotor domains of learning, it is in the affective domain along with values and beliefs" (https://thesecondprinciple.com/instructional-design/threedomainsoflearning/) [12]. While requiring more time and different approaches, being sensitive to and aware of empathetic responses can be learned. However, it is clear that clinicians can improve their empathic skills when there is a relationship in which both guide and learner (e.g., nurse or physician and patient) are engaged, finding mutual satisfaction and reciprocity. Phrases that place oneself in the space of another, such as *walking in another's shoes*, *seeing things from another's point of view*, or *taking another's perspective*, are classic definitions of empathy [13]. Empathy can be conveyed rapidly during an emergent situation where support is needed [2]. For example, a father who leans down to the eye level of an embarrassed toddler, with his hand gently resting on the child's shoulder, demonstrates an empathic response by letting the child know that her father is attempting to understand her feelings (regulating emotion). Kelley and Kelley [14] acknowledge that empathy is typically communicated through active listening and comfort skills, which are closely associated with the GP processes of joining and maintaining attention, getting and staying connected, and sharing understanding.

Kelley and Kelley [14] provide a three-step "training rubric" for focusing on empathy in a teaching/learning environment that includes reading, modeling, and practice. ***Reading*** can be accomplished through a reading list that includes examples of empathy and/or through didactic work, such as a lecture with key examples of empathic responses [8]. ***Modeling*** of empathy by a faculty member could occur through enacting a scenario that learners have generated. In PPC, the scenario might be parents expressing a strong hope that their baby will survive his or her birth so they can meet their baby alive. ***Practice*** of empathic skills by small groups of learners (two to four people) could use scenarios generated by the group members themselves or set up by the faculty. This is generally done by having two involved in a role play while one or two others observe and comment, creating an active learning situation that focuses on building empathic relationships. This strategy exemplifies the GP process of *transferring responsibility*.

Empathic responses that may be taught include NURSE statements: *Naming, Understanding, Respecting, Supporting,* and *Exploring* [15]. These skills can be quickly practiced in pairs or in a simulated scenario. GP competencies fostered are *communicating and engaging, knowing and relating, being with, doing the task, problem solving and decision making,* and *regulating emotion.*

Empathy to Action: Developing Advanced Communication Skills

Regarding teaching empathy, Back and Arnold [16] noted that it is important that the provider see emotional cues, respond by naming the emotion, and assess patient readiness to move forward by identifying goals. However, more advanced skills are needed to reach the outcome of learning a patient's "deep values that should shape goals of care." Role play using patient actors or practicing these skills with a trained observer in a real patient encounter are really the only ways to improve advanced communication skills [17]. Back and Arnold espouse that we possess both an emotional and a rational mind [16]. In a common situation with a parent whose child has a life-limiting fetal condition (LLFC), the parent may tearfully express to the clinician (i.e., using her *emotional* mind) that she knows that chances of her baby being born alive – reaching the goal of "meeting" her child while the child is alive – are slim. The clinician can acknowledge her sadness by responding, "I can see your tears and hear the sadness in your voice. You sound so fearful that your goal might not be met." Imagine that the mother says, "But what should I *do* about all of this?" That question brings forward the opportunity to engage her *rational* mind (and thus moving her to problem solving), while still acknowledging and engaging her emotions. The clinician might say, "Well, would it be helpful if we created a plan for how you want things to go that focuses on getting to know your baby even better before birth?" (e.g., she could begin a daily journal of the baby's movements or have more frequent ultrasounds to compare side-by-side with past images). This strategy uses the GP process of *structuring the task/learning*.

Compassionate Silence: *The Art of Listening*

When there really is nothing to say and words feel intrusive, simply *being with* the person is often the best approach. Back and colleagues [18] define the term *compassionate silence* as a way of being with another without using words, which refers to the GP competencies of *being with* and *knowing and relating to the other as a person*. Compassionate silence requires mindful practice [19] and is learned by keeping one's mind intently focused on what needs to happen.

Case 17.4

Imagine that you are at your roundtable at a PPC conference, and the faculty member asks you to practice compassionate silence through role play. You receive the following case on paper:

Imagine that you are a chaplain invited to the bedside of a mother in labor with a baby with anencephaly. At present, the 21-year-old single woman has her male partner and her sister in the labor and delivery suite with her. As you enter, she is crying softly, and her companions are seated next to her. Her sister is on her cellular telephone; her partner clearly does not know how to help.

1. *Rotate playing each role until everyone has had the opportunity to be the chaplain who practices compassionate silence (up to 2 minutes). Select one of the visitors as timekeeper.*
2. *The chaplain introduces herself or himself in this way: "I'm Chaplain X. I appreciate that you asked to see me. I hope to be able to bring comfort to you as you await Angelo's birth. May I sit here beside you? (Chaplain then introduces self to other of the patient's guests.)*

3. *Practice compassionate silence for 1 to 2 minutes. Concentrate on your breathing. Feel each breath coming in and then being exhaled. Work to block out all distractions. Continue to think about your chest as it rises and falls; breathe in, breathe out.*
4. *When the role play is complete, choose a facilitator to lead the group in discussing these two questions (other topics may also be covered):*
   a. *What did you learn about compassionate silence?*
   b. *As Angelo's mother, describe how you felt about the chaplain's presence.*

Relevant GP competencies are *communicating and engaging, being with,* and *regulating emotion.*

A role play around this scenario can apply the GP processes of *structuring the activity* and *getting and staying connected.*

Teaching Advanced Self-Care

Healthcare providers are very concerned and focused on caring for others but have often not been taught to care for themselves. Teaching self-care is challenging because discussion of personal practices that promote good health, although important, may not transfer to professional situations that involve intense grief, uncertainty, fear, anger, and/or self-blame. Papadatou [20] offered a way of understanding caregiver suffering by describing a dual process model of coping with loss-oriented stressors and restoration-oriented solutions. She found that caregivers frequently experience grief, stress, and sadness that alternate with a sense of hope and application of skills directed toward healing and peace. Grieving individuals at times confront, and at other times avoid, the tasks of grieving.

We provide here several ways of focusing on self-care that can be incorporated into the culture of a PPC team. Kobler [21] recommended five large-group practices that foster self-care: effective team communication, administrative acknowledgment of caregiver grief, team processing, encouraging reflective practice and self-awareness, and use of rituals (Table 17.1).

Personal self-care activities can also bring a feeling of peace and give one's mind and body a break from the intensity of working with those who are suffering. Kearney and colleagues [22] surveyed physicians to learn some of the ways they create personal spaces that help them find release from the stress that comes with routinely providing end-of-life care. Some examples are to establish a self-talk ritual on the way home; create a ritual around removing and hanging up one's lab coat or taking off one's stethoscope; meditate at the beginning of each day (even if it is brief); pause and take three to five deep breaths prior to a procedure or seeing a new patient [23]; pause in front of a window and take in what nature has to offer; or take a break to check in with a colleague who had a bad day. Devoting careful attention

Table 17.1 Workplace activities for fostering self-care [21]

Type of activity	Ways of enacting the self-care activity
Effective team communication	Use two communication point persons (for family and HCPs); among HCPs
	Guarantee uninterrupted time for completion of documentation and vital records
Administrative acknowledgment of caregiver grief	Acknowledge caregiver grief (e.g., be visible during death
	Offer 1:1 support to HCPs
	Time for team debriefing
	Time for staff self-care
Team processing	Peer or mentor support
	Reflective practice
	Promoting self-care
	Co-creating ritual
Encouraging reflective practice and self-awareness	Provide reflection room (low lighting, music, symbols, inspirational reading)
Use of rituals	Encourage in-the-moment activities that bear witness to suffering (e.g., blessing of NICU space where baby died)

Summary from Kobler [21], https://journals.lww.com/mcnjournal/Abstract/2014/05000/Leaning_In_and_Holding_On__Team_Support_with.4.aspx, with permission from Wolters Kluwer Health, Inc.

to your own list of personal self-care activities is an important topic to include in all types of PPC education.

One-Day PPC Workshop

An all-day workshop can provide a general overview of PPC, with interdisciplinary speakers addressing topics from their own fields (Table 17.2). It could also be a more focused event with numerous speakers discussing a similar topic (e.g., supporting children through the PPC process, starting a PPC program [24], or planning for eventualities in pregnancy and birth of a baby with a life-limiting diagnosis). A workshop this long calls for a planning committee to ensure relevant content, to divide the labor, and to institute a variety of teaching strategies. A liaison is needed to welcome guests and to interact with the group from the podium and during lunch and breaks. All guest speakers should be encouraged to spend the whole day at the workshop so they can engage with learners. It is optimal if speakers refer to content from previous talks to help weave together content and enable learners to see links from one aspect of a topic to another (GP process: *transferring*).

Speakers may use handouts for discussions by all participants seated at a table, who can then practice communication skills in pairs. Other methods include lecture with large-group discussion (ask speakers to allow 5–10 min at the end of their

Table 17.2 Sample agenda for a 1-day perinatal palliative care workshop for healthcare professionals

Broad topics	Specific topics
Overview of perinatal palliative care (1 hour)	Theories and/or concepts that explore, explain, and describe parent and infant relationship in the perinatal period
	Define/cite caregiving theory
	Statistics
	Barriers
	Benefits
	Characteristics
	Team members
Difficult conversations (1 hour)	Running a family meeting
	Delivering bad news
	Assessing goals of care
Parental decision-making and birth planning (1 hour)	How parents make decisions
	Creating a unified care plan (birth plan)
	The role of hope
	Regoaling
	Advances in early prenatal diagnostic testing
	Supporting a family with breastfeeding or breast milk donation
	Tissue and organ donation
Parent panel (1 hour)	Parent stories and perspectives
	Meaning-making and legacy
	Spiritual and/or religious needs
Caring for siblings (30 min)	Legacy creation with children
	The role of child life specialists for grieving children
Caring for the care team (30 min)	Team debriefing
	Strategies for education
	Individual strategies for self-care
	Spiritual and/or religious needs
	Mindfulness
	Coping with moral distress
	Understanding best interest and virtue ethics
Comfort care and symptom management (1 hour)	Pain and symptom management
	Positioning
	Temperature regulation
	Comfort through photos
Systems and organizations (1 hour)	Billing, coding
	Funding
	Weaving PPC services into an existing perinatal bereavement program
	Ongoing education for those who refer families to PPC (e.g., identifying appropriate families, opening the door to discussion, awareness of PPC services)

presentation for audience questions); an interprofessional panel; or a role play by volunteers in front of the entire group, guided by a speaker and illustrating aspects of the speaker's content. These strategies keep a full day interesting if planners change approaches and topics to keep participants engaged, but also intertwine topics to create continuity and reinforcement. GP Competencies: All.

Educational Assessment

Measurement of learning outcomes (assessing your educational activity) is essential for high-quality education. Changes in practice patterns or improvements in empathic communication skills are notoriously challenging to measure. Self-report is often the simplest way to measure, but also the least reliable.

The statement below was written by an experienced labor and delivery nurse after attending a 2-day, relationship-based training on perinatal bereavement that included content on PPC and pregnancy after loss. The participant's response, written a week later, shows evidence of changed practice after the educational experience:

> I had a patient give birth to her rainbow baby [a baby conceived and born after a pregnancy loss] this week. While everyone else was ecstatic and felt like she should be deliriously happy, I was able to sit and talk with her about the melancholy emotions this second birth evoked in her. We were able to look at pictures of both babies together and compare their similarities and differences. In short, we were able to give credence to her parenting experience of her first baby that she lost.

Qualitative data from narratives like the nurse's comment are powerful. Alternatively, a simple measure of outcomes may be included in a post-session evaluation form: "This educational experience has changed (or will change) my practice in the following ways: __________." A survey can measure the learner's comfort level or perceived self-competence before and after an educational offering. Patient interactions can be evaluated more thoroughly by others who are trained to observe specific skills (such as use of empathic statements – e.g., "I wish" statements [25]: "I wish I had different news"). Global assessment by supervisors can be helpful but fairly subjective. The most important thing is to assess your educational offering in a way that ascertains whether you are achieving your stated goals.

Clinician Training and Educational Opportunities

Fellowship Training and Board Certification (Physicians)

To become a board-certified hospice and palliative medicine (HPM) physician, one must complete a 1-year HPM fellowship program accredited by the Accreditation Council for Graduate Medical Education (ACGME) and pass the HPM Board Examination. HPM fellowships can be undertaken by physicians of many specialties [26]. Fellowship-trained physicians have intensive training in clinical skills in adult medicine, pediatrics, inpatient and outpatient settings, home care and hospice, and long-term care. They participate in quality improvement projects and work on a scholarly project. Most pediatric physicians participate in a pediatric track within an adult fellowship, although some larger children's hospitals offer pediatric-specific fellowship programs. Pediatric fellowships and tracks are available on the American Academy of Hospice and Palliative Medicine (AAHPM) website [27].

HPM fellowship guidelines do not specifically require PPC training, but most pediatric programs see many seriously ill newborns, and some also have robust prenatal/perinatal consultation services.

Non-fellowship Training for Physicians and Other Clinicians

Many clinicians cannot take time away from practice to complete a 1-year fellowship, but more general palliative care training in clinical management and difficult conversations is available in several formal settings and in local courses. Training in advanced pain and symptom management is available through workshops offered at local, regional, and national meetings and conferences (Table 17.3).

Difficult Conversation Training

The most well-known training program is VitalTalk [28], which was founded for training oncologists in communication but has been widely used by providers in other disciplines who want more experience in difficult conversations. The program offers online and in-person faculty development courses on delivering serious news and mastering tough conversations. We are not aware of courses on difficult conversations specific to PPC.

Certificate Programs for Nurses and Other Licensed Professionals

Certifications offered by the Hospice and Palliative Credentialing Center (HPCC) of the Hospice and Palliative Nurses Association include online study guides and suggested readings and education offerings, a schedule of test offerings, and instructions for preparing and registering for the examinations, among them the Certified Hospice and Palliative Pediatric Nurse (CHPPN) [29] and Certified in Perinatal Loss Care (CPLC) [30]. Recertification is also available. CPLC is the only program offered by HPCC that is interprofessional and available to all licensed professionals who care for bereaved families (e.g., nurses, social workers, chaplains, physicians, child life specialists).

Other Resources

A number of national and international organizations provide educational content at meetings and through webinars, newsletters, listservs, or interactive online platforms. The organizations and their key pediatric and PPC-specific resources are listed in Table 17.3.

Table 17.3 Resources for education and training in perinatal palliative care

Organization	Resources
American Academy of Hospice and Palliative Medicine (AAHPM) [31]	Pediatrics special interest group (SIG)
	Pediatric topics at annual assembly
	Pediatrics-specific conference
	Connect page for pediatric SIG members
	Fellowship director special interest group
	Fellowship-director pre-conference workshop at annual assembly
	Connect page for fellowship director SIG members
	Education special interest group
	Interactive educational exchange at annual assembly
	Connect page for education SIG members
American Academy of Pediatrics (AAP) [32]	Section on hospice and palliative medicine (SOHPM)
	Listserv for palliative care providers (all professions), families
	Advocacy, position statements
Center to Advance Palliative Care (CAPC) [33]	Provides essential tools, training, technical assistance, and metrics to build and sustain palliative care in all healthcare settings Website, conferences, and webinars available
End-of-life nursing education consortium (ELNEC) [34] EPEC (education in palliative and end-of-life care) [35]	The ELNEC project is a national education initiative to improve palliative care
	Partnership between the American Association of Colleges of nursing (AACN), Washington, DC, and the City of Hope, Duarte, CA
	The project provides undergraduate and graduate nursing faculty, CE providers, staff development educators, specialty nurses in pediatrics, oncology, critical care, and geriatrics, and other nurses with training in palliative care so they can teach this essential information to nursing students and practicing nurses
	Over 22,500 nurses and other health professionals trained through national programs
	Taken from http://www.aacnnursing.org/Portals/42/ELNEC/PDF/FactSheet.pdf [34]
	Offers online and in-person training curriculum, train-the-trainer courses Pediatric-specific adaptation to core curriculum
National Hospice and Palliative Care Organization (NHPCO) [36]	ChiPPS newsletter: free, regular contributions on palliative care, available online

Pediatric Palliative Care and End of Life Treatment (Boston Children's Hospital/Harvard Medical School Teaching Hospital) [37]	3.5-hour course for practitioners who treat pediatric palliative care patients
Pediatric Palliative Care Research Network (PPCRN) [38]	Organization of pediatric palliative care providers who are involved in pediatric PC research. Mission to foster collaboration, advanced research questions, increased investigators, enable evidence-based practice
Perinatal Hospice and Palliative Care [39]	Website founded by Amy Kuebelbeck, author of *Waiting With Gabriel* and coauthor of *A Gift of Time*
	Lists over 300 PPC programs worldwide
	Provides examples of care plans and other relevant documents to assist those who are beginning or expanding PPC programs or services
	Keeps updated list of recent publications
Pregnancy Loss and Infant Death Alliance [40]	Biennial International Perinatal Bereavement Conference
	Website with Ask PLIDA and position statements as member benefits
	Interprofessional membership organization
	Strong focus on PPC and evidence-based practice
	Provides numerous opportunities for volunteers
	Consists of board of directors and the following committees: Education, development, governance, conference planning, and others
Resolve Through Sharing [41]	PPC education as part of perinatal bereavement and neonatal/pediatric trainings
	Train-the- Trainer education available (RTS Coordinators)
	PPC toolkit
	Parent resources (reading material, memory boxes)
	PPC Position Paper (www.resolvethroghsharing.org)
	Bereavement trainings across the lifespan (perinatal; neonatal and pediatric; adult)
State-Wide Coalitions	On-site conferences, webinars (state-dependent)

Acknowledgements The authors are grateful to Cathy Mikkelson Fischer, MA, ELS, for her assistance with this chapter. She is Managing Editor/Writer for the Department of Medical Research, Gundersen Medical Foundation, Inc., La Crosse, Wisconsin.

Appendix: Supplementary Materials/Additional Readings

Exemplary Articles to Prepare for Designing Relationship-based Education, Programs, and Services in Perinatal Palliative Care

Title of article	Major points
Davies B, Steele R, Krueger G, Albersheim S, Baird J, Fibirie M, et al. Best practice in provider/parent interaction. Qual Health Res. 2017;27:406–20 [42]	Using grounded theory methodology, researchers of this unique study identified the conceptualization of "best practice healthcare providers (BPHCPs)" (p. 406). The results were published with categories of Connecting Behaviors (p.411–2); Direct Care Activities (p. 412–5); and Personal and Contextual Influencing Factors (p. 415–6). For example, they identified eight connecting behaviors: trust, listening, empathizing, suspending judgment, pacing, maintaining hope, focusing on the positive, and showing kindness. Conversely, failing to care for a patient's heart in the way described above lives on in one's memory, likely causing suffering and the inability to undo the pain
	These connecting behaviors, although seemingly simple, have not previously been seen as a necessary combination in caring for patients and families. These types of relationships remain in one's memory, often throughout life. Expert communication skills in professional education affect the one cared for – and those doing the caring – holistically. The way the authors write about relationship is a lesson in caring for the patient's heart, something rarely addressed in depth
Browning DM, Solomon MZ. Relational learning in pediatric palliative care: transformative education and the culture of medicine. Child Adolesc Psychiatr Clin N Am. 2006;15:795–815 [43]	Although published over a decade before the reported findings by Davies and colleagues (above), the "pedagogy and process" (p. 797) of the Initiative for Pediatric Palliative Care (IPPC) bear strong similarities to other relational pedagogy models covered in this chapter. The authors offer practical suggestions for educating that incorporate the everyday social processes typically in place in a center that provides interprofessional staff education. They emphasize the following points: target a few units at a time (e.g., labor and delivery and NICU); piggyback on existing education such as grand rounds, staff meetings, noon conference, maternal or pediatric morbidity conferences, and interprofessional debriefings. Most if not all these opportunities will function as higher-quality relational learning provided they have "relational teachers" (p. 806). Browning and Solomon consider the integration of patients and families into any or all these relational learning opportunities as essential. They consider "real family-centered care," "real partnerships with parents," and "real listening to children" as requiring organizational commitment (p. 808)

Title of article	Major points
Limbo R. Resolve Through Sharing bereavement education model. La Crosse, WI: Gundersen Medical Foundation, Inc.; 2008, 2017, 2018. Retrieved from http://www.gundersenhealth.org/resolve-through-sharing/resources/ [44]	This position statement summarizes much of what has been written in this manuscript. Effective education is relationship-based and offers a variety of methods. One unique strategy is parallel process. For example, if teaching is done by a two-person team, learners watch the instructors relate to each other and thereby use observations to create their own ways of teaching and/or caring for patients and families in a relational way
Limbo R, Kobler K. The tie that binds: relationships in perinatal bereavement. MCN: Am J Matern Child Nurs. 2010;35:316–21 [45]	Relationship is highly relevant in education and clinical practice. The authors identify numerous examples of relationships in perinatal bereavement, which includes PPC. Examples include baby and parents, parents with each other, parents and HCP, HCP and baby, and siblings and parents, reinvesting in relationship through self-care, continuing and maintaining relationship through follow-up
Ballantine A, Feudtner C. The 10 R's of clinician education: a checklist. Arch Pediatr Adolesc Med. 2010;163:389–90 [46]	Written for physicians, but equally relevant to all PPC professionals, a sample of the 10 Rs of clinical education include relevant, researched, relational, reflective, and repetition. The authors emphasize that the "sage on the stage" (meaning lecturer serving as the expert, transmitting knowledge to an audience of learners using animated slides and video and Web links) model is insufficient and requires the relatively new discipline of "instructional design" (p. 389)
Pridham K, Limbo R, Schroeder M, editors. Guided participation in pediatric nursing practice: relationship-based teaching and learning with parents, children, and adolescents. New York, NY: Springer Publishing; 2018 [2]	Chapters 1, 2, 22, 23
	Chapter 1: Guided participation theory for teaching and learning in clinical practice (Pridham K, Scott A, Limbo R). "Clinicians may assume they are doing guided participation when initiating and maintaining open-ended discussion about what is going on for parents, what is on their minds, and what they are doing about it. Guided participation, however, is a practice (Lave, 1993). In addition to expectation of active engagement of parents [of babies with a life-limiting fetal condition], guided participation is oriented to the learner's life circumstances or issues and, in that context, is directed to increasing competencies for addressing these circumstances with improved, maintained, or promoted health" (p. 11)

(continued)

Title of article	Major points
	Chapter 2: Relationship-based approach to caring for children with serious illness (Kobler K)
	Professional self-assessment is critical for understanding what one brings to a relationship. Dr. Kobler described *PRAM* (*P*ause, *R*eflect, *A*cknowledge, and be *M*indful) as a way of doing so. For example, one could pause and reflect on "How does this child's situation remind me of past experiences with other children?" (the GP process of bridging) (p. 22)
	Chapter 22: Using principles of guided participation to develop and maintain a bereavement program [Resolve Through Sharing – RTS] (Hensel M, Limbo R)
	Relationship was central to RTS at its inception: among team members, in structure and process of the program, through design of materials, and most importantly in communication skills between care provider and patient, pre- and post-training assessments showed statistically significant positive change in participants' comfort, skills, and knowledge, all designed to focus on relationship
	Chapter 23: Case examples: Using "holding in mind" and "joining attention" as relational strategies (Limbo R).
	"Holding in mind" (or being held in mind) refers to a way of being in relationship. Essentially, holding someone in mind is thinking about that person in their absence. This is a powerful process and may be unfamiliar to those who may live in a deprived or even abusive environment. Saying, "I've been thinking about you" is a simple way of describing holding someone in mind
	Many who learn guided participation initially are intrigued by the idea of "joining attention" or "joint attention." Think of times when you have heard someone describe another as being "noncompliant" or "failing treatment." More accurately, the HCP failed to make the instructions clear enough (i.e., failed to gain joint attention) or the treatment failed the patient. These descriptions of joint attention highlight relationship and respect
Hinsdale MJ. Relational pedagogy. Oxford Research Encyclopedia of Education (Published online December 2016) [47]	"The words *care* and *caring* often arise in discussions of teaching, and perhaps not surprisingly, we can trace the roots of relational pedagogy to the literature on caring
	Carol Gilligan's landmark work *In a Different Voice* [48] offers a woman's perspective on moral responsibility, one based on caring and relationship" (p. 3)

Guidelines for Preparing Letters to Bereaved Parent Educators Inviting Them to Participate on a Parent Panel

1. Address the invitees and their baby by name (extend this to the actual presentation by using name tents with names in large, dark-colored font)
2. Explain what is expected of them
3. Describe the audience

4. Include complete directions, parking instructions, what time to arrive, where to wait, and who will meet them. Ask them to arrive approximately a half hour before the session begins
5. Assure them that they will be reimbursed for mileage, tolls, and parking
6. Define the amount of time they will be asked to talk
7. Describe the facilitator's role
8. Invite them to bring photos, cards, and/or other keepsakes
9. Assure them that they are not expected to answer any questions that they are not comfortable with and that the facilitator will help move the discussion forward if needed
10. Define a short list of questions you would like them to address in their presentation
11. To ensure anonymity, remind them to *avoid* giving any personal identifying information. This includes organization names, names of all HCPs, and names of other parents
12. Ask that they help participants learn how to give high-quality care by describing what things were the most helpful and what were the least helpful in all interactions with HCPs. This could include how the news was delivered, how the ultrasound went, how advance care planning was completed, and how their baby's comfort care was delivered
13. Be certain the parent(s) has a telephone number and email address to connect with the contact person

References

1. King A. From sage on the stage to guide on the side. Coll Teach. 1993;41(1):30–5. https://doi.org/10.1080/87567555.1993.9926781.
2. Pridham KF, Limbo R, Schroeder MM, editors. Guided participation in pediatric nursing practice: relationship-based teaching and learning with parents, children, and adolescents. New York: Springer Publishing Company, LLC; 2018.
3. Pridham KF, Scott A, Limbo R. Guided participation theory for teaching and learning in clinical practice. In: Pridham KF, Limbo R, Schroeder MM, editors. Guided participation in pediatric nursing practice: relationship-based teaching and learning with parents, children, and adolescents. New York: Springer Publishing Company, LLC; 2018. p. 3–19.
4. Koloroutis, M. Overview. Advancing Relationship-based Cultures, Koloroutis, M., & Abelson, D. (Eds.). Minneapolis, MN: Creative Health Care Management 2017;3–18.
5. Nurse-Clarke N, DiCicco-Bloom B, Limbo R. Application of caring theory to nursing Care of Women Experiencing Stillbirth. MCN Am J Matern Child Nurs. 2019;44(1):27–32. https://doi.org/10.1097/NMC.0000000000000494.
6. Kitzman HJ. Foreword. In: Pridham KF, Limbo R, Schroeder MM, editors. Guided participation in pediatric nursing practice: relationship-based teaching and learning with parents, children, and adolescents. New York: Springer Publishing Company, LLC; 2018. p. xix–xxii.
7. Gundersen Lutheran Medical Foundation. (n.d.). Resolve through sharing.
8. Hinsdale MJ. Relational pedagogy. In: Noblit GW, editor. Oxford research encyclopedia of education. New York: Oxford University Press; 2016.
9. Limbo R. Case examples: using "holding in mind" and "joining attention" as relational strategies. In: Pridham KF, Limbo R, Schroeder MM, editors. Guided participation in pediatric

nursing practice: relationship-based teaching and learning with parents, children, and adolescents. New York: Springer Publishing Company, LLC; 2018. p. 403–10.
10. Adams G, Green A, Towe S, Huett A. Bereaved caregivers as educators in pediatric palliative care: their experiences and impact. J Palliat Med. 2013;16:609–15. https://doi.org/10.1089/jpm.2012.0475.
11. Baile WF, Buckman R, Lenzi R, Glober G, Beale EA, Kudelka AP. SPIKES-A six-step protocol for delivering bad news: application to the patient with cancer. Oncologist. 2000;5:302–11. https://doi.org/10.1634/theoncologist.5-4-302.
12. The Second Principle. (n.d.). https://thesecondprinciple.com/instructional-design/threedomainsoflearning/. Accessed 7-19-19.
13. Basch MF. Empathic understanding: a review of the concept and some theoretical considerations. J Am Psychoanal Assoc. 1983;31:101–26. https://doi.org/10.1177/000306518303100104.
14. Kelley KJ, Kelley MF. Teaching empathy and other compassion-based communication skills. J Nurses Prof Dev. 2013;29:321–4. https://doi.org/10.1097/01.NND.0000436794.24434.90.
15. VitalTalk. Responding to emotion: articulating empathy using NURSE statements; 2018. Available from: https://www.vitaltalk.org/guides/responding-to-emotion-respecting/.
16. Back AL, Arnold RM. "Yes it's sad, but what should I do?" Moving from empathy to action in discussing goals of care. J Palliat Med. 2014;17:141–4. https://doi.org/10.1089/jpm.2013.0197.
17. Dadiz R, Spear ML, Denney-Koelsch E. Teaching the art of difficult family conversations. J Pain Symptom Manag. 2017;53:157–61.e2. https://doi.org/10.1016/j.jpainsymman.2016.12.322.
18. Back AL, Bauer-Wu SM, Rushton CH, Halifax J. Compassionate silence in the patient-clinician encounter: a contemplative approach. J Palliat Med. 2009;12:1113–7. https://doi.org/10.1089/jpm.2009.0175.
19. Cacciatore J. When the unthinkable happens: a mindfulness approach to perinatal and pediatric death. In: Black BP, Wright PM, Limbo R, Nieginski E, editors. Perinatal and pediatric bereavement in nursing and other health professions. New York: Springer Publishing Company; 2016. p. 97–110.
20. Papadatou D. In the face of death: professionals who care for the dying and the bereaved. New York: Springer Publishing Company; 2009.
21. Kobler K. Leaning in and holding on: team support with unexpected death. MCN Am J Matern Child Nurs. 2014;39:148–54. https://doi.org/10.1097/NMC.0000000000000028.
22. Kearney MK, Weininger RB, Vachon ML, Harrison RL, Mount BM. Self-care of physicians caring for patients at the end of life: "being connected… a key to my survival". JAMA. 2009;301:1155–64., E1. https://doi.org/10.1001/jama.2009.352.
23. Kobler K. Relationship-based approach to caring for children with serious illness. In: Pridham KF, Limbo R, Schroeder MM, editors. Guided participation in pediatric nursing practice: relationship-based teaching and learning with parents, children, and adolescents. New York: Springer Publishing Company; 2018. p. 21–32.
24. Kobler K, Limbo R. Making a case: creating a perinatal palliative care service using a perinatal bereavement program model. J Perinat Neonatal Nurs. 2011;25:32–41.; quiz 42–3. https://doi.org/10.1097/JPN.0b013e3181fb592e.
25. Quill TE, Arnold RM, Platt F. "I wish things were different": expressing wishes in response to loss, futility, and unrealistic hopes. Ann Intern Med. 2001;135:551–5.
26. Hospice and palliative medicine fellowship training. Chicago: American Academy of Hospice and Palliative Medicine; 2018. Available from: http://aahpm.org/career/clinical-training#fellowship-directory.
27. Pediatric palliative care fellowships and pediatric tracks. Chicago: American Academy of Hospice and Palliative Medicine; 2018. Available from: http://aahpm.org/uploads/Pediatric_Palliative_Care_Fellowships_and_Pediatric_Tracks_Update_7.24.18.pdf.
28. VitalTalk. (n.d.). Available from: http://vitaltalk.org/courses/.
29. Certified Hospice and Palliative Pediatric Nurse (CHPPN). (n.d.). Available from: https://advancingexpertcare.org/HPNA/Certification/Credentials/RN_Peds_CHPPN/HPCC/CertificationWeb/CHPPN.aspx?hkey=b14562c3-d628-4641-9f41-29c3736aefa9.

30. Certified in Perinatal Loss Care (CPLC). (n.d.). Available from: https://advancingexpertcare.org/HPNA/Certification/Credentials/Perinatal_Loss_CPLC/HPCC/CertificationWeb/CPLC.aspx?hkey=a9579be5-a0fa-4518-a359-f91ef4aedb29.
31. American Academy of Hospice and Palliative Medicine. (n.d.) (AAHPM) Available from: http://aahpm.org/.
32. American Academy of Pediatrics. (n.d.). Available from: https://www.aap.org/en-us/Pages/Default.aspx.
33. Center to Advance Palliative Care (CAPC). (n.d.). Available from: www.capc.org.
34. End-of-Life Nursing Education Consortium (ELNEC). (n.d.). Available from: https://elnec.academy.reliaslearning.com/http://www.aacnnursing.org/Portals/42/ELNEC/PDF/FactSheet.pdf.
35. Education in Palliative and End-of-Life Care (EPEC). (n.d.). Available from: http://bioethics.northwestern.edu/programs/epec/.
36. National Hospice and Palliative Care Organization (NHPCO). (n.d.). Available from: https://www.nhpco.org/.
37. Pediatric Palliative Care and End-of-Life Treatment (Boston Children's Hospital/Harvard Medical School Teaching Hospital). (n.d.). Available from: https://www.openpediatrics.org/course/pediatric-palliative-care-and-end-life-treatment.
38. Pediatric Palliative Care Research Network (PPCRN). (n.d.). Available from: https://www.dana-farber.org/research/departments-centers-and-labs/departments-and-centers/department-of-psychosocial-oncology-and-palliative-care/research/pediatric-palliative-care-research-network/.
39. Perinatal Hospice & Palliative Care. (n.d.). Available from: www.perinatalhospice.org.
40. Pregnancy Loss and Infant Death Alliance. (n.d.). Available from: www.plida.org.
41. Resolve Through Sharing. (n.d.). Information available at gundersenhealth.org/resolve-through-sharing/bereavement-training/andresolvethroughsharingonline.org.
42. Davies B, Steele R, Krueger G, Albersheim S, Baird J, Fibirie M, et al. Best practice in provider/parent interaction. Qual Health Res. 2017;27:406–20. https://doi.org/10.1177/1049732316664712.
43. Browning DM, Solomon MZ. Relational learning in pediatric palliative care: transformative education and the culture of medicine. Child Adolesc Psychiatr Clin N Am. 2006;15:795–815. https://doi.org/10.1016/j.chc.2006.03.002.
44. Limbo R. Resolve through sharing bereavement education model. La Crosse: Gundersen Medical Foundation, Inc; 2008, 2017, 2018. Available from: http://www.gundersenhealth.org/resolve-through-sharing/resources/
45. Limbo R, Kobler K. The tie that binds: relationships in perinatal bereavement. MCN Am J Matern Child Nurs. 2010;35:316–21. https://doi.org/10.1097/NMC.0b013e3181f0eef8.
46. Ballantine A, Feudtner C. The 10 R's of clinician education: a checklist. Arch Pediatr Adolesc Med. 2010;163:389–90. https://doi.org/10.1001/archpediatrics.2010.3.
47. Hinsdale MJ. Relational pedagogy. Oxford Research Encyclopedia of Education. [Published online December 2016]. doi:https://doi.org/10.1093/acrefore/9780190264093.013.28
48. Gilligan C. In a different voice: psychological theory and Women's development. Cambridge, MA: Harvard University Press; 1982. p. 216.

Advancing the Field of Perinatal Palliative Care: Needs and Strategies

18

Erin M. Denney-Koelsch, Kathie Kobler, Rebecca A. Kirch, Steven R. Leuthner, Karen Kavanaugh, and Denise Côté-Arsenault

Introduction

The purpose of perinatal palliative care (PPC) is to help parents faced with a life-limiting fetal condition (LLFC) make the time with their baby the best it can possibly be, optimizing patient and family quality of life and supporting shared decision-making to minimize regret [1]. To achieve this goal, parents need to be well-informed and understand their options, be empowered to make critical decisions, and feel supported and cared for to help them cope with their child's condition and the challenges they may confront. Anticipating continued expansion of the field of PPC, in this chapter, we will take a high-level view describing the current state of the field, opportunities to support its further maturation and increase reliable PPC access for all the families. From the *clinical perspective*, strategies are needed to facilitate and empower parents in informed decision-making on behalf of their

E. M. Denney-Koelsch (✉)
University of Rochester Medical Center/Strong Memorial Hospital, Department of Medicine, Division of Palliative Care, Rochester, NY, USA
e-mail: erin_denney@urmc.rochester.edu

K. Kobler
Advocate Children's Hospital, Center for Fetal Care, Park Ridge, IL, USA

R. A. Kirch
National Patient Advocate Foundation, Policy Department, Washington, DC, USA

S. R. Leuthner
Children's Hospital of Wisconsin, Medical College of Wisconsin, Department of Pediatrics, Wauwatosa, WI, USA

K. Kavanaugh
Children's Hospital of Wisconsin, Nursing Research, Milwaukee, WI, USA

D. Côté-Arsenault
St. Louis University, Trudy Busch Valentine School of Nursing, St. Louis, MO, USA
e-mail: denise.cotearsenault@slu.edu

E. M. Denney-Koelsch, D. Côté-Arsenault (eds.), *Perinatal Palliative Care*,
https://doi.org/10.1007/978-3-030-34751-2_18

infants, help providers achieve effective self-care, and structure patient-centered and family-focused PPC services. In addition, a focused strategy is needed for the field to achieve *key programmatic goals*: (1) improve access to programs and services in various settings; (2) integrate PPC into mainstream pediatric and palliative care medicine, sharing the benefits of continuing medical advances in all fields; (3) develop the evidentiary foundation for delivery of high-quality PPC; and (4) create a national agenda for PPC advocacy and policy.

PPC Clinical Approaches and Strategies

Focus on Relationships Between Patients and Providers

The field of PPC needs a clear foundation of principles and a framework to unify its unique approach to care. These must reflect values specific to the perinatal period that extend the basic principles of palliative care. The *relationship-based care model provides an ideal framework to ground PPC* because it helps to shape caring relationships of healthcare professionals (HCPs) with self, with each other as colleagues, and with families [2]. Practicing relationship-based care (RBC) requires of HCPs "a consciousness of purpose, clarity about their roles and those of their colleagues, competency in managing relationships, and a commitment to touching each patient and family in ways that are meaningful to them" [2]. Working within a caring philosophy creates positive and hopeful space for patients and for HCPs. We hear the compassion of experts in this field in every chapter of this book.

Everyone who works in PPC should *understand and apply relationship-based care (RBC) and its principles* (https://chcm.com/solutions/relationship-based-care/) [2], as described in detail in Chaps. 15 and 17. RBC is based in part on Swanson's Theory of Caring (see Chap. 2), in which the caring process is grounded in "maintaining belief in persons and their capacity to make it through events and transitions and face a future with meaning" by maintaining a hope-filled attitude [3]. Caring depends on knowing and understanding a circumstance through the eyes of parents, being emotionally present with them, doing for them what they cannot do for themselves, and enabling them to care for their child and themselves through informing, supporting, advocating, and preparing them for the future.

Professionals who use relationship-based care approach all individuals and parents with respect, with a desire to seek and understand their unique perspective and inform them of their options [2]. The conversations in which parents explain their understanding of their baby's condition, the meaning of this baby in their lives, and what is most important to them, inherently lead to a deeper interpersonal understanding between the HCPs and the family. HCPs often receive satisfaction from these conversations, in which they can help parents be the best parents they can be, make the most of the bad situation, and ultimately have no regrets about the outcome. As Swanson explains in her Theory of Caring [3], the HCP provides caring through *knowing, being with, enabling, and doing for: these are the fundamental principles of clinical care in PPC.*

Curricula that Foster Relationship-Building Skills

Relationships are created and nurtured through communication, so training programs need to teach advanced communication skills specific to PPC. Obstetrical, neonatal, and palliative care team members should practice non-judgmental listening and empathic therapeutic responses to support parents' information-seeking and decision-making processes, as well as helping parents listen to each other and find common ground when their points of view or needs differ. Many PPC training programs provide communications training that is applicable to all interprofessional disciplines that care for seriously ill infants, children, and their families (see Chap. 17).

Curricula for PPC professionals should teach that pregnancy is a developmental process that should inform providers as they create a caring relationship with parents. Understanding this developmental process is specific to PPC, different from providing palliative care for seriously ill adults. As discussed in Chap. 2, Fig. 2.3 (Tasks of Pregnancy), parents have a developing relationship with their baby; even if the fetus is in jeopardy, most parents see that baby as a person and call the baby by a name. HCPs need to recognize fetal personhood when parents have expressed it; respect for the baby as a person also validates the couple as parents. They can be empowered to parent their unborn baby as they make difficult decisions that are consistent with their revised tasks of pregnancy [1]. Hearing what is important to parents at a particular point in the pregnancy often reveals where the parents are developmentally. Ultimately, when HCPs listen to parents' goals and values in the context of a caring relationship, they can help to assure that parents are able to do all that they can for their child and for themselves so they will have no regrets when all is said and done [1, 4].

Using Clear and Consistent Messaging with Families and Colleagues

Developing relationships with parents is the key to all aspects of PPC integration. In particular, open and effective communications between the HCPs and the mother are essential. Although the fetus is the patient at risk, the mother is the most affected physically and emotionally, as well as being the default decision-maker for the baby. Mothers need to be introduced to PPC using key guiding points explaining that these services will help them navigate the care complexities and difficult decisions they are forced to confront. *Parents who know that they have a right to ask questions and control the flow of information will feel more confident in their role of making care decisions on behalf of their child.*

When confronting a LLFC, parents are trying to navigate unfamiliar territory and often don't even know what they don't know. Initially, the offer of supportive or palliative care may feel to them like just one more appointment in an already overwhelming array of specialist visits, especially if the term palliative care is unfamiliar to them. As they try to ingest and adjust to the news of their unborn child's diagnosis, they need compassion, knowledge, support, and advocacy. They will likely be open to assistance with any or all of these things, if they understand what services are being offered and the benefits of those services. In the future, wherever PPC is available, *a standard goal should be to give parents a seamless introduction to PPC concurrent with or shortly after the fetal diagnosis, and in coordination with various specialist visits*.

Ideally, parents find out about PPC through their HCPs, but many learn from other sources, such as websites, social media, or parent groups. The perspectives of other parents can be very helpful for some parents when their baby's situation is similar and the advice is given nonjudgmentally. But opinions expressed on social media may also be misinformation, content irrelevant to the particular case of their child, or advice to advocate for care that is not appropriate or desired by the family. PPC teams should assist parents in obtaining accurate, relevant, and timely information based on their needs and wishes.

Up until the time of the fetal diagnosis, the mother has been reliant on an obstetrician or midwife, with anticipated access to a pediatrician after birth. Then screens and tests plunged her into a world of unexpected specialists who may work in dispersed locations and may not interact with each other. In addition to the disease specialists, the mother may be introduced to PPC using varied and non-descriptive terms: the "supportive care team," "advanced care team," or "the butterfly team" (all common alternative names for the palliative care team). HCPs can inadvertently further contribute to the confusion about these services, often erroneously conflating perinatal hospice and PPC. Hospice by definition is an insurance benefit for those in the last 6 months of life that discontinues life-prolonging interventions and focuses on comfort care. While pediatric hospice allows disease-directed treatment to continue concurrent with hospice care under a provision enacted through the Affordable Care Act [5], many misunderstandings persist among HCPs about how to apply concurrent care and bill appropriately for concurrent services. A helpful implementation toolkit is available from the National Hospice and Palliative Care Organization at https://www.nhpco.org/sites/default/files/public/ChiPPS/CCCR_Toolkit.pdf [6]. *To alleviate this confusion and promote PPC awareness and understanding, we urge the field to advocate for and use clear and consistent messaging to parents and colleagues describing palliative care and its benefits:PPC focuses on coordinating care and comfort for their baby while also honoring parents' needs and preferences, providing an extra layer of support optimizing quality of life for the entire family.*

Critical Role of the PPC Care Coordinator

Because of the need for PPC teams to provide complex support for families over a long period, we believe that *PPC coordinators are an essential part of the interdisciplinary PPC team*. This individual can provide consistent support and contact for families, helping to create a safe place where no judgments will be made and all questions and concerns will be addressed. Even a normal pregnancy is inherently uncertain. With the addition of a serious fetal diagnosis in pregnancy, shock and trauma can occur for parents; the world no longer feels safe [7]. A PPC care coordinator can develop a longitudinal relationship with the family and use familiar routines and rituals to create a comforting sense of predictability for parents [8].

Palliative care is provided to and through the parents while the fetus is in utero, accompanied by development of a birth plan that anticipates neonatal care needs following birth. Ideally, birth planning is guided by the care coordinator, who introduces topics and questions that parents need to consider, presented as an opportunity to learn about options. A PPC care coordinator might provide parents with a list of questions to ask their providers, thereby giving parents permission to ask what they want to know at the time and pace of their choosing, thereby giving control over the flow of information. Some parents may choose not to make many decisions but rather to let nature, God, or the baby, lead the way.

Care coordinators can also help families navigate the complex and fragmented world of healthcare specialists, bridge between maternal care and neonatal care, and provide a consistent presence to answer questions and offer support. Care coordinators should be integral to an interdisciplinary PPC team, coordinate visits with subspecialists, share information among healthcare professionals and family, facilitate access to services, and conduct advanced planning and documentation of a plan of care. Parents report that receiving care from one key person from diagnosis through birth and bereavement provides invaluable emotional support [10].

Currently, the roles of PPC coordinators are highly variable, and training programs specifically for these key members of the PPC team have not been developed. To maximize the care coordinator's effectiveness, *training programs should facilitate the creation of job descriptions that specify the context of care and needed competencies and develop curricula based on those competencies.*

Perspectives on Prenatal Palliative Care in the Healthcare System

Access to Perinatal Palliative Care Services

Our vision for the field is that *every family confronting a serious or life-limiting fetal condition (LLFC) will have access to high-quality PPC close to home.* For this goal to be realized, parents need easier and more reliable access to programs and services, with better supports at local institutions and an increased number of more comprehensive programs at large academic centers. A 2015 national survey of 75 programs showed that 70% of PPC programs were <10 years old and that location, structure, personnel, and funding were highly variable [11]. Many existing programs reported that they were understaffed and underfunded, held together by one or two passionate people trying to meet many families' complex needs [11] (See Chap. 13).

To build new programs, key stakeholders must understand the value of and need for PPC, institutional leaders must be convinced that delivery of PPC services helps to achieve institutional objectives, and evolving PPC teams need guidance on how to structure an effective and sustainable program. Obtaining essential funding requires political acumen combined with access to financial data. Hence program leaders need leadership and financial skills and tools to support them in making the case for their programs. The Center to Advance Palliative Care [12] has a number of helpful resources and toolkits relevant to these field educational needs in building and sustaining successful business plans and programs. Data should be gathered about the PPC population and demonstrate the potential for meaningful outcomes such as parental satisfaction and lack of regrets.

PCC service models are variable, depending on geography and proximity to a tertiary care center. One model adopted by tertiary care centers is a multidisciplinary consultation day, in which parents come, sometimes from long distances, to meet with multiple providers: e.g., an ultrasonographer followed by a maternal-fetal-medicine physician, a neonatologist, a genetic counselor, and a member of the palliative care team. This model has the advantage of limiting travel for families coming from long distances and providing an opportunity for providers to talk to a parent in an interdisciplinary setting. On the other hand, the long day can be overwhelming for some families, and the “all at once” approach is inconsistent with what is known about a family’s psychological developmental tasks when continuing pregnancy with LLFC [1] (See Chap. 2). Parents often need time to process new information away from the hospital and discuss issues with their loved ones and, in some cases, spiritual care leaders. When feasible, scheduling multiple visits over time better accommodates the way parents obtain and process information. When single, longer visits are the most pragmatic, it helps to give parents a quiet room and downtime for processing information and emotions. Follow-up conversations by telephone or text can also help bridge time and distance gaps. Use of telemedicine for long-distance consultations with specialists has been used successfully in adult palliative care [13]. In addition, community-based programs that “meet patients where they are” can provide continuity of care and parent support during the pregnancy and into the bereavement and family transition periods (See Chap. 14). These can be coordinated by a PPC coordinator to reduce parent burden.

Staffing options are also variable. Having a team of PPC specialists in every hospital is not realistic, but at a minimum, *all clinicians and staff who care for families coping with life-limiting fetal and neonatal conditions should have basic training in palliative care communication and care coordination core competencies. PPC communication and coordination core competencies can be learned and done by obstetricians and maternal-fetal-medicine physicians, neonatologists, nurses in all areas, social workers, and genetic counselors.* For HCPs in all disciplines, training programs are needed to teach core PPC competencies grounded in relationship-based care. Anyone who interacts with patients with LLFCs can get continuing professional training through a variety of programs, as discussed in Chap. 17.

The variability in program structures, staffing, and HCP training are mirrored in the wide differences in types of fetal diagnoses seen across programs [11]. Confusion has been created by the sometimes interchangeable use of the names "perinatal hospice" and "perinatal palliative care," as discussed above. In many areas, no hospice programs are available for either children or infants. Where they do exist, perinatal hospice programs may care only for patients who have a clearly lethal condition *and* are following a purely comfort-oriented approach to care, because of insurance restrictions. Other programs may see any patient who *might* die of their illness at some point in the future and are seeking all possible life-sustaining treatments. We believe that PPC should support both infants very likely to die at birth and those who may have a longer life with chronic illness and will need long-term support and symptom management. Both conditions are associated with a high likelihood of intense family distress, symptom burden, the potential for death, and the need for complex medical decision-making. The supportive services of PPC are highly appropriate and consistent with the care provided to both palliative care populations. *We encourage delivery of PPC services for a broad population of eligible patients, in keeping with the palliative care model, which encourages early access to care, concurrent palliative and life-sustaining care, and inclusion of any patient who has a serious and symptomatic illness.*

Medical Advances and Their Implications for PPC

Fetal Testing and Prognostication For adult and pediatric populations, palliative care is being introduced early in a disease process and concurrently with therapy. *It is time for palliative care to also be provided perinatally for all fetuses with high-risk conditions and their families.* Fletcher and Evan wrote in 1983, "Just as many centuries of cultural and biological evolution were required before childhood was viewed as a differentiated stage of life…ultrasound and a host of other fetal technologies could become part of a more complex evolutionary story. Perhaps a new stage of human existence, 'prenatality'…" [14]. More recently, Michael Harrison echoed this message: "Powerful new imaging and sampling techniques have stripped the veil of mystery from the once secretive fetus" [15].

Development of fetal imaging, particularly MRI, and of methods for genetic evaluation of the fetus has been rapid. These technologies will continue to develop and improve and certainly become more mainstream and hopefully affordable. However, whether or how these advances will change the practice of palliative care is hard to predict. If they help to make more specific diagnoses and thereby narrow the expected range of prognoses, they may clarify which cases can be helped by fetal or neonatal interventions. Throughout medical history, diagnostic modalities have been improving, yet prognostic certainty eludes us. For example, the current standard is to obtain an MRI of a fetus with congenital diaphragmatic hernia (CDH). The data supports that this technology has more accuracy in prognostication than prenatal ultrasound measurements [16]. However, MRI remains a screening tool that is not definitive. Some babies with very poor MRI findings do quite well, and others with good prognostic indicators are born with severe hypoxia and pulmonary hypertension that are incompatible with life. The best predictor of survival remains how the infant responds to neonatal care.

Genetic testing, like fetal imaging, is not always definitive. Historically, genetic testing was limited to chromosomal abnormalities, but advances in genetic microarray testing are now providing much more detail on individual gene mutations, some of which have unknown implications. These studies often predict a range of phenotypic possibilities, from mild to very severe or lethal effects. Hence while some genetic tests improve prognostic certainty, others may add uncertainty.

With neonatal therapeutic advances or parental advocacy requesting full, aggressive care, the field should anticipate caring for fetal diagnoses that were once considered lethal. Meeting with the palliative care team during the prenatal period helps to foster relationships and a smooth transition from the perinatal to neonatal setting that may include a trial of therapy to allow the uncertainty to play out.

Despite these ambiguities, it is important to recognize that *uncertainty should be considered a trigger for palliative care discussions, not a barrier*. Improved technologies can still help members of a PPC team by providing useful information for ethical decision-making on maternal risks, such as delivery mode, and levels and limits of care for the newborn. In the end, improved prognostication will not change the need for spiritual care or bereavement care but knowing what is most likely to happen may help parents and providers to make value-aligned decisions.

Even when fetal imaging or genetic testing suggest a poor fetal outcome, many parents choose a plan for initial aggressive support and evaluation. In this case, the goal for palliative care is to develop a caring relationship with the parents during pregnancy in case the baby struggles to survive and parents raise questions about care limitations after birth. *We recommend initiating PPC as early as possible to support all parents whose baby has an uncertain prognosis*, not only when they are faced with imminent death.

Fetal Surgery and Other Invasive Procedures Historically, fetal interventions were only performed for a fetus who was otherwise going to die in utero or shortly after birth. For example, in a fetus with nonimmune hydrops secondary to a large lung mass (a congenital cystic adenomatoid malformation), in utero resection of the mass may reverse the hydrops, allowing the potential for successful neonatal resuscitation. If the procedure works, a viable baby may be born. If the procedure does not work, the fetus will die, and the bereaved family is left to navigate the loss. Palliative care discussions should precede such interventions to provide support for the family, regardless of the outcome. *We believe that early palliative care should be offered routinely to families experiencing fetal surgery.*

Palliative care discussions prior to in utero fetal surgery should include exploring the parents' hopes and fears. While the family may consent to treatment with the hope and goal of cure, that family will also benefit from resources and relationships to support them if the fetal intervention is not successful. In the case of death despite fetal intervention, they can consider the option to allow natural death without neonatal resuscitation. Comfort care, spiritual care, and memory-making can provide support and offer a full spectrum of options for the family. If the procedure goes well, the PPC service can celebrate with the family.

Despite the best intentions, the reality in many cases is that the fetal procedure may work well enough to help a baby survive, but perhaps also result in a significant health risk and/or a chronic condition. A PPC service is a good resource for counseling families who are weighing these decisions prenatally, so they are not forced to make an unexpected, difficult decision in the NICU about whether to continue life-sustaining medical interventions.

Ethical Considerations in Supporting Parental Decision-Making Consideration of issues of the ethics and beneficence of medical interventions are moving from the NICU to the perinatal period. In contrast to a neonate, any parental decision to undergo a fetal intervention for the unborn baby requires at some level an intervention on the pregnant woman. Underlying these maternal-fetal decisions are ethical concerns of weighing maternal and fetal risks and benefits. For example, when HCPs share with a family the diagnosis of fetal renal agenesis, they have the option of choosing an investigational procedure of serial amniotic fluid infusions to facilitate fetal lung development. The maternal burden of serial procedures and the risk of infection require that she be the one with the ultimate authority to decide. From the fetal perspective, mechanical replacement of vital fluid may allow for some lung tissue development, but the absence of viable fetal kidneys remains [17]. Prior to pursuing such treatment, it is essential to ascertain whether a family is willing and able to pursue neonatal peritoneal dialysis as a bridge to eventual kidney transplant when the baby is older. If the family does not wish to pursue transplant, then there is no ethical reason for the mother to undergo the risks of such an invasive prenatal procedure. PPC counseling is highly appropriate no matter what the parental decision. If they decide not to begin amniotic fluid infusions, the disorder is a lethal condition, and classical PPC can proceed. If they do want to embark on the procedure, they need to know that the path is fraught with complications and possible causes of pain, suffering and even possible death of the infant in the NICU or beyond, as well as maternal risk. *Applying palliative care concepts and developing relationships early and over time in this and similar scenarios will help to provide the best care and decision-making support for the child down the road.*

Consideration of interventions for a fetus who is likely to survive, but only with aggressive neonatal care, also offers opportunities to use palliative care counseling strategies, clear delineation of goals and limits of care, consideration of maternal safety, and family support. For example, with some forms of hypoplastic left heart syndrome (HLHS), a family might be offered a fetal aortic balloon valvuloplasty, with the hope of preventing HLHS. The goal would be to prevent their baby from having to undergo the lifelong burdens of a single ventricle heart condition, because they perceive that the outcome of life with a single ventricle is poor enough that they would risk the life of the fetus. However, the procedure itself risks fetal demise, premature birth, or failure to fix the problem. Palliative care support could help to facilitate consistency in conversations and decision-making as a family weighs the options for their baby [18]. Is life quality with a single ventricle poor enough that they would not want their infant to proceed down the path of multiple surgical interventions, including eventual cardiac transplantation? Instead, is palliative care from birth to keep the infant comfortable a better option for them? Even if that family pursues cardiac interventions, the palliative care team is poised to support the family and be present if things take a turn for the worse.

Directions for Future Research

State of the Science

PPC programs to serve families have been proliferating over the last decade, and there is an increasing body of evidence on which to base high-quality practice. Research has shed light on a growing number of topics of palliative and end-of-life care for the perinatal population (see Table 18.1) including PPC program characteristics and parent and provider experiences, although much remains unexplored.

Limitations in the evidence for PPC practice are clearly revealed in a recent systematic review of palliative care interventions [32]. No studies specific to PPC were included in the review. Research is needed about decision-making surrounding the numerous choices faced by parents. Much of the prior research on parental

Table 18.1 Examples of selected PPC-related studies 2009–2019

Topics	References
Distribution, structural models, and personnel of PPC programs nationally	Wool, Côté-Arsenault, Black, Denney-Koelsch, Kim, Kavanaugh, 2015 [11]
	Denney-Koelsch, Black, Côté-Arsenault, Wool, Kim, Kavanaugh, 2016 [19]
Parents' experiences with perinatal palliative care	Côté-Arsenault, Denney-Koelsch, McCoy, and Kavanaugh, 2019 [20]
	Kamrath, Osterholm, Stover-Haney, George, O'Connor-Von, and Needle, 2019 [21]
Parents' experiences when they learn prenatally of a serious condition in their unborn infant	Black & Sandelowski, 2010 [22]
	Chitty Barnes, and Berry, 1996 [23]
	Côté-Arsenault and Denney-Koelsch 2011 [24], 2016 [1]
	Côté-Arsenault, Krowchuk, and Denney-Koelsch, 2015 [4]
	Denney-Koelsch, Côté-Arsenault and Lemcke-Berno, 2015 [25]
	Lalor, Begley, and Galaven, 2009 [26]
PPC and counseling parents at risk for a very preterm delivery	Kavanaugh, Roscigno, Swanson, Savage, Kimura, Kilpatrick, 2015 [27]
Clinician comfort with providing PPC care	Wool, 2013 [28]
Parents' perception of satisfaction with PPC	Wool, Black, and Woods, 2016 [29]
	Wool, Repke, Woods, 2017 [30]
	Wool, Kain, Mendes, and Carter, 2018 [31]

behaviors has been limited to the immediate post loss period. Studying the long-term effects of loss in this population of parents is critical because of reported poor long-term parental outcomes in parents who experience a perinatal loss: depression has been reported up to 4 years after the loss [33] and symptoms of post-traumatic stress up to 18 years after such an experience [34, 35]. *Future research studies of parental outcomes should also include a population of parents and families diverse in race, ethnicity, culture, gender identity, and family structure and those whose treatment decisions vary.*

Overcoming Challenges

Numerous challenges exist when conducting palliative and end-of-life research. Participants are inherently vulnerable, and prognostic uncertainty makes adherence to standard study designs difficult [36]. For example, the duration of data collection could be highly variable across research participants. Perinatal palliative and end-of-life research requires great sensitivity in approaching parents, given that for many, the birth and death of their infant often overlap in a short period of time. Another challenge to conducting studies of PPC is that PPC is often provided along with aggressive interventions. Several authors have been successful in conducting prospective longitudinal studies beginning in the prenatal period [1, 27] by conducting the study based on a model of caring as described by Swanson [3] and translated for research purposes [37]. Using this approach, >80% recruitment and retention was achieved. Parents who participated in bereavement research appreciated having a way to find meaning in loss by honoring their infant and helping other parents [38].

Another challenge for conducting PPC research is the limited access to an adequate sample of research participants. Although perinatal deaths are not uncommon, the incidence is far less than occurs in other research populations, making it challenging to recruit an adequate sample in any one setting. Recruitment from a number of clinical sites is often needed. *The feasibility of conducting future studies will also be dependent upon having accessible health records and data for identifying eligible parents as potential research participants, recruiting them, and collecting relevant data from the health records.* Several researchers have been successful in recruiting perinatal programs for their survey research [11] by partnering with other advocates for improving PPC, such as Amy Kuebelbeck, the manager of an internationally accessed website perinatalhospice.org [39]. They have also made use of existing pediatric palliative care listservs. Working with professional organizations like the Pregnancy Loss and Infant Death Alliance (PLIDA; plida.org [40]) is another strategy to increase collaboration, nationally and internationally such as the international collaboration among Wool and her colleagues [31]. Use of emerging technology-based strategies developed successfully in other sensitive research should be considered to broaden the reach of PPC research. Internet recruitment [41] and e-mail interviewing [42] have been used successfully.

Development of Tools

The development of valid and reliable tools to measure parent outcomes after receiving PPC, as well as effects of care on PPC interdisciplinary team members, is essential to advance the science on which the field relies. To date, several tools specific to PPC have been created including the *Quality Indicators and Parental Satisfaction of Perinatal Palliative Care Instrument* [43, 44] and the *Perinatal Palliative Care Perceptions and Practice Barriers Scale* [45]. Although not specific to PPC, other instruments have been used to measure the quality of decisions made surrounding treatment choices and parents' mental health outcomes after perinatal loss. These tools include:

- Decision Regret Scale [46]
- User Manual-Decision Regret Scale [47]
- Decision Evaluation Scale [48]
- Impact of Event Scale – Revised [IES-R] [49]
- Beck Anxiety Inventory [50]
- Perinatal Grief Intensity Scale [PGIS] [51]
- Perinatal Grief Scale [52]
- Hospital Anxiety and Depression Scale (HADS)[53]

Because of the complexity and intensity of parents' experiences of perinatal loss, better definition of the range of parent outcomes is needed. These might include constructs other than mental health diagnoses that reflect ways that parents cope and adapt after the loss. For example, the *Grief and Meaning Reconstruction Inventory* (GMRI) [54], which was developed with a population in which 15% were bereaved parents, measures positive health outcomes after a loss. Measures of resilience are important because we know that when bereaved parents try to make sense of their loss through meaning-making and seek something good from their tragedy, they can experience positive personal growth [22] that leads to less maladaptive grief [55]. Measuring constructs like meaning-making in understanding parental response to loss could contribute realistic measures of adaptive outcomes to enhance PPC research. Future research should extend beyond satisfaction with care and mental health conditions and focus on identifying and describing constructs that reflect resilience. Another topic that has emerged from recent research is the parents' stated goal to "have no regrets" despite their devastating experience with perinatal loss [1]. Testing strategies to improve the process of counseling around parental decision-making is likely to help parents achieve this important goal. *PPC is a relatively new field, and opportunities for new areas of research are likely to emerge frequently as our research program evolves.*

Opportunities for Research Collaboration

Several national groups can serve as a resource for PPC researchers. The Palliative Care Research Cooperative Group (PCRC) is a collaborative funded by the National Institutes of Nursing Research (NINR). This group was established in 2010 to facilitate research on the quality of life of patients with advanced and/or potentially life-limiting illnesses, and their caregivers and providers (http://palliativecareresearch.org/about-us/) [56]. As of April 2018, approximately 10% of PCRC members identified with a pediatric focus and many of those members are likely to be involved in PPC. The group's recently funded research grant will provide more opportunities for pediatric palliative care researchers to pursue multi-site and collaborative studies. With a national presence and participation in the PCRC, PPC researchers can build a network for future collaboration and access to research participants, as is currently done with adult palliative care investigators in the PCRC. Another goal for PPC researchers is to expand the instrument library in the PCRC to include tools for PPC research, with the ultimate goal of expanding the PCRC data repository to include PPC data. Therefore, *membership in the PCRC should be a priority for PPC researchers.*

Another resource for PPC research funding, mentorship and development is the National Palliative Care Research Center (NPCRC) (http://www.npcrc.org/) [57]. Its mission is to strengthen the evidence base needed for strong health policy and high-quality clinical practice in palliative care medicine by supporting the growing community of palliative care research scientists and stimulating expanded research and innovation. The NPCRC provides mechanisms to establish research priorities, develop new investigators, and coordinate studies on palliative care. In partnership with the Center to Advance Palliative Care, the NPCRC's goal is to rapidly translate research findings into clinical practice.

Funding

Currently there are several mechanisms for funding PPC research. The NIH Office of End-of-Life and Palliative Care Research (OEPCR) is a major program whose purpose is to coordinate the development, implementation, and evaluation of palliative care research in direct collaboration with other NIH Institutes and Centers, federal research agencies, and outside constituencies (https://www.ninr.nih.gov/researchandfunding/desp/oepcr) [58]. Currently, studies that focus on neonatal palliative and end-of-life care can be considered for funding. Investigators whose studies include the prenatal or the neonatal period can seek funding from the Eunice Kennedy Shriver National Institute of Child Health and Human Development.

A number of sources offer pilot funding. The PCRC provides funding for pilot studies; one investigator must be a member and there must be a PCRC senior investigator who serves as a mentor for the proposed study. The NPCRC also offers several funding mechanisms, including career development awards, research design and statistical support grants, and infrastructure support for collaborative studies. Numerous professional organizations and private sources such as The Greenwall Foundation (http://www.greenwall.org/index.php) [59] also offer pilot funding. For international research, the Fulbright Global Scholar Award enables US professionals to conduct multi-country projects (https://www.cies.org/program/fulbright-global-scholar-award) [60].

For the future, more attention should be paid to the importance of funding PPC research. One way to raise awareness and garner funding support is through development of policy statements, such as the one prepared by members of the American Academy of Nursing [61]. Another strategy for raising awareness is the inclusion of PPC in NIH sponsored programs, such as the summit on The Science of Compassion: Future Directions in End-of-Life and Palliative Care (https://www.ninr.nih.gov/researchandfunding/scienceofcompassion) [62] or through the many other advocacy initiatives described in this chapter.

Political and Social Climate for Perinatal Palliative Care

Legal and Political Debates About Abortion and Fetal Life

Changes in laws about the pregnant woman and her fetus and ongoing political discussions inevitably influence PPC practices. Early writings on PPC clearly portrayed it as an alternative to termination of a pregnancy [63]. For women and families who are opposed to undergoing an abortion, PPC after LLFC continues to provide supportive obstetrical and neonatal services as the family continues the pregnancy and delivers their baby. *Although advanced fetal imaging may provide information that leads parents to decide on termination of the pregnancy, PPC is there to support the fetus, mother, and family.* In recent years, PPC has matured into a full interdisciplinary care model and now provides care for more than lethal conditions alone.

At the time of this writing, there are political processes at national or state levels proposing to restrict or eliminate abortion through challenges to Roe v Wade [64]. Some state laws specify fetal conditions that make abortion illegal, including gestational age, presence of pain [32], and presence of a heartbeat. These laws have different levels of exceptions to protect the life and well-being of the mother. Other laws are aimed at protecting the fetus after birth [65]. Some have argued that fetal protections should be added to the Emergency Medical Treatment and Labor Act (EMTALA) [66] or the Child Abuse Prevention and Treatment Act (CAPTA) [67] to create mandates for neonatal resuscitation and care [68, 69]. Some newer state laws are adding language to criminalize or punish practitioners whose actions end fetal life; it is beyond the scope of this writing to predict how the legal debates will conclude in the future. *The field of PPC must stay abreast of abortion and fetal life policy issues in order to advocate for families, practitioners, and good medical care and adapt as needed to care for pregnant women.*

PPC Advocacy: An Essential Accelerant for Advancing the Field

Growth in Recognition of the PPC Field Advocacy amplifies patient, parent, and professional voices to move beyond individual solutions and create broader systemic change. Taking collective action is an essential step in advancing the PPC field, both to improve access and to enhance the regulatory, accreditation, and payment landscape for PPC services, whether they occur in hospital, ambulatory, or home settings and are covered by either private or public insurance.

More people are recognizing the benefits of palliative care and its person-centered approach to maximizing quality of life for patients and families. This growing recognition comes from a decade of deliberate and strategic investment in coordinated research, program development, and advocacy initiatives [70, 71]. Pediatric palliative care has also experienced notable growth over the past decade [72, 73]. As a result, momentum is building for improving access and adherence to high-quality palliative care, and enhanced evidence-based clinical guidelines have expanded the field's reach across all care settings. The expanding recognition of palliative care across the lifespan has positioned PPC and the interprofessional clinicians providing perinatal services to receive deserved credit for their work in providing essential skilled communication, symptom management, and care coordination for families navigating complex conditions confronting their unborn child.

Clarifying the Identity of PPC To achieve this objective, the field must address palliative care's persisting identity challenges. Conflation of palliative care with end-of-life and hospice care is common within the medical community and among the public. This identity challenge is a major barrier to achieving improved access and quality care experiences. Advocacy is needed to build recognition for PPC as an integral component of seamless care and as a standard of practice during pregnancy and in the neonatal period. *Advancing consistent messaging about PPC and broadcasting a corresponding call to action are needed to connect communities of professionals engaged in caring for women who experience prenatal diagnoses of a serious fetal condition.*

A consumer research study commissioned by the Center to Advance Palliative Care (CAPC) in 2011 revealed that seven in ten Americans are "not at all knowledgeable" about palliative care. Yet when palliative care was explained to them, using key messages that were developed through focus groups and interviews with patients and caregivers, an overwhelming majority of people polled (92%) said that they would want palliative care for themselves or their loved ones and believed it should be accessible in our nation's hospitals [74]. Using the same consumer-derived messages to describe pediatric palliative care, the American Childhood Cancer Organization informally surveyed its pediatric parent constituency in October 2014 to reveal similar findings. Among 275 responding parents, 86% would be likely to consider pediatric palliative care for their child during cancer treatment, and 89% indicated that it is important that pediatric palliative services are available in all hospitals caring for children [75].

Consumer-driven research showed that the public needs to learn the following specific messages.

Palliative care:

- Helps to provide the best possible quality of life for patients and their families
- Helps patients and families manage the pain, symptoms, and stress of serious illness

- Is a partnership of patient, family, and all medical specialists
- Provides an extra layer of support for patients and families with serious illness
- Is appropriate at any age and any stage of a serious illness and can be provided alongside curative treatment

Using these consistent messages, customized and adapted to address the particular needs of perinatal patients, can help the field improve and expand parent and practitioner awareness, thereby driving increased demand. As a jumpstart for this effort, the National Institute for Nursing Research offers specific Conversations Matter® pediatric palliative care messaging resources [76] and CAPC has produced a helpful pediatric palliative care field guide that features a comprehensive table of key messaging resources available from various organizations [77].

Dialogue and Action Through collaborative outreach and leadership, PPC has an opportunity to partner in and personalize advocacy efforts happening in the broader pediatric and palliative care fields to bring palliative care everywhere [71]. Specific strategic options for PPC to consider include:

- *Define.* Identify clear, consensus language that the field can use to describe PPC and its benefits. It can build off existing palliative care messaging resources and be customized to perinatal needs.
- *Disseminate.* Share this consensus definition and description of interprofessional services to build PPC awareness, understanding and availability among various stakeholders, using communication channels available through patient advocacy and professional organizations, state palliative care advisory councils, pediatric palliative care coalitions, and related community outreach initiatives.
- *Deploy.* Expand education and training opportunities for frontline clinician colleagues to clarify their understanding of PPC services and integrate core palliative care competencies into their interprofessional skills development.
- *Participate.* Embed PPC interprofessional perspectives and parent/patient voices consistently in current and future national palliative care initiatives. Provide data in the National Palliative Care Registry™[78] and through ongoing activities of the Quality Care Roundtable for People with Serious Illness of the National Academies of Science, Engineering and Medicine [79]. Participate in palliative care public policy activities advanced by the Patient Quality of Life Coalition [80].

Collaborations Among Palliative Care Organizations We believe the field of PPC will benefit greatly from focused collaborative efforts among the communities of maternal-fetal medicine, fetal therapy, obstetrics/labor and delivery, neonatology, palliative care, perinatal bereavement, and family advocacy, to determine shared goals and strategies in the care of families. Bringing leaders in the perinatal, neonatal, and palliative specialties together is essential to address access limitations, deepen care provision standards, establish quality measures, and enhance reimbursement models. To foster collective dialogue and identify optimal starting places, these collaborations can draw upon the learned experiences and opinion research outcomes already completed by adult palliative initiatives, such as the CAPC sponsored consumer research study described above, which developed consistent messages to define palliative care.

At present, a handful of national organizations have published statements about the importance of providing PPC, including the:

- Institute of Medicine's *Dying in America* report (2015) [81]
- National Association of Neonatal Nursing palliative care guidelines (2015) [82]
- American Academy of Nursing's perinatal palliative policy statement (2017) [61]
- International Fetal Medicine and Surgical Society's and the North American Fetal Therapy Network's joint statement outlining critical components (including palliative care) for fetal therapy centers (2017) [83]
- American College of Obstetricians and Gynecologists, Committee on Ethics; American Academy of Pediatrics, Committee on Bioethics. Clinical report – Maternal-fetal intervention and fetal care centers [17]

More recently, the National Academies of Sciences, Engineering and Medicine reinforced these statements by convening its multi-year Roundtable on Quality Care for People with Serious Illness. Inspired by previous work at the Academies, including the 2014 Dying in America Institute of Medicine report, this Roundtable fosters an ongoing dialogue about critical policy and research issues to accelerate and sustain progress in care for seriously ill infants, children, and adults across all ages. The initiative focuses stakeholders on five priority areas that align with needs of perinatal populations:

- Delivery of person-centered, family-oriented care
- Communication and advance care planning
- Professional education and development
- Policies and payment systems
- Public education and engagement

Roundtable membership includes patient advocates, healthcare professional organizations, healthcare providers and insurers, foundations, federal agencies, researchers, and others interested in improving care for seriously ill populations. The perspectives of parents caring for seriously ill infants and children and pediatric/perinatal palliative care professionals have been represented in many of the Roundtables' workshops and publications, such as its first workshop on Integrating the Voices of Patients and Caregivers in Serious Illness Care [79]. *The PPC field will benefit from continuing its collective advocacy and intentional inclusion in future opportunities to integrate perinatal perspectives and needs into the broader discourse about advancing a national strategy for palliative care.*

PPC can also position itself in prime time through program participation in the National Palliative Care Registry™ [78]. The National Registry collects annual data on process and operational features of palliative care programs across the country as a project of CAPC and the NPCRC. CAPC has worked directly with pediatric palliative care experts from diverse programs over the past year to improve the survey's relevance and reach for pediatric and perinatal programs [84]. Registry data provide a crucial resource for program development, policy, and advocacy to advance the PPC field. Perinatal and pediatric teams can use the Registry to measure their progress and track their operational capacity and reach. There is no cost to participate or to receive data reports. *Robust program participation in the National Palliative Care Registry will strengthen our ability to create perinatal- and pediatric-specific reports and enable further evolution of the database over time to better address the needs of programs serving families with seriously ill infants and children.*

Development of Evidence-Based Guidelines In 2018 the National Consensus Project (NCP) published the fourth Edition of their Clinical Practice Guidelines for Quality Palliative Care, containing evidence-based perinatal, neonatal, and pediatric-focused criteria and clinical practice examples in all guideline domains. It is the hope of NCP writers of the fourth Edition (2018) [85] that the perinatal and neonatal communities will see their work more clearly reflected in the updated guideline criteria, which have been endorsed by more than 80 national organizations and supported by a companion systematic evidence review published in the *Journal of Pain and Symptom Management* [86]. These Clinical Practice Guidelines provide a solid framework for the development of specific PPC standards of care and outcome measurements. For example, Guideline 6.3.3 (NCP, 2018, pg. 41) highlights the importance of PPC clinicians assessing the meaning of the pregnancy to parents, how parents define their role during pregnancy, and their childbirth preferences. This guideline could subsequently be translated into standardized assessment questions that PPC teams could use to study how parents' answers to such questions are incorporated into the fetal plan of care.

Current and future PPC practice will also require the *continued refinement and measurement of strategies to honor the parent/child relationship while supporting the unique psychosocial needs of pregnant women (and their families).* Understanding parents' preferences and respecting the family's needs as the baby's living and dying unfolds is essential to high-quality PPC [87, 88]. Accomplishing this goal requires harnessing the collective wisdom and skills of all interdisciplinary team members.

Resources should be readily available for PPC teams and families to ensure access to evidence-based information about fetal serious illness, morbidity, and mortality, a process that is challenged by continuing advances in prenatal diagnostic and genetic testing [88, 89]. Specialists in maternal-fetal medicine, obstetrics, fetal surgery, and neonatology will benefit from the development and use of multi-modal strategies, such as communication simulations, to deepen their skills in bidirectional information sharing and guiding prenatal decision-making. *Sharing evidence-based strategies, standards, and measures to inform PPC professionals will foster individual clinician and team well-being* [85].

This call to collaborative advocacy action and development of standards will challenge the PPC professional community to hone and use their advocacy skills on top of their busy work schedule. HCPs and advocacy experts must be able to nimbly navigate the politically charged landscape surrounding the unborn in this country and describe the need for PPC with wisdom and eloquence. We hope that this chapter serves as a rallying call for PPC clinicians to actively participate in national palliative initiatives, including strategic planning, research, advocacy, palliative care registry enhancement, and other initiatives [90].

Conclusion

PPC specialists are solidifying their place in the larger field of palliative care, with growing numbers of programs and increasing national recognition of its importance. However, we need to continue our work to help all stakeholders see its value. Parents deserve reliable access to the relationship-based support, programs should be deepened to improve and measure high-quality care through research that can be translated into consensus documents. Meaningful outcomes measurement is needed to demonstrate the many benefits of PPC, including satisfaction with care, quality of care, and respect for babies and parents. While we cannot control the political landscape of fetal status and women's rights, we can use clear language about what PPC is and what it provides, so that parents are open to receiving care and support from the interdisciplinary teams ready to help them.

It is a privilege to enter into a family's story [91] as they anticipate welcoming a baby with serious illness. Their needs can continue to motivate and unify our collective efforts to advance the field of perinatal palliative care.

References

1. Côté-Arsenault D, Denney-Koelsch E. "Have no regrets:" parents' experiences and developmental tasks in pregnancy with a lethal fetal diagnosis. Soc Sci Med. 2016;154:100–9. https://doi.org/10.1016/j.socscimed.2016.02.033.
2. Felgen J. Chapter 1 a caring and healing environment, pages 23-52, in relationship-based care. In: Koloroutis M, editor. Relationship-based care: a model for transforming practice. Minneapolis: Creative Health Care Management; 2004.
3. Swanson KM. Empirical development of a middle range theory of caring. Nurs Res. 1991 May–Jun;40(3):161–6.
4. Côté-Arsenault D, Krowchuk H, Denney-Koelsch E, Jenkins Hall W. "We want what's best for our baby": prenatal parenting of babies with lethal conditions. J Prenat Perinat Psychol Health. 2015;29(3):157–76.
5. Your Child's Health Care and the Affordable Care Act (ACA): Concurrent Care for Children. (n.d.). https://medicalhomeinfo.aap.org/tools-resources/Documents/ACA-Concurrent Care%20FINAL.pdf/. Accessed 7/8/19.
6. National Hospice and Palliative Care Organization at (n.d.). https://www.nhpco.org/sites/default/files/public/ChiPPS/CCCR_Toolkit.pdf/. Accessed 7/8/19.

7. Janoff-Bulman R. Overview of developmental theories looking at humans over time. In: Shattered assumptions: towards a new psychology of trauma. New York: The Free Press, Sage; 1992. https://us.sagepub.com/sites/default/files/upm-binaries/43318_3.pdf.
8. Limbo R, Kobler K. Ritual and reflection: when a child dies. LaCrosse: Resolve Through Sharing; 2013.
9. Strupp J, Dose C, Kuhn U, Galushko M, Duesterdiek A, Ernstmann N, et al. Analysing the impact of a case management model on the specialized palliative care multi-professional team. Support Care Cancer. 2018;26(2):673–9. https://doi.org/10.1007/s00520-017-3893-3.
10. Denney-Koelsch E, Côté-Arsenault D, Jenkins Hall W. Feeling cared for versus experiencing added burden: parents' needs from health care in Pregnancy with a lethal fetal diagnosis. Illn Crisis Loss. 2016;26(4):293–31.5; Print: October 1, 2018. https://doi.org/10.1177/1054137316665817.
11. Wool C, Côté-Arsenault D, Black B, Denney-Koelsch E, Kim S, Kavanaugh K. Provision of services in perinatal palliative care: a multicenter survey in the United States. J Palliat Med. 2015;19(3):279–85. https://doi.org/10.1089/jpm.2015.0266.
12. Center to Advance Palliative Care. (n.d.). www.capc.org/. Accessed 7/8/19.
13. Menon PR, Stapleton RD, McVeigh U. Telemedicine as a tool to provide family conferences and palliative care consultations in critically ill patients at rural health care institutions: a pilot study. Am J Hospice Palliat Med. 2014;32(4):448–53.
14. Fletcher JC. The fetus as patient: ethical issues. JAMA. 1981;246(7):772–3.
15. Harrison MR, Evans MI, Adzick NS, Holzgreve W., editors. The unborn patient: the art and science of fetal therapy. 3rd ed. Philadelphia: W.B. Saunders Company; Copyright 2001.
16. Akinkuotu AC, Cruz SM, Abbas PI, Lee TC, Welty SE, Olutoye OO, et al. Risk-stratification of severity for infants with CDH: prenatal versus postnatal predictors of outcome. J Pediatr Surg. 2016;51(1):44–8. https://doi.org/10.1016/j.jpedsurg.2015.10.009. Epub 2015 Oct 22
17. American College of Obstetricians and Gynecologists, Committee on Ethics; American Academy of Pediatrics, Committee on Bioethics. Clinical report – maternal-fetal intervention and fetal care centers. Pediatrics. 2011;128(2):e473–8. https://doi.org/10.1542/peds.2011-1570. Epub 2011 Jul 25
18. Leuthner SR. Ethical issues in managing fetal and neonatal cardiac lesions. In: Rao PS, Vidyasagar D, editors. Perinatal cardiology: a multidisciplinary approach. Minneapolis: Cardiotext Publishing, LLC; 2015: Chapter 7.
19. Denney-Koelsch E, Black B, Côté-Arsenault D, Wool C, Kim S, Kavanaugh KA. Survey of perinatal palliative care programs in the US: structure, process, and outcomes. J Palliat Med. 2016;19(10):1080–6.
20. Côté-Arsenault D, Denney-Koelsch E, McKoy TP, Kavanaugh K. African American and Latino bereaved parent health outcomes after receiving perinatal palliative care. Appl Nurs Res 2019.
21. Kamrath HJ, Osterholm E, Stover-Haney R, George T, O'Connor-Von S, Needle J. Lasting legacy: maternal perspectives of perinatal palliative care. J Palliat Med. 2019;22:310–5.
22. Black B, Sandelowski M. Personal growth after severe fetal diagnosis. West J Nurs Res. 2010 Dec;32(8):1011–30.
23. Chitty LS, Barnes CA, Berry C. Continuing with pregnancy after a diagnosis of lethal abnormality: experience of five couples and recommendations for management. BMJ. 1996 Aug 24;313(7055):478–80.
24. Côté-Arsenault D, Denney-Koelsch E. "My baby is a person:" family experiences with life-threatening fetal diagnosis. J Palliat Med. 2011;14(12):1302–8.
25. Denney-Koelsch EM, Côté-Arsenault D, Lemcke-Berno E. Parents' experiences with ultrasound during pregnancy with a lethal fetal diagnosis. Glob Qual Nurs Res. 2015;2:1–8.
26. Lalor J, Begley CM, Galavan E. Recasting hope: a process of adaptation following fetal anomaly diagnosis. Soc Sci Med. 2009 Feb;68(3):462–72.
27. Kavanaugh K, Roscigno CI, Swanson KM, Savage TA, Kimura RE, Kilpatrick SJ. Perinatal palliative care: parent perceptions of caring in interactions surrounding counseling for risk of

delivering an extremely premature. Palliat Support Care. 2015 Apr;13(2):145–55. https://doi.org/10.1017/S1478951513000874.

28. Wool C. Clinician confidence and comfort in providing perinatal palliative care. J Obstet Gynecol Neonatal Nurs. 2013 Jan–Feb;42(1):48–58. https://doi.org/10.1111/j.1552-6909.2012.01432.x.
29. Wool C, Black BP, Woods AB. Quality indicators and parental satisfaction with perinatal palliative Care in the Intrapartum Setting after Diagnosis of a life-limiting fetal condition. ANS Adv Nurs Sci. 2016;39(4):346–57. https://doi.org/10.1097/ANS.0000000000000147.
30. Wool C, Repke JT, Woods AB. Parent reported outcomes of quality care and satisfaction in the context of a life-limiting fetal diagnosis. J Matern Fetal Neonatal Med. 2017 Apr;30(8):894–9. https://doi.org/10.1080/14767058.2016.1195362.
31. Wool C, Kain VJ, Mendes J, Carter BS. Quality predictors of parental satisfaction after birth of infants with life-limiting conditions. Acta Paediatr. 2018 Feb;107(2):276–82. https://doi.org/10.1111/apa.13980.
32. Lee SJ, Ralston HJP, Drey EA, Partridge JC, Rosen MA. Fetal pain: a systematic multidisciplinary review of the evidence. JAMA. 2005;294(8):947–54. https://doi.org/10.1001/jama.294.8.947.
33. Cacciatore J. Psychological effects of stillbirth. Semin Fetal Neonatal Med. 2013 Apr;18(2):76–82.
34. Christiansen DM, Olff M, Elklit A. Parents bereaved by infant death: sex differences and moderation in PTSD, attachment, coping and social support. Gen Hosp Psychiatry. 2014 Nov;36(6):655–61.
35. Gravensteen IK, Helgadóttir LB, Jacobsen E-M, Rådestad I, Sandset PM, Ekeberg Ø. Women's experiences in relation to stillbirth and risk factors for long-term post-traumatic stress symptoms: a retrospective study. BMJ Open. 2013;3(10):1–10.
36. Kavanaugh KL, Campbell ML. Conducting end-of-life research: strategies for success. Nurs Sci Q. 2014 Jan;27(1):14–9. https://doi.org/10.1177/0894318413509711.
37. Kavanaugh K, Moro TT, Savage T, Mehendale R. Enacting a theory of caring to recruit and retain vulnerable participants for sensitive research. Res Nurs Health. 2006;29(3):244–52. PMCID: PMC2818299
38. Kavanaugh K, Hershberger P. Perinatal loss in low-income African American parents. J Obstet Gynecol Neonatal Nurs. 2005;34(5):595–605. PMCID: PMC1388191
39. Perinatal Hospice & Palliative Care. (n.d.). www.perinatalhospice.org/. Accessed 7-8-19.
40. Pregnancy Loss and Infant Death Alliance (PLIDA). (n.d.). www.plida.org/ Accessed 7-8-19.
41. Akard TF, Gerhardt CA, Hendricks-Ferguson V, Given B, Friedman DL, Hinds PS, Gilmer MJ. Facebook advertising to recruit pediatric populations. J Palliat Med. 2016;19:692–3. https://doi.org/10.1089/jpm.2016.0128.
42. Hershberger PE, Kavanaugh K. Comparing appropriateness and equivalence of email interviews to phone interviews in qualitative research on reproductive decisions. Appl Nurs Res. 2017;37:50–4. https://doi.org/10.1016/j.apnr.2017.07.005.
43. Wool C. Instrument psychometrics: parental satisfaction and quality indicators of perinatal palliative care. J Palliat Med. 2015;18:872–7. https://doi.org/10.1089/jpm.2015.0135.
44. Wool C. Instrument development: parental satisfaction and quality indicators of perinatal palliative care. J Hosp Palliat Nurs. 2015;17(4):301–8. https://doi.org/10.1097/NJH.0000000000000163.
45. Wool C, Northam S. The perinatal palliative care perceptions and barriers scale instrument©: development and validation. Adv Neonatal Care. 2011 Dec;11(6):397–403. https://doi.org/10.1097/ANC.0b013e318233809a.
46. Brehaut JC, O'Connor AM, Wood TJ, Hack TF, Siminoff L, Gordon E, Feldman-Stewart D. Validation of a decision regret scale. Med Decis Mak. 2003 Jul–Aug;23(4):281–92.
47. O'Connor AM. User Manuel – decision regret scale [document on the internet]. Ottawa: Ottawa Hospital Research Institute: 1996. [modified 2003].
48. Stalmeier PF, Roosmalen MS, Verhoef LC, Hoekstra-Weebers JE, Oosterwijk JC, Moog U, et al. The decision evaluation scales. Patient Educ Couns. 2005 Jun;57(3):286–93.

49. Weiss D, Marmar C. The impact of event scale - revised. In: Wilson J, Keane T, editors. Assessing psychological trauma and PTSD. New York: Guilford Press; 2004.
50. Beck AT, Steer RA. Manual for the Beck anxiety inventory. San Antonio: Psychological Corporation; 1990.
51. Hutti MH, de Pacheco MR, Smith M. Development and validation of the perinatal grief intensity scale. J Obstetr Gynecolog Neonatal Nurs. 1998;27(5):547–55. https://doi.org/10.1111/j.1552-6909.1998.tb02621.
52. Potvin L, Lasker J, Toedter L. Measuring grief: a short version of the perinatal grief scale. J Psychopathol Behav Assess. 1989;11(1):29–45.
53. Bjelland I, Dahl AA, Haug TT, Neckelmann D. The validity of the hospital anxiety and depression scale: an updated literature review. J Psychosom Res. 2002;52(2):69–77.
54. Gillies JM, Neimeyer RA, Milman E. The grief and meaning reconstruction inventory (GMRI): initial validation of a new measure. Death Stud. 2015 Feb 7;39(2):61–74.
55. Keesee NJ, Currier JM, Neimeyer RA. Predictors of grief following the death of one's child: the contribution of finding meaning. J Clin Psychol. 2008 Oct;64(10):1145–63.
56. Palliative Care Research Cooperative Group (PCRC). (n.d.). http://palliativecareresearch.org/about-us//. Accessed 7-8-19.
57. National Palliative Care Research Center (NPCRC). (n.d.). http://www.npcrc.org//Accessed 7-8-19.
58. NIH Office of End-of-Life and Palliative Care Research (OEPCR). (n.d.). https://www.ninr.nih.gov/researchandfunding/desp/oepcr/. Accessed 7-8-19.
59. The Greenwall Foundation. (n.d.). http://www.greenwall.org/index.php/. Accessed 7-8-19.
60. Fulbright Global Scholar Award. (n.d.). https://www.cies.org/program/fulbright-global-scholar-award/accesssed. 7-8-19.
61. Limbo R, Brandon D, Cote-Arsenault D, Kavanaugh K, Kuebelbeck A, Wool C. American Academy of Nursing on policy: perinatal palliative care as an essential element of childbearing choices. Nurs Outlook. 2017;65:123–5.
62. The Science of Compassion: Future Directions in End-of-Life & Palliative Care. (n.d.). https://www.ninr.nih.gov/researchandfunding/scienceofcompassion/. Accessed 7-8-19.
63. Hoeldtke NJ, Calhoun BC. Perinatal hospice. Am J Obstet Gynecol. 2001;185(3):525–9. https://doi.org/10.1067/mob.2001.116093.
64. Roe v. Wade, 410 U.S. 113. (1973).
65. Born Alive Infant Protection Act. Pub L No. 107–207, 116 Stat 926. (2002).
66. Examination and treatment for emergency medical conditions and women in labor 42 U.S.C. § 1395dd (1994).
67. Office on Child abuse and neglect. 42 U.S.C. 5101(g) (1994).
68. Sayeed SA. Baby doe redux? The Department of Health and Human Services and the born-alive infants protection act of 2002: a cautionary note on normative neonatal practice. Pediatrics. 2005;116:e576–85. URL: www.pediatrics.org/cgi/doi/10.1542/peds.2005-1590
69. Partridge JC, Sendowskia MD, Drey EA, Martinez AM. Resuscitation of likely nonviable newborns: would neonatology practices in California change if the born-alive infants protection act were enforced? Pediatrics. 2009;123:1088–94.
70. Kirch R. Building a quality of life National movement: igniting advocacy to integrate palliative care in our US health system. Health Affairs Blog. 2015; http://healthaffairs.org/blog/2015/03/30/building-a-quality-of-life-national-movement-igniting-advocacy-to-integrate-palliative-care-in-our-us-health-system/
71. Meier DEBA, Berman A, Block SD, Corrigan JM, Morrison SMA. National strategy for palliative care. Health Aff. 2017;36(7):1265–73.
72. Kirch R, Reaman G, Feudtner C, et al. Advancing a comprehensive cancer care agenda for children and their families: Institute of Medicine Workshop highlights and next steps. CA Cancer J Clin. 2016;66(5):398–407.
73. Positioning Pediatric Palliative Care in Prime Time: Progress highlights. ChiPPS E-Journal Issue 50; 45–47 (February 2018). http://www.houstonhospice.org/ChiPPSejournalIssue50.pdf.

74. Public Opinion Strategies Market Research Findings Summary. (n.d.). https://media.capc.org/filer_public/3c/96/3c96a114-0c15-42da-a07f-11893cca7bf7/2011-public-opinion-research-on-palliative-care_237.pdf
75. Palliative Care in Oncology ASCO Symposium poster presentation on Putting Pediatric Palliative Care in Prime Time. (n.d.). https://meetinglibrary.asco.org/record/103464/poster
76. National Institute of Nursing Research Conversations Matter Campaign Materials. (n.d.). https://www.ninr.nih.gov/newsandinformation/conversationsmatter/conversations-matter-newportal
77. Center to Advance Palliative Care Pediatric Palliative Care Field Guide. A catalog of resources, tools and training to promote innovation, development and growth. (2016).
78. National Palliative Care Registry. (n.d.). https://registry.capc.org/.
79. National Academies of Science, Engineering and Medicine Quality Care for Serious Illness Roundtable. (n.d.). http://nationalacademies.org/hmd/Activities/HealthServices/QualityCareforSeriousIllnessRoundtable.aspx
80. Patient Quality of Life Coalition. (n.d.). http://patientqualityoflife.org/.
81. Dying in America: Improving Quality and Honoring Individual Preferences Near the End of Life. Institute of Medicine report (2014).
82. National Association of Neonatal Nurses. Position statement: palliative and end-of-life Care in Newborns and Infants. Chicago: National Association of Neonatal Nurses; 2015. Retrieved from: http://nann.org/uploads/About/PositionPDFS/1.4.5_Palliative%20and%20End%20of%20Life%20Care%20for%20Newborns%20and%20Infants.pdf
83. Moon-Grady AJ, Baschat A, Cass D, Choolani M, Copel JA, Crombleholme TM, et al. Fetal treatment 2017: the evolution of fetal therapy centers – a joint opinion from the international fetal medicine and surgical society (IFMSS) and the north American fetal therapy network (NAFTNet). Fetal Diagn Ther. 2017;42(4):241–8. https://doi.org/10.1159/000475929.
84. Rogers M, Kirch R. Spotlight on pediatric palliative care: National landscape of hospital-based programs 2015–2016. 13 July 2017. https://www.capc.org/blog/palliative-pulse-palliative-pulse-july-2017-spotlight-pediatric-palliative-care-national-landscape-hospital-based-programs-2015-2016/
85. National Consensus Project for Quality Palliative Care. Clinical practice guidelines for quality palliative care. 4th ed. Richmond: National Coalition for Hospice and Palliative Care; 2018. https://www.nationalcoalitionhpc.org/ncp.
86. Ahluwalia SC, Chen C, Raaen L, Motala A, Walling AM, Chamberlin M, et al. A systematic review in support of the National Consensus Project Clinical Practice Guidelines for quality palliative care, fourth edition. J Pain Symptom Manag. 2018 Dec;56(6):831–70. https://doi.org/10.1016/j.jpainsymman.2018.09.008
87. Cole JCM, Moldenhauer JS, Jones TR, Shaughnessy EA, Zarrin HE, Coursey AL, Munson DA. A proposed model for perinatal palliative care. J Obstet Gynecol Neonatal Nurs. 2017 Nov–Dec;46(6):904–11. https://doi.org/10.1016/j.jogn.2017.01.014.
88. Hasegawa SL, Fry JT. Moving toward a shared process: the impact of parent experiences on perinatal palliative care. Sem Perinatol. 2017;41:95–100.
89. Carter BS. Pediatric palliative care in infants and neonates. Children (Basel). 2018;5(2):pii: E21. https://doi.org/10.3390/children5020021.
90. Community Palliative Care Mapping Project. (n.d.). https://mapping.capc.org/.
91. Carter BS. More than medication: perinatal palliative care. Acta Paediatr. 2016;105:1255–6.

Index

E. M. Denney-Koelsch, D. Côté-Arsenault (eds.), *Perinatal Palliative Care*,
https://doi.org/10.1007/978-3-030-34751-2

MIX
Papier aus verantwortungsvollen Quellen
Paper from responsible sources
FSC® C105338

If you have any concerns about our products,
you can contact us on
ProductSafety@springernature.com

In case Publisher is established outside the EU,
the EU authorized representative is:
Springer Nature Customer Service Center GmbH
Europaplatz 3, 69115 Heidelberg, Germany

Printed by Libri Plureos GmbH
in Hamburg, Germany